W9-CXP-325

ATLAS OF REPLANTATION AND TRANSPLANTATION OF TEETH

ATLAS OF REPLANTATION AND TRANSPLANTATION OF TEETH

Jens O. Andreasen

Associated Director of Oral Surgery and Oral Medicine,
University Hospital (Rigshospitalet),
and
Research Associate, Departments of Oral Pathology and Oral
and Maxillofacial Surgery,
Royal Dental College,
Copenhagen, Denmark

Odont. Dr. h.c., Karolinska Institute,
Stockholm Sweden

F.R.C.S., London, England

Lennart Håkansson

Coordinator

1992
W.B. Saunders Company
Harcourt Brace Jovanovich, Inc.
Philadelphia London Toronto
Montreal Sydney Tokyo

Medical drawings
Poul Buckhöj
Med. Dr. h.c.
Lund University

Authorized English edition copublished
1992 by Mediglobe SA, Fribourg and
W.B. Saunders, Philadelphia.

W.B. Saunders Company
Harcourt Brace Jovanovich, Inc.

The Curtis Center
Independence Square West
Philadelphia, PA 19106

ISBN 0-7216-6711-2 (Saunders)
LC catalog card number 83-50513

Copyright © 1992 Mediglobe SA

Mediglobe SA
Beauregard 12
Case postale 286
CH-1700 Fribourg 1, Switzerland

ISBN 2-88239-015-X (Mediglobe)

All rights reserved. This book, or any
parts thereof, may not be used or reproduced in any manner without written permission from the copyright holder.

Printed by

KIN KEONG PRINTING CO PTE LTD
SINGAPORE

Foreword

It is an honor and a pleasure to write a foreword to this outstanding volume on "Replantation and Transplantation of Teeth" by Dr. Jens O. Andreasen. This volume is truly at the cutting edge of research and clinical practice in this area. It surely will serve as the definitive reference source for many years to come. The incredible attention to detail, the magnificent illustrations in outstanding color, the superb radiographs, the efficient organization, and the very complete references make this a volume that all dentists should have and that all who deal with facial dental injuries must have. The chapters on wound healing and replantation of avulsed teeth are based on the great clinical experience of the author. All other chapters are equally authoritative. As an orthodontist, I find Chapter 10 on orthodontic treatment planning and autotransplantation and transplantation of teeth by Drs. Paulsen and Zachrisson again exceedingly accurate and to the point. As an author and as an editor of an international journal, it gives me the greatest pleasure to be able to introduce this outstanding contribution.

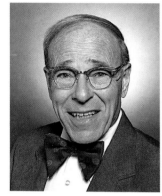

T.M. Graber

D.M.D., M.S.D., Ph.D., D. Sc., Odont. Dr. (Sweden)

Professor and Past Chairman, Department of Orthodontics, University of Chicago

Director, Kenilworth Dental Research Foundation

Research Scientist, American Dental Research Association

Editor, American Journal of Orthodontics and Dentofascial Orthopedics

Bodily injury is an incalculable cause of human suffering in developed and underdeveloped societies around the world. Health expenditures have risen much faster annually than the gross national product of most countries during recent years. Fortunately, injury control measures are now being given painstaking thought and responsible medical, dental, political, and social address in many countries, but people are still being seriously hurt in unbelievable numbers and they require expert, immediate care and rehabilitation. Each bodily part has unique anatomic, functional, and emotional considerations, but no physical component is more entwined with passionate anxiety than injury about the maxillofacial area. Without giving weight to relevance of injury to the frontal, nasal, orbital, auricular, or oral areas, each has meticulous requirements for early management and ultimate final repair. No element of the oral mechanism is more tied to function, esthetics, and powerful emotion than the state of the dentition. For this reason, a superb understanding of the fastidious essentials in salvaging and ultimately restoring fractured and avulsed teeth and the supporting bone is a necessity for anyone dealing with this offended area. "Replantation and Transplantation of Teeth" is not wanting in any detail regarding wound healing, the inflammatory response, replantation of teeth, preoperative and postoperative care, the factors involved in resorption of teeth or bone, and restoration in form of the teeth; it is a much needed and most useful work.

This remarkable book has no comparison in the world today to its extraordinary completeness in study and management of dental injury. Dr. Jens O. Andreasen has firmly established himself as the final global authority relative to the multiple factors involved in the cause, response, management, and outcome of this unique injury. One can only hope that every injured anatomic part receives as close scrutiny and explanation as Dr. Andreasen has given to the traumatized tooth and its supporting components of periodontium and bone. The final hope is that trauma control persistence as a requirement by every nation of its citizenry will lessen the number of serious injuries which occur each day, hour, minute, and second around the world. Until that magic time occurs, injuries must be cared for in the finest professional and skilled manner. This book will be the definitive resource and guide in control of dental injury. It is one important part of the total trauma control thrust being made around the world.

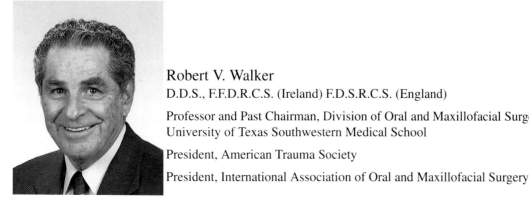

Robert V. Walker

D.D.S., F.F.D.R.C.S. (Ireland) F.D.S.R.C.S. (England)

Professor and Past Chairman, Division of Oral and Maxillofacial Surgery,
University of Texas Southwestern Medical School

President, American Trauma Society

President, International Association of Oral and Maxillofacial Surgery

Preface

Dental replantation and transplantation of teeth have had a long and troublesome history. They have been practiced for centuries, but have usually failed due to healing complications. Thus, despite experimental investigations initiated by Hunter as early as 1771, the time was not ripe for a breakthrough in this area, primarily because of a lack of knowledge about the etiology of root resorption and control of infection. However, extensive research particularly in the past two decades into the etiology and pathogenesis of root resorption, wound healing processes in the pulp and periodontium, and how these relate to infection, has made replantation and transplantation of teeth predictable and usually reliable clinical procedures. These operations can thus be added to the dental armamentarium, while at the same time challenging the various dental specialties to broaden their horizons for new treatment potentials.

In **orthodontics,** autotransplantation of teeth can add a new dimension to treatment planning. Instead of considering limited tooth movements within one segment of the dental arch, a freedom of movement has been achieved in many situations where teeth can be placed exactly where the need dictates, whether it be in remote regions of the same jaw or in the opposing dental arch. Furthermore, banking for later use of premolars which must be extracted is now possible, for example where doubt exists about the prognosis of traumatized or endodontically treated anterior teeth. The orthodontic profession is thus challenged to outline indications for these new treatment possibilities.

In **pedodontics,** replantation of avulsed teeth has been an unreliable procedure. Recent advances in the knowledge of wound healing which takes place after replantation of teeth has improved the predictability of these procedures and significantly increased their success rate. In addition, the unfortunate situation often faced that traumatized anterior teeth cannot be saved can now often be remedied by autotransplantation of premolars and later recontouring with a composite technique, a treatment which in some cases is to be preferred over fixed or removable prosthetic appliances.

In **endodontics,** intentional replantation has been the last chance for teeth which could not be treated adequately by conventional or surgical endodontic procedures. Another treatment approach, namely autotransplantation of premolars and third molars as replacements for unsalvageable teeth with endodontic complications, is now another feasible alternative.

In **prosthodontics**, teeth can now in selected cases be placed exactly where the need dictates. In this context, the auto- or allotransplant must be carefully evaluated in light of various implant techniques. The latter procedure, however, is usually not indicated in young individuals due to the interference with growth of the alveolar process.

In **oral surgery** traditional techniques for the removal of impacted teeth have aimed at not traumatizing the alveolus in order to promote socket healing. These techniques have for obvious reasons given no consideration to the preservation of a vital pulp, periodontal ligament, or dental follicle and as such must be altered radically when teeth are to be transplanted. A great challenge now in oral surgery is, therefore, the development of techniques which allow maximum cell survival in and around the potential transplant.

The prerequisite for successful replantation and autotransplantation of teeth is a thorough knowledge of responses of the pulp and periodontium to injury and the healing capacities of both of these tissues. In a sense, autotransplantation of teeth can be considered as an intentional, controlled dental trauma. The knowledge accumulated over the years in dental traumatology can in most situations be applied directly to autotransplantation of teeth. Thus, dental traumatology and dental transplantation are in fact two sides of the same coin, one being forced upon an individual, causing more or less damage, the other being an intentional trauma used to repair the earlier damage or remedy a difficult treatment problem. Especially the latter situation requires a thorough cost-benefit analysis to ensure that the advantages of this type of therapy outweigh the potential complications.

The emphasis in this book is to present a detailed description of the responses of the various cellular systems to replantation and autotransplantation and to describe suitable surgical techniques which will optimize the chances for successful healing. In this context, artistic drawings have been used to a great extent instead of actual microphotographs. It should be noted that anatomic and cellular structures have been simplified including both their number and size, in order to facilitate understanding of the general buildup of tissues and their response to trauma.

A very important fact to consider is that replantation and autotransplantation of teeth are the most powerful tools in the dental armamentarium and as such should only be used after thorough consideration of all facets of the treatment problem and solution possibilities. And if decided upon, these procedures must be performed with professional skill and due respect to the healing potential of all cellular systems involved.

Finally, the author wants to express his gratitude to the entire staff at the Department of Oral Medicine and Oral Surgery, University Hospital, Copenhagen, for their help and support in treating transplant and trauma patients. Separate thanks to our photographers for their painstaking efforts in producing the illustrative material in this text. A special thank to Dr HE Schroeder, Detal School, Zürich, Switzerland, for valuable discussions concerning anatomic details. Finally, thanks to my wife, Dr. F.M. Andreasen, Departments of Pediatric Dentistry and Oral and Maxillofacial Surgery, Royal Dental College, Copenhagen, for professional criticism and language correction, and Lene and Dorte for typing the manuscript.

Copenhagen, July 1991

Jens O. Andreasen

Authors

Background information

The treatment procedures described in this book are based on documented follow-up of approximately 4000 replantations and transplantations carried out at different research centers in Scandinavia over a 20-year period. In the observation period, standardized clinical and radiographic controls have been performed at regular intervals, whereby it has been possible to disclose the long-term prognosis of these treatments.

The details of the various replantation and transplantation procedures have all been developed experimentally. Thus over the past 10 years, 45 experiments have been carried out to examine the influence of various treatment procedures upon the outcome of pulpal and periodontal healing after replantation and transplantation. Due to improvements in surgical technique resulting from animal experiments and in graft selection, a good long-term prognosis of tooth transplants has been achieved. These improvements in prognosis have now made transplantation an integral part of treatment planning in the correction of malocclusions and/or missing teeth by many orthodontists.

Successful replantation after accidental avulsion is now becoming more frequent due to several improvements in the extraoral handling of the avulsed teeth. This treatment procedure has therefore become an important part of the pedodontic service.

All participants in this book have been involved in experimental and/or clinical investigations of replantation and transplantation since the mid 1960s. Throughout a joint research program it has been possible to detect the most important predictors for success or failure in both replantation and transplantation situations.The academic position of the authors in this textbook is as follows:

J.O. Andreasen. Odont. Dr. h.c., Associated Director of Oral Surgery and Oral Medicine, University Hospital (Rigshospitalet), and Research Associate, Departments of Oral Pathology and Oral and Maxillofacial Surgery, Royal Dental College, Copenhagen, Denmark

O. Schwartz. Associate Professor, Ph. D., Department of Oral Surgery, The Royal Dental College and Research Associate, Tissue Typing Laboratory, University Hospital, Copenhagen

H.U. Paulsen. Head of the Orthodontic Service, Peder Lykke School, Department of Orthodontics, Municipal Dental Care, Copenhagen, Denmark

B. U. Zachrisson. Odont. Dr., Professor and Former Head of the Department of Orthodontics, Dental School, University of Oslo, Norway

Table of contents

Chapter 10 Autotransplantation of teeth and orthodontic treatment planning

HU. Paulsen & BU. Zachrisson.

Chapter 11 Restoration of transplanted teeth

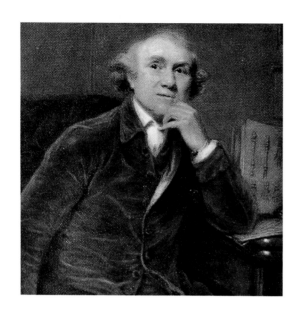

Dedicated to John Hunter (1728-1793), founder of scientific dental replantation and transplantation.

John Hunter was the founder of experimental medical and dental surgery and also had a number of other achivements to his name.

During a series of various organ transplantations he demonstrated that a human tooth heterotransplanted into a cock´s comb "adhered everywhere to the comb by vessels similar to the union of a tooth with the gums and sockets".

In addition he described root resorption phenomena after allotransplantation of teeth in humans.

Reproduced by kind permission of the President and Counsil of the Royal College of Surgeons of England.

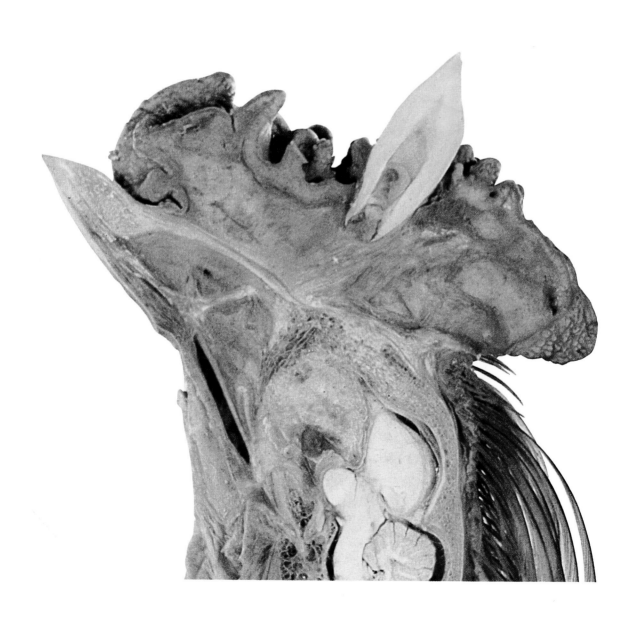

Chapter 1
Surgical anatomy and wound healing

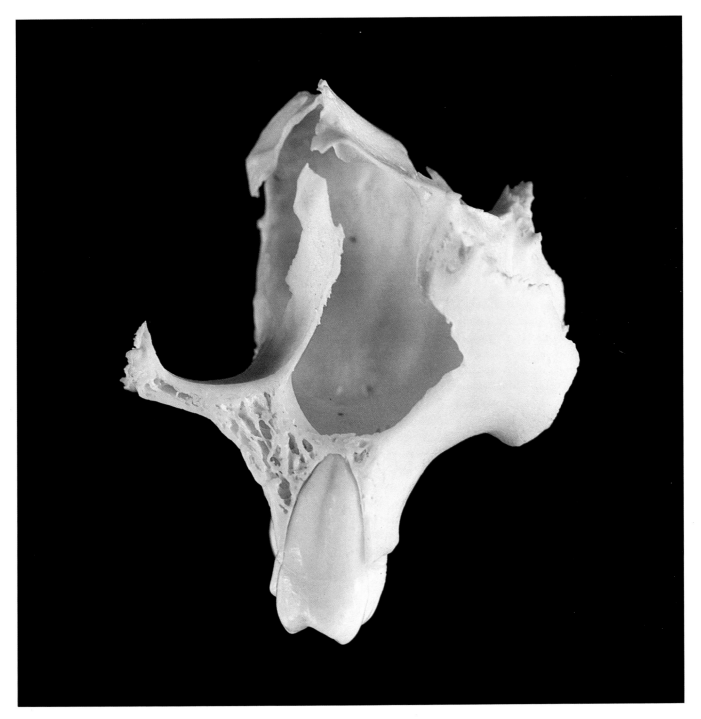

Surgical anatomy and wound healing related to replantation and transplantation of teeth

In the performance of replantation and transplantation procedures and monitoring subsequent pulpal and periodontal healing it is essential to know not only the healing capacity of individual cell types, but also the healing capacity of tissue compartments. In the delineation of these compartments, anatomic borders have been chosen which are typically the result of incisions or separation lines during graft removal. The following surgical anatomic zones evolve in removal of teeth with completed root development: *gingiva and periosteal complex, cementum-periodontal ligament-alveolar bone complex, and the pulp-dentin complex.* In developing teeth the following structures are also involved: the *dental follicle* and *Hertwig´s epithelial root sheath.*

For each tissue compartment, a short description will be given of its healing capacity with respect to surgical injury and infection.

Dental follicle

The dental follicle (dental sac) is the connective tissue separating the developing tooth from the alveolus. Functionally it is considered the formative organ of the periodontal attachment [i.e., cementum, periodontal ligament (PDL) and alveolar bone proper] and it plays a decisive role during tooth eruption. [1-18]

The anatomy of the follicle varies considerably according to the stage of tooth development, a fact which dictates various surgical approaches for transplantation of tooth germs at various stages of root development (Fig. 1.1). Thus in the design of suitable surgical procedures for atraumatic graft removal, the architecture of the collagenous fibers in the follicle is of utmost importance. Their number and insertion sites can cause problems in atraumatic tooth removal due to the creation of compression zones arising during the extraction procedure and subsequent death of cells in the follicle or PDL. Depending on the extent of this cell kill, root resorption and/or eruption disturbances may result (see p. 45).

Crown formation completed, initial (stage 0) or one-quarter root development (stage 1)

(Fig. 1.1)
In stage 0 the tooth-forming tissues are very sensitive to injury. Transplantation is not indicated at this stage as such a procedure will traumatize the enamel organ and result in severe enamel hypoplasia. [19-20]

When stage 1 is reached collagen fibers are found cervically emanating perpendicular to a thin layer of newly formed cementum. These fibers then change direction and course coronally and apically, parallel to the tooth germ Fig. 1.2a. [21,22]

As the tooth moves coronally, the parallel fibers of the follicle blend with fibers of the PDL of the primary tooth.

The anatomy of the follicle dictates that the following surgical precautions be taken for successful graft removal: If a primary tooth is present, it is extracted. Then a buccal or lingual flap is raised whereafter the maximum extent of the crown is exposed, preferably using chisels or alternately using a bur while the follicle is shielded by a thin periosteal elevator or an amalgam carver. The coronal part of the follicle is then separated from the socket with an amalgam carver, whereafter the tooth can be lifted out of its socket with minimal resistance.

Fig. 1.1a. Development of second maxillary permanent premolars

Stage 0: Initial root formation. The tooth germ is placed between the roots of the primary molar and the sinus. The tooth germ is separated from the primary molar by bone.

Stage 0

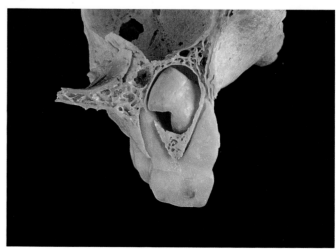

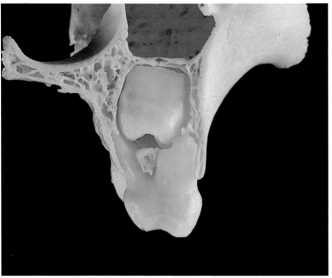

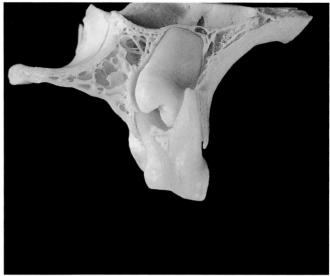

Stage 1   Stage 3

Fig. 1.1b-e. Development of second maxillary permanent premolars

Stage 1: One-quarter formation. The tooth has moved slightly coronally and is now in contact with the PDL of the primary molar. Physiologic root resorption of the primary molar has started. Note the lingual tilt of the premolar.

Stage 3: Three-quarters´ root formation. Almost all intraradicular bone has been resorbed, and root resorption has progressed.

Stage. 4: Almost full length and the apex is wide open. The tooth is partly erupted.

Stage 6: Full root length; the apical foramen is constricted.

Stage 4   Stage 6

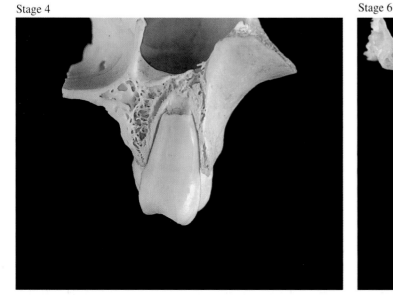

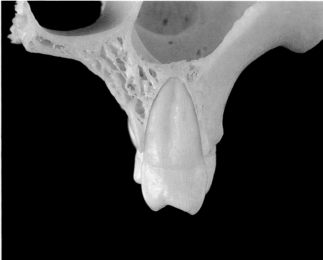

One-half (stage 2) to three-quarters' root formation (stage 3), tooth unerupted

(Fig. 1.1)

The erupting tooth is now approaching the alveolar mucosa. The most cervically inserted fibers are seen fanning out coronally and blending with the gingival fibers. Apically, a few principal fibers are seen uniting cementum and bone (Fig. 1.2b). Further apically of the root, fiber direction is still parallel to the root surface.

The following procedures for graft removal should be used: If a primary tooth is present, it is extracted. Thereafter, flaps are raised buccally and/or lingually to ensure that the collagen fibers of the coronal part of the follicle are not included in the flaps. The buccal and/or lingual parts of the bony socket surrounding the crown of the graft are then removed as described for the previous stage of root development. With an amalgam carver, the follicle is completely separated from adjacent bone immediately below the cementoenamel junction. The tooth is then removed with elevators and forceps.

Three-quarters' root formation (stage 3), initial eruption but no occlusion (Fig. 1.1)

Penetration of the tooth into the oral cavity significantly alters the amount of PDL insertion. Instead of principal fibers inserting only cervically, fiber insertion is now also seen in the coronal half of the root and a few fibers are present in the apical area.[21,22] Otherwise, fiber arrangement is identical to that described for stages 2 and 3 (Fig. 1.2c).

Surgical removal of the erupting tooth implies the following procedures: An incision is made with a thin, pointed scalpel blade which includes the marginal gingiva and which ends at the crest of the alveolar process. Thereafter, the scalpel blade is inserted parallel and as deep as possible into the PDL in order to sever the marginal principal fibers. The tooth is then grasped coronally with forceps and luxated with slight rotating movements.

Root formation complete, apical foramen wide open (stage 4), half-closed (stage 5), or constricted (stage 6). Eruption complete and full occlusion (Fig. 1.1)

The classical fiber arrangement of the PDL is now seen.[21,22] This consists of the circular gingival fibers and the dentogingival, dentoperiosteal, and transseptal fibers. In the PDL, the horizontal, oblique, and apical fibers are recognized (Fig. 1.2d) (see also p. 21).

Atraumatic extraction should include the following. The gingival tissues and the cervical portion of the periodontal ligament are incised as described in Stage 3. The preservation of the attached gingiva will prevent epithelial downgrowth along the tooth surface. Finally, the tooth is removed with forceps using slight rotating movements.

Reaction to surgical injury and infection

Under experimental conditions, it has been shown that when larger parts of the dental follicle are removed, an ankylosis is formed between the tooth surface and the crypt, and eruption is arrested.[14,23,24] The extent to which a follicle can be damaged without leading to these complications is not known at the present time. Finally the dental follicle appears to be very resistant to infection.[25,26]

Fig. 1.2a. Collagen fiber insertion during tooth development
Stage 1. The tooth germ is surrounded by a few circumferential collagen fibers. There is no fiber insertion in cementun and bone.

Fig. 1.2b. Collagen fiber insertion during tooth development
Stage 2. A few fibers emanate from the cervical cementum, but there is no insertion into the bone.

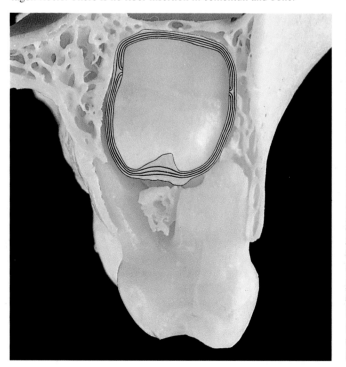

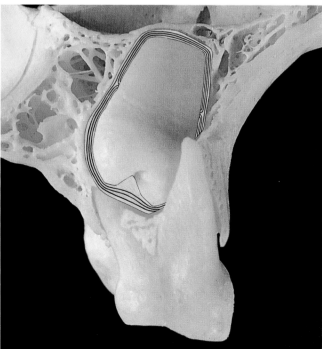

Fig. 1.2c. Collagen fiber insertion during tooth development
Stage 3. A number of principal fibers are now found in the cervical half of the root and a few in the apical area.

Fig. 1.2d. Collagen fiber insertion during tooth development
Stage 4. The classical fiber arrangement of the PDL is now established.

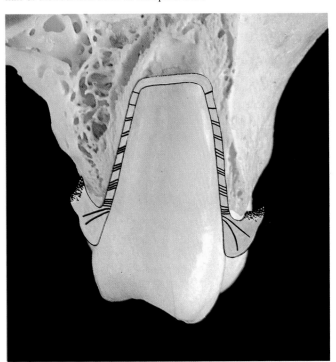

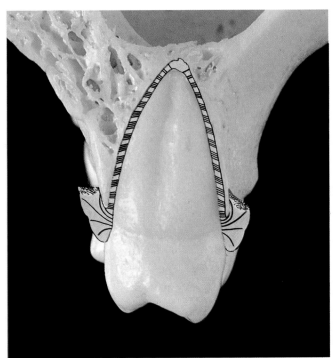

Gingiva and periosteal complex

The function of the free gingiva is to seal, maintain, and defend the critical area where the tooth penetrates its connective tissue bed and enters the oral cavity. The *junctional epithelium* represents the seal between the periodontium and the oral cavity whereas the *sulcular epithelium* faces the tooth without being in direct contact with it. The *fibrillar system* of the gingiva is very complex, being built up of groups of collagen fibers with different sites of insertion (Fig. 1.3).[28-33]

Fig. 1.3. Anatomy of the gingiva and periosteal complex

1. Sharpey´s fibers
2. Dentoperiosteal fibers
3. Alveologingival fibers
4. Dentogingival fibers
5. Junctional epithelium
6. Gingival epithelium
7. Sulcular epithelium
8. Periosteogingival fibers
9. Intergingival fibers
10. Circular fibers

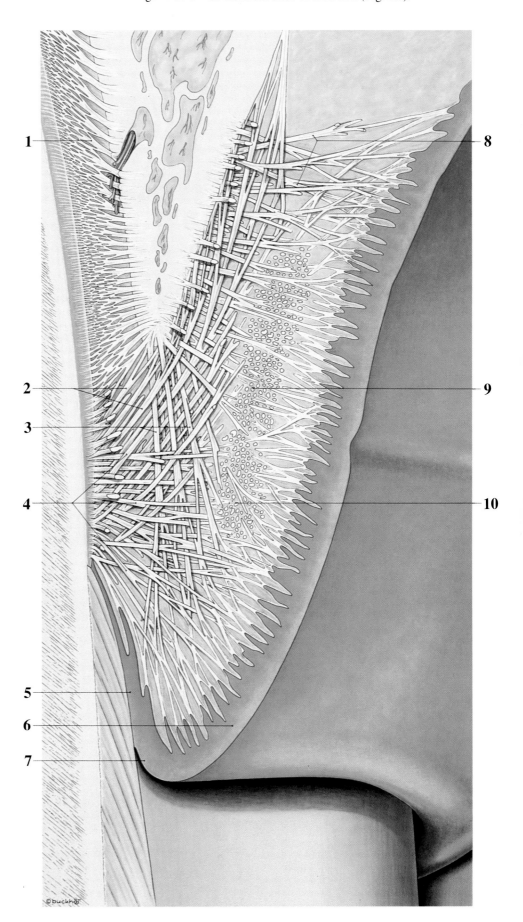

The *periosteum* covers the alveolar process and serves an important function in appositional bone growth, remodeling, and bone repair after injury.[34-37] Furthermore, it anchors tendons and carries blood and lymphatic vessels and nerves.

Reaction to surgical injury and infection

Seven days after replantation or autotransplantation a new junctional epithelium is formed. In the connective tissue, the ruptured gingival and transseptal collagen fibers are usually also united by this time (Fig. 1.4).[37,40]

Fig. 1.4. Gingival response to surgical or traumatic injury
Laceration (A) or loss of a part of the gingival seal (B) is usually followed by complete regeneration of this structure (C).

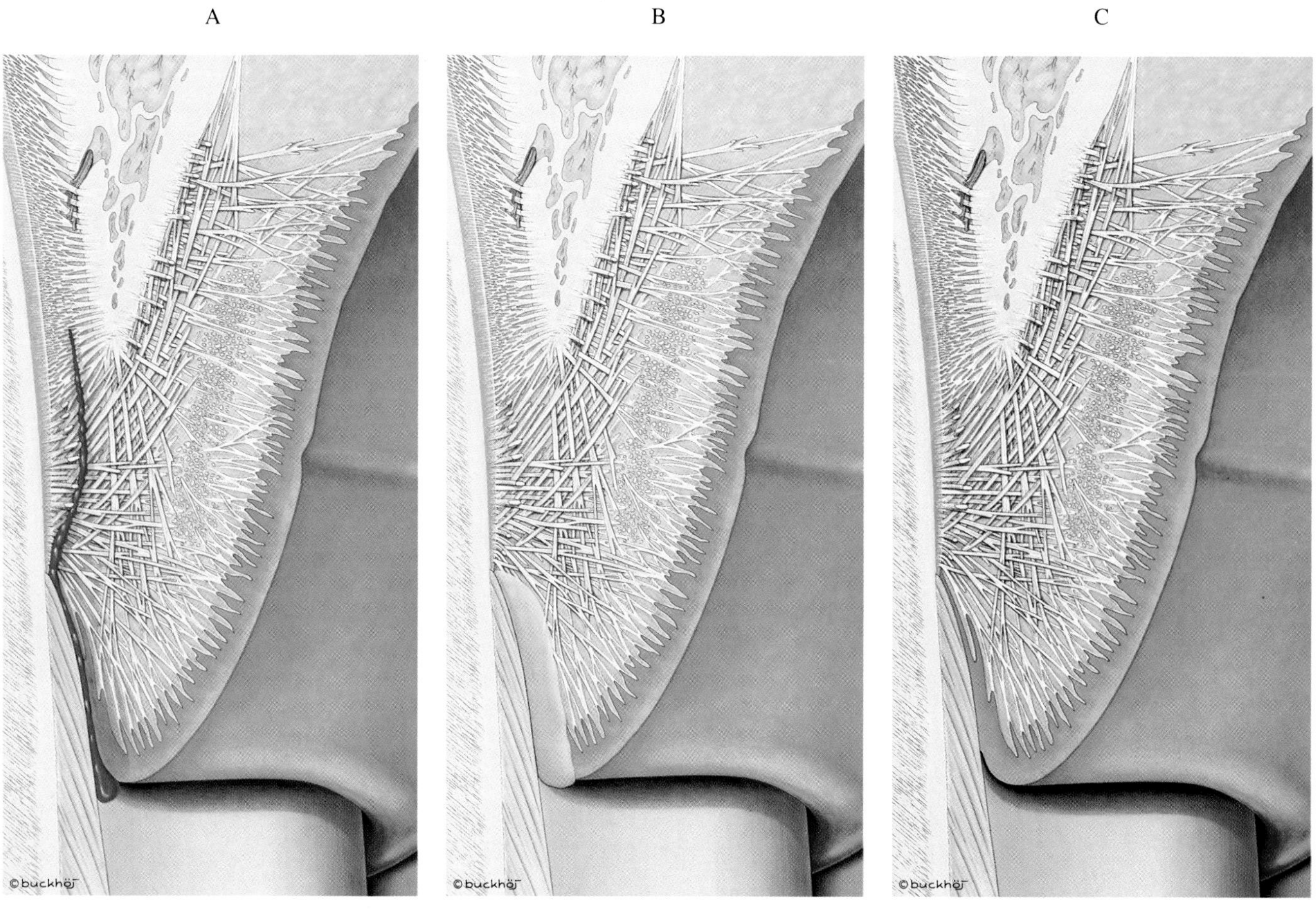

A   B   C

The relation between infection and gingival attachment after replantation or transplantation has not yet been examined.

Elevation of flaps involves injury to the periosteum and the underlying bone, leading to an initial resorption of the bony surface.[41-44] This is, however, later followed by bone deposition which more or less repairs the initial loss. In addition to the bone lost due to the flap procedure, bone may also have to be surgically removed, as during graft removal or in connection with preparation of the recipient site. In that case the osteogenic potential of the flap becomes essential. Thus in young individuals a considerable osteogenic potential exists whereby the bony contour is often fully repaired[45-49] whereas in adults this capability is restricted or absent.

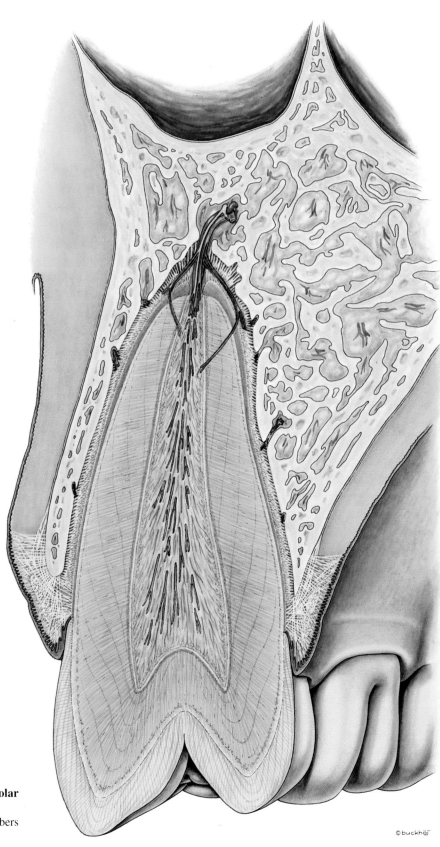

Fig. 1.5. Anatomy of the cementum-PDL-alveolar bone complex
Note the varying orientation of the principal fibers around the fully erupted tooth.

Cementum-periodontal ligament-alveolar bone complex

The PDL is a specialized connective tissue which responds specifically to surgical and traumatic injuries as well as to bacterial insults. The main function of the PDL is to support the tooth in its socket during function.

The anatomic border for the PDL is the most cervically located principal fibers (Sharpey's fibers) which insert in cementum and bone (Figs. 1.3 and 1.5). *Cementoblasts* form the organic matrix of cementum (i.e., intrinsic collagen fibers and its ground substance),[50-52] while the extrinsic fibers (i.e., Sharpey's fibers) are formed by fibroblasts from the PDL. If cementoblasts become incorporated in the mineralizing front, cellular cementum is formed. The deposition of cementum appears to occur rhythmically throughout life at a speed of approximately 3 μm per year.[52]

Periodontal fibroblasts are the predominant cells in the PDL. They are positioned parallel to Sharpey's fibers and envelop the principal fiber bundles. Through multiple contacts they form a cellular network (Fig. 1.6A).[53,54] This intricate relationship between fibroblasts and Sharpey's fibers is possibly of importance for the rapid remodeling of the PDL and the rapid healing after injury.[55,56] *Undifferentiated mesenchymal cells (progenitor cells)* are found paravascularly, and play a significant role during wound healing in the PDL.[57-60]

The vast majority of collagen fibers in the PDL are arranged in distinctive fiber bundles, the so-called principal fibers (Sharpey's fibers) (Fig. 1.6). In their course from cementum to alveolar bone the majority of the principal fibers span the entire periodontal space, although they usually branch and join adjacent fibers, creating a ladder-like architecture in the PDL (Fig. 1.6).[61-73] Whenever functional demands are changed, corresponding adjustments take place in the architecture of the PDL whereby the orientation, the amount, and the insertion pattern changes.

Osteoblasts line the alveolar socket wall, the marrow spaces, and the haversian canals and are responsible for formation of new bone. They participate together with osteoclasts in the remodelling of bone (Fig. 1.6).

Blood supply to the PDL arises from branches of the superior or inferior alveolar artery. Before these arteries enter the apical foramen, they give off branches to the apical part of the PDL interdental bone.[74-78] On their way to the alveolar crest, they give off multiple branches to the midportion of the PDL which perforate the socket wall and form a plexus which surrounds the root surface. Cervically anastomoses are formed with gingival vessels. In general, the *nerve supply* to the periodontium follows the same pathways as the blood supply.

Fig. 1.6. Anatomy of the PDL
A. Sharpey´s fibers start as minor bundles in cementum and then join to assure a ladder-like configuration in the middle portion and enter the socket wall in larger bundles.
B. The PDL cells form a dense network around the Sharpey´s fibers.

A

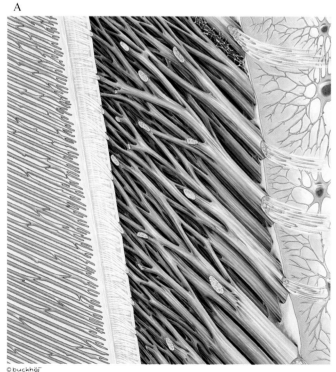

B

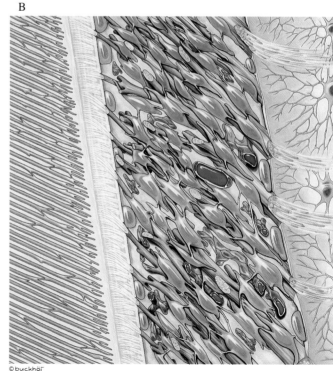

Reaction to surgical injury and infection

The most common surgical injury to the alveolar bone is the extraction wound. The following *overlapping* stages have been found based on biopsies from healing of normal extraction wounds in humans.[79-84]

Stage I. Once bleeding has stopped, a coagulum is formed, consisting of erythrocytes and leukocytes in the same ratio as in circulating blood, entrapped in a mesh of precipitated fibrin.

Stage II. *Granulation tissue* is formed along the socket walls 2 - 3 days postoperatively and is characterized by proliferating endothelial cells, capillaries, and many leukocytes. Within one week, granulation tissue has usually replaced the coagulum.

Stage III. *Connective tissue* formation begins peripherally and has within 3 weeks replaced the initial granulation tissue.

Stage IV. *Bone development* can be seen after 1 week, starting peripherally, at the base of the alveolus. The major contributors to alveolar healing appear to be cancellous bone and bone marrow, while the remaining PDL apparently plays only an insignificant role.[85,86] After 6 weeks the socket is completely occupied by immature bone. Within 2-3 months, this bone is mature and forms trabeculae. After 3-4 months, maturation is complete.[87]

The reaction to *severance* of the PDL has recently been studied in monkeys. It appears that after luxation a rupture of the PDL fibers usually occurs in the middle of the PDL or close to the alveolar wall or root surface. One week after repositioning, union of the principal fibers has taken place in isolated areas (Fig. 1.7).[39] After 2 weeks larger amounts of healed principal fibers are seen and the mechanical properties of the injured PDL are now restored to about 50%-60% that of un-

injured PDL.[88] After 8 weeks, the injured PDL cannot be distinguished histologically from an uninjured PDL.

During avulsion and subsequent replantation or autotransplantation, *contusion* of the PDL can be seen (Figs. 1.8-1.11). In these locations the resulting cell necrosis results in wound healing processes whereby necrotic PDL is removed by macrophages and sometimes also cementum by osteoclastic activity. The latter will then lead to either surface or inflammatory resorption depending on the pulp status, the age of the patient, and the stage of root development[89] (see p. 28). When large areas of the PDL are traumatized, competitive wound healing begins between bone marrow-derived cells destined to form bone and PDL-derived cells which are programmed to form PDL fibers and cementum. The outcome of this competition can result in transient or permanent ankylosis[89] (see p. 30).

The cell populations in the PDL appear to be rather resistant to infection. Thus, when infection has been eliminated, the PDL usually returns to normal.[90-92]

Finally it should be mentioned that a vital PDL cover on the root has a certain bone-inducing potential (see p. 45).[89]

Healing events after replantation

Healing with vital PDL (Fig. 1.7).

The histologic events after replantation of teeth where efforts have been made to preserve a *vital* PDL include the following:

24 hours: The torn ligament fibers are separated by a blood clot. The separation line is generally positioned at the midline of the PDL.

Fig. 1.7. PDL response to surgical or traumatic injury in the midportion of the ligament.
Laceration of the PDL (A) is repaired with new Sharpey's fibers after 2 weeks (B).

A
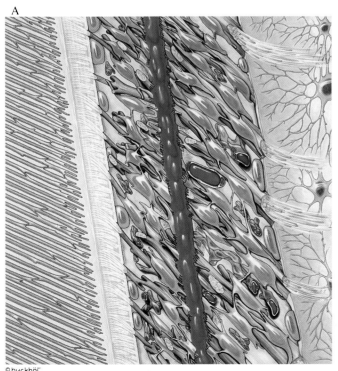

B
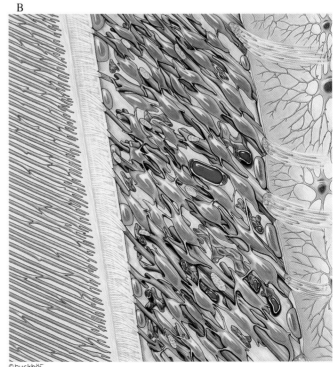

3-4 days: Many areas in the PDL show hyalinization, with disappearance of cells from both the alveolar and the cemental aspects. These areas represent the compression zones from extraction. There is no blood circulating in the vessels of the cemental aspect of the PDL at this time.

1 week: While gingival collagen fibers are generally united, only a few areas in the infrabony part of the PDL demonstrate healed principal fibers. Circulation in the blood vessels is seen in both the cemental and the alveolar aspects of the PDL. Both *surface resorption* and *inflammatory resorption* can be seen.[99-101]

2 weeks: In most areas the separation line in the PDL is not recognizable. Principal periodontal fibers extending from the cemental surface to the alveolar surface are common. Ankylosis sites can now be found.

2 months: The arrangement of the principal fibers appears normal in both amount and orientation.

Healing with an avital PDL

This occurs typically after extensive drying or after intentional removal of the PDL.[102-106] The healing processes lead to a normal appearing gingival attachment cervically, while intra-alveolar healing consists of an extensive ankylosis. Depending on the endodontic status of the tooth, inflammatory resorption may also be seen (see p. 28).

Healing events after autotransplantation

Periodontal ligament healing after *autotransplantation* has been examined in a number of experimental studies. The following healing events appear from these studies.[107-115]

4 days: The blood clot surrounding the tooth starts to become organized into granulation tissue.

7 days: The gingival fibers on the graft have united with the gingiva at the recipient site. A few intra-alveolar ligament fibers on the tooth appear to be united with the socket.

3-4 weeks: A new socket has been formed, including new Sharpey's fibers

In the following a synopsis will be given of the present knowledge about the different etiology and pathogenesis of the different external root resorption types and bone resorption which may occur after replantation and autotransplantation due to injury to various components of the PDL.

Fig. 1.8 A. Surface resorption elicited by surgical or traumatic injury to the cemental part of the ligament
Injury has affected a relatively small tissue compartment next to the root surface.

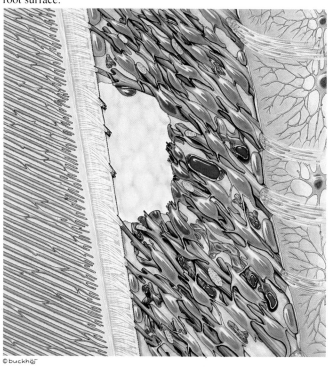

Fig. 1.8 B. Ingrowth of new tissue
New connective tissue repopulates the injury site.

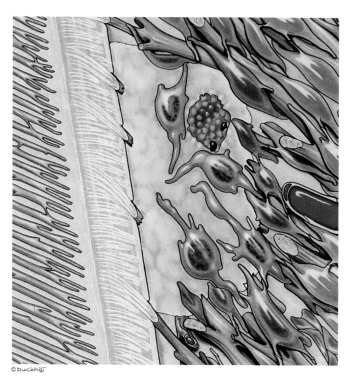

Surface resorption (Fig. 1.8)

This resorption type results from small injuries to the innermost layer of the PDL and possibly also the cementum, which elicits a superficial osteoclastic attack on the root surface. Healing takes place from adjacent vital PDL, whereby the initial resorption cavity is more or less completely repaired with new cementum.[99,100,116-117]

Surface resorption can be demonstrated histologically as early as 1 week after replantation.[99] Damage to cells in the PDL along the root surface can be due to the extraction trauma, physical removal, or drying of the PDL. Surface resorption is not primarily related to root canal content, as long as the resorption cavity does not penetrate cementum.[105]

Surface resorption cavities usually cannot be seen *radiographically* because of their small size. In rare instances, however, they show up initially as shallow cavities affecting both the root and the lamina dura of adjacent bone. Later, repair takes place whereby a normal PDL space is established, usually along the original outline of the defect (see Chapter 4, p. 78).

Fig. 1.8 C. Resorption attack
Osteoclasts attack the damaged root surface superficially.

Fig. 1.8 D. Repair of the PDL
New cementum with insertion of PDL fibers is deposited in the resorption lacunae.

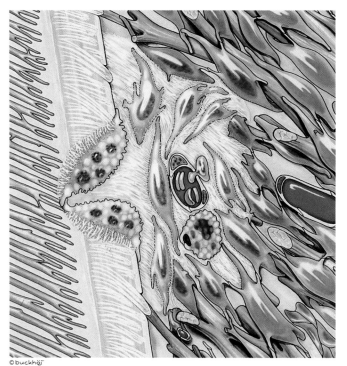

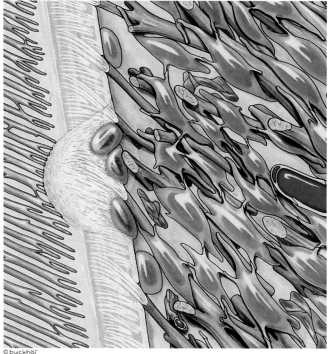

Inflammatory resorption (Fig. 1.9)

Inflammatory resorption is the result of injury to the innermost layer of the PDL and possibly also the cementum eliciting a deep osteoclastic attack on the root surface, exposing dentinal tubules. When these tubules communicate with bacteria of pulpal origin, continuous activation of the resorption process takes place. If the bacterial stimulus is weak or endodontic treatment is performed, repair can occur; otherwise the resorption will continue until granulation tissue has penetrated into the root canal.[99,100,105,106,118, 119,120] Inflammatory resorption can be demonstrated *histologically* 1 week after replantation.[99] Development of inflammatory root resorption is dependent upon at least four conditions. The first is an injury to the PDL eliciting resorption. The second and third conditions are that the initial resorption process exposes dentinal tubules and that these tubules communicate with necrotic pulp tissue or a leukocyte zone harboring bacteria. Finally, an age or maturation factor is also in operation.[105] Thus inflammatory root resorption is more frequent in replanted immature and young mature teeth than in older mature teeth.[120,121] Inflammatory resorption may also be caused by an inflammatory process originating from sources other than infected pulpal tissue. Thus, marginal periodontal inflammation is sometimes related to cervical inflammatory resorption.

Radiographically inflammatory resorption is seen as bowl-shaped resorption cavities on the root surface and in the adjacent bone (see also Chapter 4, p. 79).[120]

Fig. 1.9 A. Inflammatory resorption elicited by surgical or traumatic injury to the cemental part of the ligament
Injury has affected a tissue compartment next to the root surface.

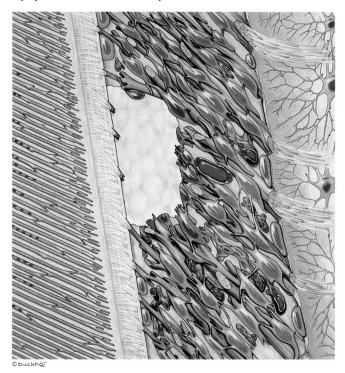

Fig. 1.9 B. Ingrowth of new tissue
New connective tissue repopulates the injury site.

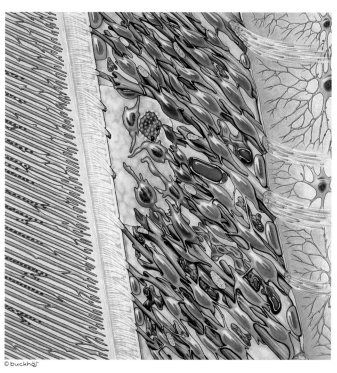

Fig. 1.9 C. Resorption attack
Osteoclasts attack the damaged root surface, whereby dentinal tubules are exposed. These tubules may harbor bacteria or lead to bacteria located in the root canal.

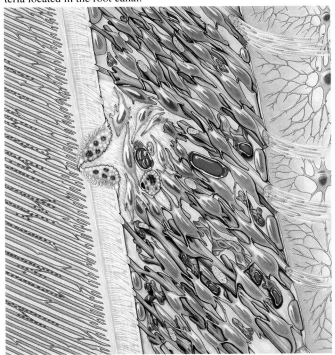

Fig. 1.9 D. Progression of root resorption
The presence of bacteria stimulates further osteoclastic activity as well as an intense inflammatory response.

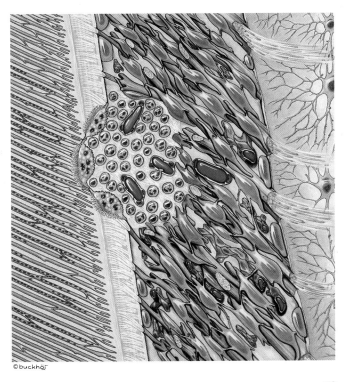

Replacement resorption (ankylosis) (Fig. 1.10)

Replacement resorption is the result of extensive injury to the innermost layer of the PDL and possibly also the cementum. Healing then takes place from the adjacent bone, whereby an ankylosis is formed.[99,101,106,119] Due to the normal remodeling cycle of bone, the tooth becomes an integral part of that system and the root is gradually transformed to bone at the same rate as in other parts of the body. This remodeling is especially prominent in children and diminishes significantly in adults.[122]

Ankylosis can be demonstrated histologically 2 weeks after replantation.[99] The pathogenesis of replacement resorption is manifested in two ways - either *permanent replacement resorption* which gradually resorbs the entire root or *transient replacement resorption*, in which a once-established ankylosis later disappears.[119,123] The permanent form is always elicited when the entire PDL is removed before replantation. Transient replacement resorption is related to minor areas of damage on the root surface. In these cases, an ankylosis is initially formed and later resorbed by adjacent normal areas of the PDL.[119,123]

Radiographically ankylosis will *initially* be seen as an obliteration of the PDL space. Replacement of root substance with bone is a later finding (see also Chapter 4, p. 81).

Fig. 1.10 A. Replacement resorption (ankylosis) elicited by a surgical or traumatic injury to the cemental part of the ligament
Injury has affected a large tissue compartment next to the root surface.

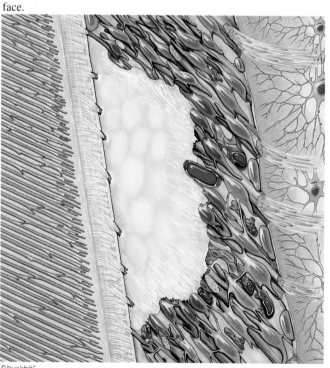

Fig. 1.10 B. Ingrowth of new tissue
New connective tissue, presumably recruited from bone marrow or the alveolar portion of the PDL, repopulates the injury site.

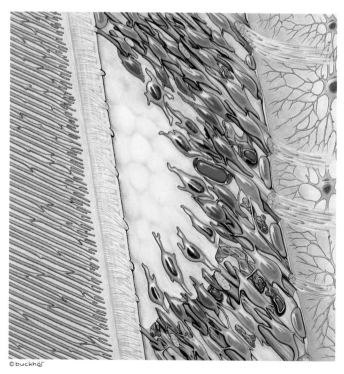

Fig. 1.10 C. Resorption attack
Osteoclasts may attack the root surface.

Fig. 1.10 D. Formation of an ankylosis
The healing tissue bridges the PDL with immature bone.

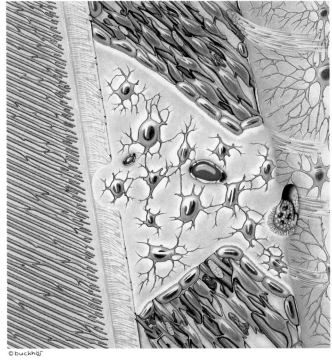

Bone resorption (Fig. 1.11)

If an injury occurs to the tissue compartment next to the bone surface, new connective tissue will repopulate the injury zone. During this process osteoclastic resorption of the socket wall usually takes place.

However, this resorption is later arrested, and the resorption cavity filled in with new bone. At the same time new principal fibers are anchored in the socket wall.

Fig. 1.11 A. PDL response to a surgical or traumatic injury in the alveolar part of the ligament
An injury has traumatized the tissue compartment adjacent to the bone surface.

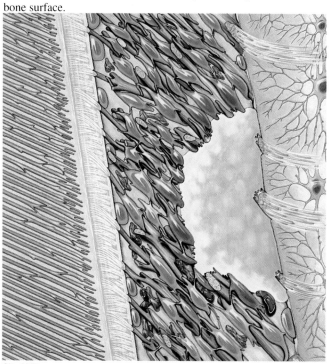

Fig. 1.11 B. Ingrowth of new tissue
New connective tissue repopulates the traumatized area.

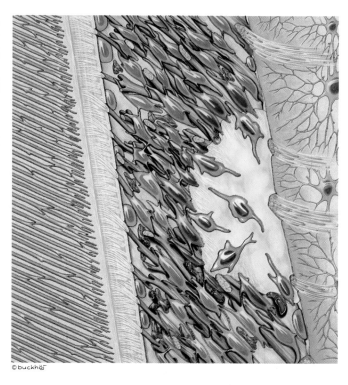

Fig. 1.11 C. Resorption attack
Damaged bone surface is resorbed by osteoclasts.

Fig. 1.11 D. Full regeneration of the PDL
Architecture and function of the PDL has been reestablished.

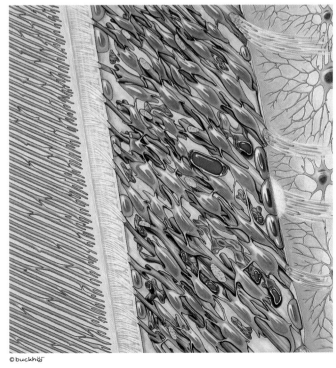

©buckhöj

©buckhöj

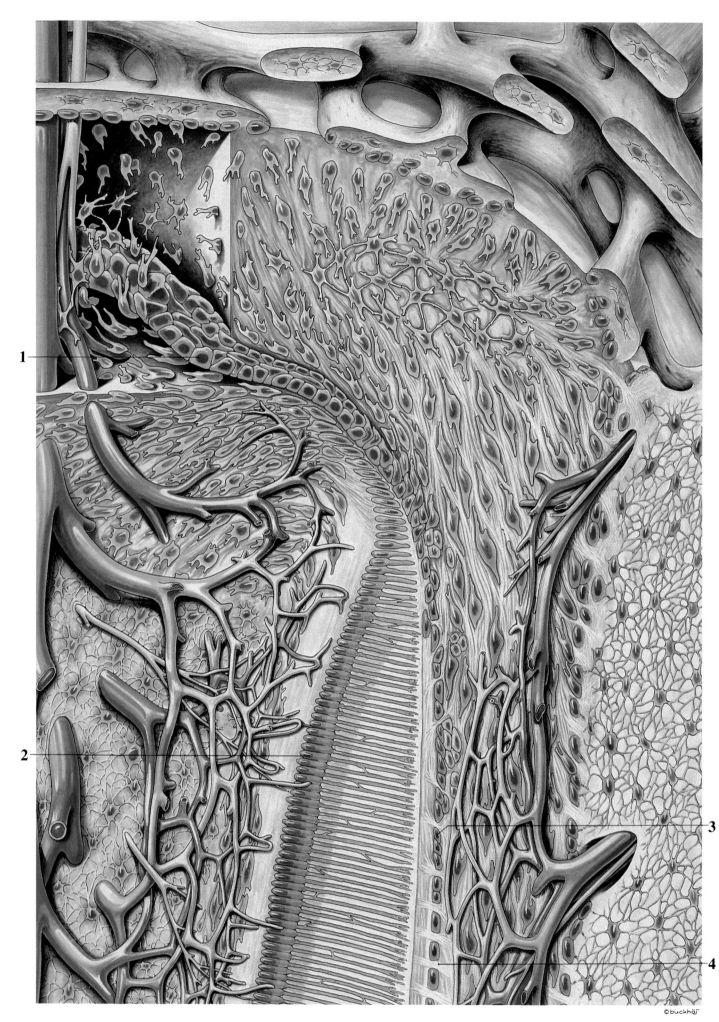

34

©buckhöj

Pulp-dentin complex

The pulp is a specialized loose connective tissue which responds specifically to surgical and traumatic injuries as well as bacterial insults. The predominant cells in the pulp are the fibroblasts (Fig. 1.12). *Undifferentiated mesenchymal cells (progenitor cells)* are located paravascularly. The latter cells probably play an important role in pulpal healing after injury.[125] The *odontoblasts* are elongated cells adjacent to the dentin and with processes which extend some distance into the dentinal tubules (Fig. 1.13).[125-127] Dentinal ground substance and collagen is secreted by the odontoblasts while pulp collagen is secreted by the fibroblasts. The average production of primary dentin in man appears to be 3 μm per day during eruption.[128] When eruption is complete, dentin formation decreases in the pulp chamber whereas it continues in the root.

The *vascular supply* to the immature human dental pulp consists of multiple thin-walled arterioles and venules passing through the apical foramen (Fig. 1.12).[129-132] The number of vessels entering the apical foramen appears to be related to maturity of the tooth, with a decreasing number found in mature teeth. A well, developed capillary network is formed in relation to the odontoblasts (Fig. 1.13).

The *pulpal nerves* generally follow the course of the blood vessels. The nonmyelinated nerves are responsible for vasoconstriction and dilation and possibly also monitoring the activity of the odontoblasts whereas the myelinated nerves respond to pain stimuli. The number of myelinated fibers increases with tooth maturity, corresponding to a lowering of the threshold for electrometric pulp stimulation.[133-137]

The function of the pulp-dentin complex is multiple. First, together with Hertwig's epithelial root sheath, root formation is ensured. Later, the function becomes a protective and reparative one against noxious stimuli, such as dentin exposure due to attrition, cavity preparation, trauma, or the progression of caries.

Fig. 1.12. Anatomy of the pulp

1. Hertwig´s epithelial root sheath.
2. Odontoblasts.
3. Cementoblasts.
4. Periodontal ligament fibers.

Fig. 1.13. Anatomy of the odontoblast layer
Note the close proximity of the terminal vascular network and the odontoblasts.

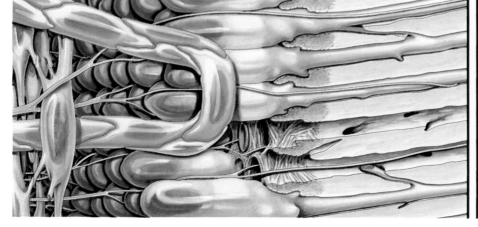
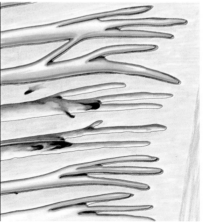

©buckhøj

Reaction to surgical injury and infection

During replantation and autotransplantation, pulpal tissue is ruptured close to or at the apical foramen, implying severance of the neurovascular supply and subsequent involvement of all cell populations in the pulp. Healing processes begin apically by the ingrowth of vascular connective tissue which moves coronally and gradually replaces the injured avascular pulp tissue. A successful revascularization is first of all dependent upon the size of the pulpal-periodontal interface (i.e., stage root development), being usually successful in cases with a wide open apex and usually unsuccesful in cases with a narrow apical foramen.[121] The second decisive factor is infection.[200,201] Thus if bacteria gain access to the avascular pulp tissue, revascularization will be permanently arrested. The way bacteria gain access to the pulp is not fully understood. Possible paths are the extraoral handling, bacteria entrapped in the coagulum, or bacteria proliferating from the gingival crevice along the coagulum to the pulp. Furthermore, bacteria can invade the pulp via exposed dentin.[200-201]

Dentin formation after replantation and autotransplantation is usually very extensive and soon leads to massive pulp canal obliteration.[202-203] In replanted or transplanted monkey incisors observed for 9 months, it was thus found that the average daily dentin production was 4 µm.

Finally, it should be realized that necrotic pulp tissue can persist over a prolonged period without becoming infected so that infection is not inevitable.[204]

Healing of pulp after replantation and autotransplantation

This can be divided into the reactions encountered in *immature* teeth and in *mature* teeth, as healing events appear to be closely related to stage of root development. To date no significant difference in the pattern of healing has been found between replantation[138-148] and autotransplantation.[108-110,113,142-146]

Pulpal healing after replantation and autotransplantation of *immature* teeth (Fig. 1.14)

3 days: Extensive pulpal change is found as early as 3 days after replantation where pulpal necrosis is evident, especially in the coronal part of the pulp.

4 days: A revascularization process is initiated from the apical foramen, whereby damaged pulp tissue is gradually replaced by proliferating mesenchymal cells and capillaries.

4 to 5 weeks: The revascularization process is usually complete. However, in a few cases where an end-to-end anastomosis has occurred between ingrowing new vessels and the existing vessels, a complete revascularization can be seen as early as 1 week after replantation. The healing process leads to the formation of a new cell layer along the dentinal wall. Initially hard tissue is formed without dentinal tubules, but with occasional cell inclusions (osteodentin). In some cases the cells along the pulp canal walls begin to resemble odontoblasts with cytoplasmic processes within the newly formed matrix whereafter tubular dentin is formed. In animals and in humans, regenerating and functioning nerve fibers have been found at between 1 and 2 months.[206,207]

Fig. 1.14a. Revascularization of a replanted tooth with an open apical foramen
Condition is shown immediately after replantation.

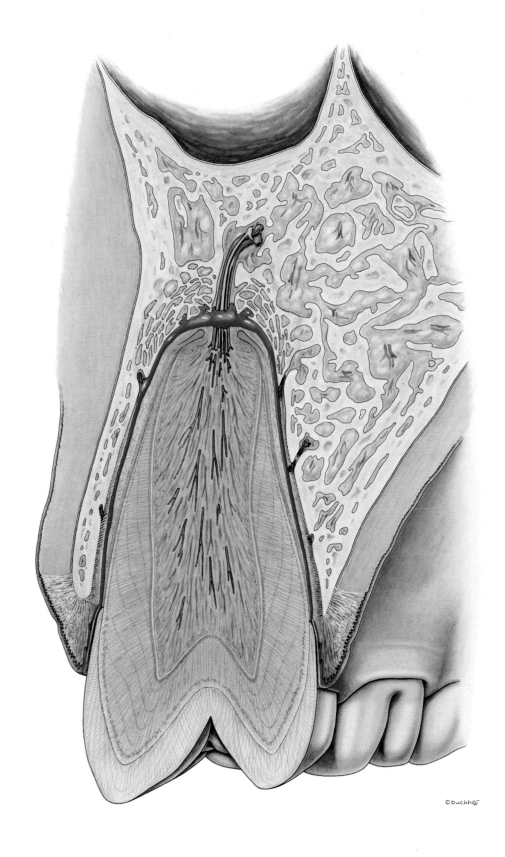

©buckhöj

Fig. 1.14b. Condition after 4 days
Initial revascularization in the apical aspect of the pulp. The coronal aspect has suffered extensive ischemic injury.

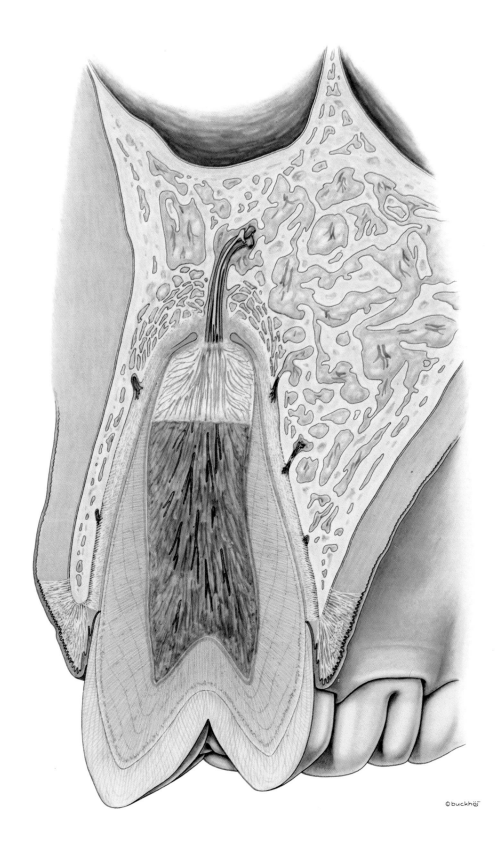

©buckhöj

Fig. 1.14c. Condition after 4 weeks
The pulp is revascularized and reinnervated. A new odontoblastic layer has been formed.

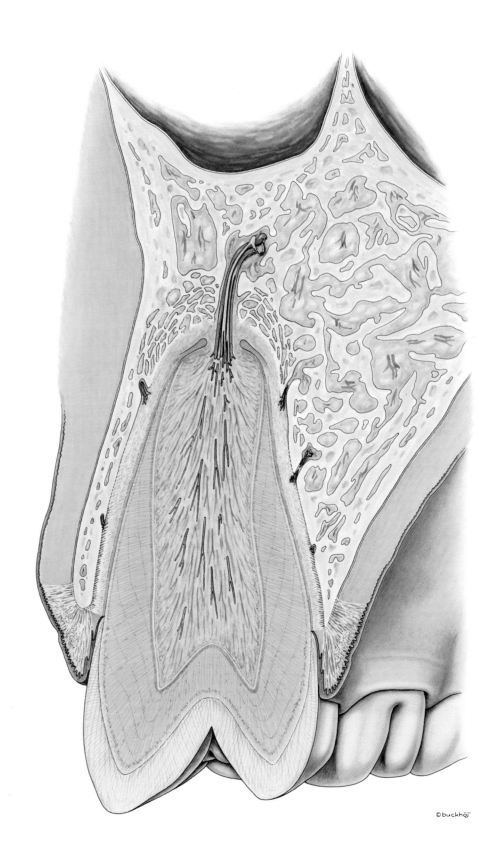

©buckhöj

Pulpal healing after replantation and autotransplantation of *mature* teeth (Fig. 1.15)

Usually the major part of the pulp becomes necrotic and revascularization ceases 1 or 2 mm. into the canal.[105,113,118,121,144-146,149] In rare cases, however, the entire pulp may become revascularized and in these cases an extensive canal obliteration occurs with cellular hard tissue (osteodentin or cementum).

Fig. 1.15a. Revascularization of a replanted tooth with a narrow apical foramen
Condition is shown immediately after replantation.

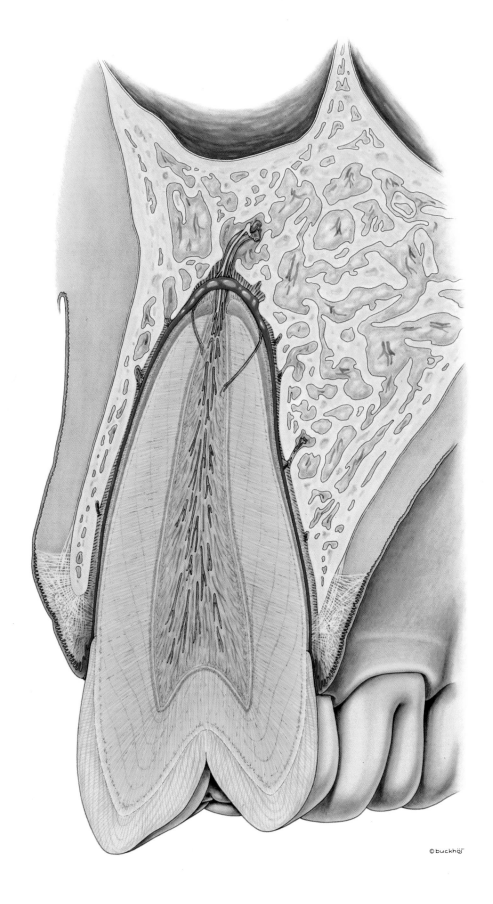

©buckhöj

Fig. 1.15b. Condition after 4 days
Very limited revascularization apically. The coronal part suffers from the effects of ischemia.

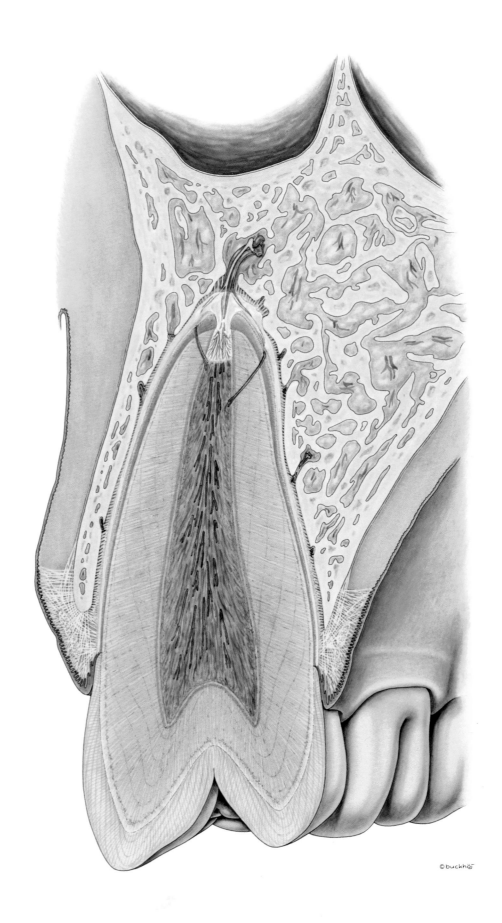

©buckhøj

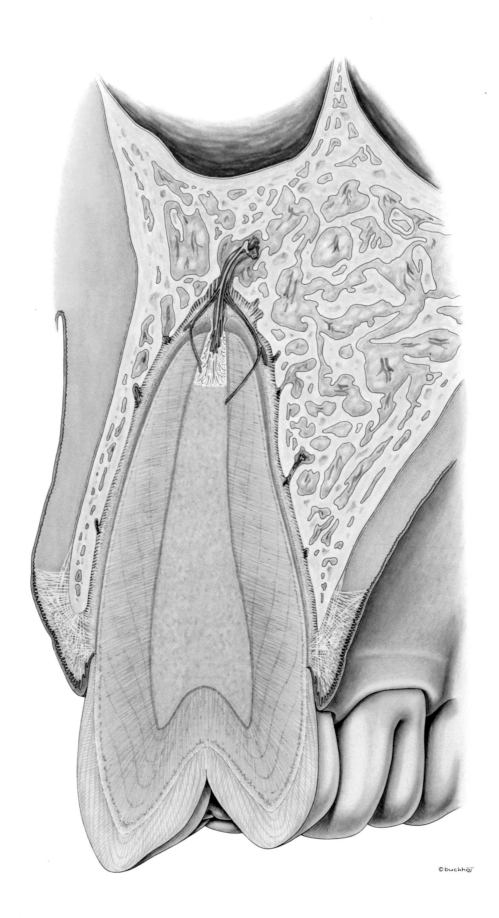

©buckhøj

Hertwig´s epithelial root sheath

The root sheath is a continuous sleeve of epithelial cells which separates the pulp from the dental follicle.[150] *Root growth* is determined by its activity (Fig. 1.16).[151-158]

Fig. 1.16. Anatomy of Hertwig´s epithelial root sheath
Note how the root sheath disintegrates when cementum formation starts.

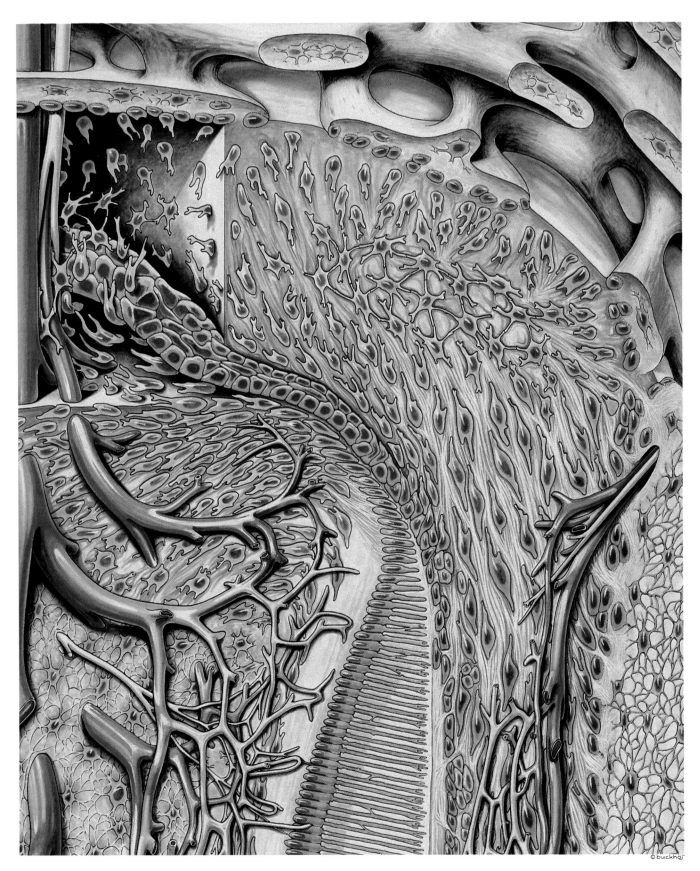

Reaction to surgical injury and infection

In a replantation or transplantation situation, the root sheath may be injured or severed from the base of the pulp either during the avulsion or extraction phase or by repositioning.[158] If this happens, further root growth will be partially or totally arrested and bone from the fundus of the socket will invade the root canal, but will be separated from the root canal wall by an internal PDL (Fig. 1.17).[158]

The epithelial root sheath is remarkably resistant to inflammation due to partial pulp necrosis.[158,160-165], and restricted root formation has sometimes been found to take place in cases with partial pulp necrosis irrespective of whether endodontic therapy is instituted or not (see also Chapter 2, p. 90). The fact that the epithelial root sheath can continue to function despite inflammation elicited by a partial pulp necrosis demonstrates that root development as such cannot be taken as a criterion for pulpal vitality.

Fig. 1.17. Hertwig´s epithelial root sheath, response to surgical or traumatic injury
In the event extensive damage to the Hertwig´s epithelial root sheath, an influx of bone and PDL-derived cells into the pulpal lumen takes place, whereby an "internal" PDL is created.

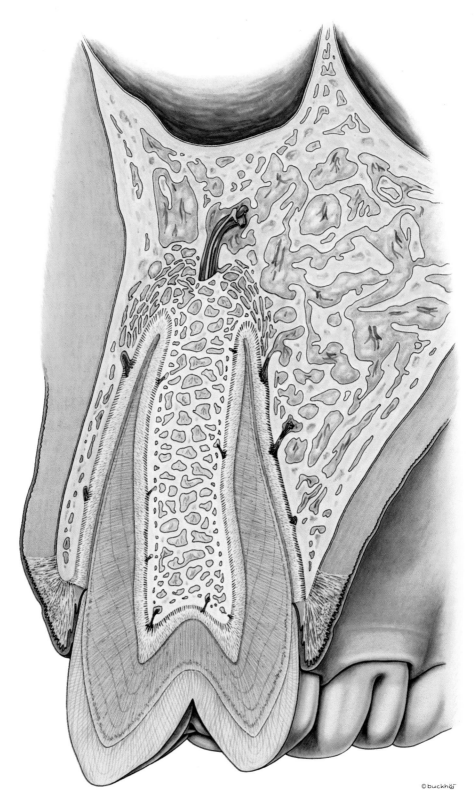

©buckhoj

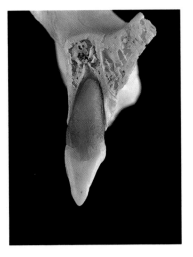
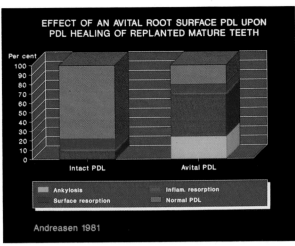
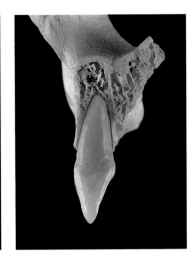

Fig. 1.18. Effect of loss of vitality of the cemental aspect of the PDL in mature replanted monkey teeth. From Andreasen, 1981.[112]

Factors influencing periodontal and pulpal healing after replantation and autotransplantation

In the following a synopsis will be given of the effect of damage to various anatomic structures as well as the effect of different treatment procedures upon pulpal and periodontal healing for teeth with complete or incomplete root formation.

The role of damage to the follicle

If larger areas of the follicle are damaged, ankylosis will occur and the teeth will not erupt after autotransplantation.[23] The minimum area of damage which can elicit these disturbances is not known at present.

The role of the PDL on the root in periodontal healing (Fig. 1.18)

The presence and vitality of the PDL upon replanted or autotransplanted teeth is decisive for periodontal healing.[93,103,166-169] Hence removal of the PDL leads to extensive root resorption. Furthermore the storage of teeth in non-physiologic media or damage to the PDL by the extraction procedure may also damage or kill periodontal cells resulting in the same root resorption phenomena.

The role of the alveolar socket wall in periodontal healing (Fig. 1.19)

Tooth germs as well as mature teeth with a vital PDL have a certain osteogenic potential.[171-179] Preliminary findings in humans indicate that reformation of bone will take place after autotransplantation of human third molars and premolars with incomplete root formation (see Chapter 4, p. 122 and Chapter 5, p. 143). Whether this healing mode will also be seen after replantation or transplantation of teeth with completed root formation is yet to be examined.

Fig. 1.19. Effect of removal of labial socket upon PDL healing of mature replanted monkey teeth. From Andreasen, 1981.[172]

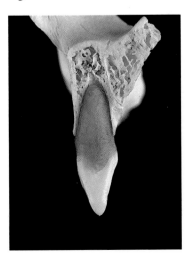
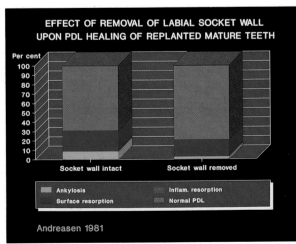
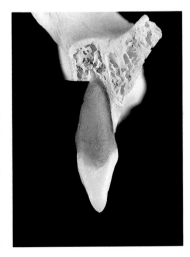

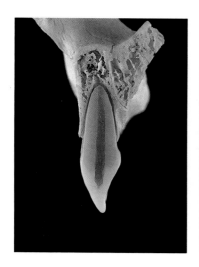
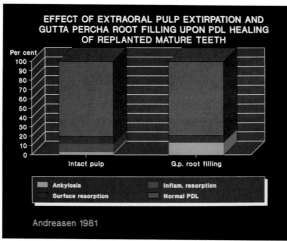
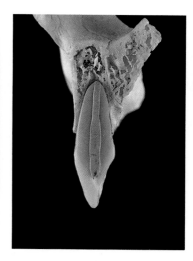

Fig. 1.20. Effect of extraoral pulp extirpation and gutta-percha root filling of replanted mature monkey teeth. From Andreasen, 1981.[180]

The role of pulpal status in periodontal healing (Figs. 1.20 and 1.21)

Extraoral root filling of mature teeth will significantly reduce the amount of inflammatory resorption compared to non-endodontically treated teeth.[114,121,180] However, at the same time, replacement resorption increases significantly in the apical area.[180] Thus immediate replantation or autotransplantation and a postponed root filling is the method of choice (Figs. 1.20 and 1.21). It may be argued that this procedure can lead to an increase in the extent of inflammatory resorption. However, clinical evidence indicates that this resorption type can be treated successfully by subsequent pulp extirpation and root filling with calcium hydroxide (see Chapter 2).[180-184] A postponement of the endodontic procedure by 7-10 days in replantation and 3 weeks after replantation seems optimal when considering the rate of PDL repair and its time relationship to inflammatory resorption.[99]

Fig. 1.21. Effect of extraoral pulp extirpation and gutta-percha root filling upon PDL healing in mature autotransplanted monkey teeth. From Andreasen, 1981.[114]

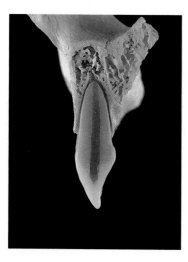
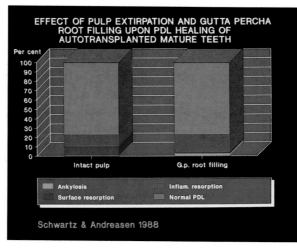
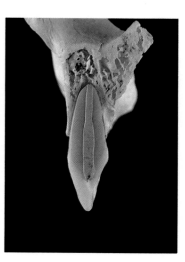

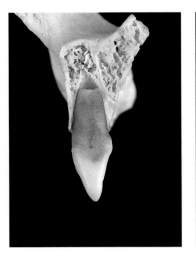
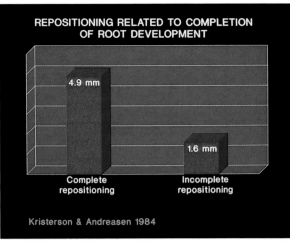
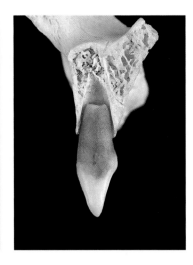

Fig. 1.22. Effect of repositioning upon root growth of autotransplanted immature monkey teeth. From Kristerson & Andreasen, 1984.[113]

The role of storage media and storage period in periodontal and pulpal healing

In most clinical cases, avulsed teeth have been stored either in the oral cavity (i.e., saliva) or in other media, such as physiologic saline or tap water before replantation. As these storage media differ considerably, especially with regard to electrolyte concentration, one might assume that the choice of storage medium could influence pulpal healing and the development of different types of root resorption. A strong relationship has been found between dry storage and storage in non physiologic media (e.g., tapwater) and periodontal healing and root resorption.[96,104,106,118,121,122,141,166-168,183,186-192] This relationship is described in Chapter 2, p. 76.

The role of positioning in periodontal and pulpal healing (Fig. 1.22).

If tooth germs are placed too superficially in the socket, the revascularization of the pulp leads to severe damage to the Hertwig´s epithelial root sheath.[113] The result is usually absent or diminutive root formation and sometimes ingrowth of bone in the root canal with an internal PDL.[113,202,203]

The role of splinting and functional stimuli in periodontal and pulpal healing

(Figs. 1.23-1.27)
Recent experimental studies indicate that rigid splinting does not improve periodontal healing after *replantation*, but actually results in an increase in ankylosis sites (Fig. 1.23).[193-196] It should be mentioned that in one experimental study no difference was found between splinting and no splinting.[205] In autotransplantation of immature and mature teeth, rigid splinting has a negative effect on pulpal revascularization and periodontal healing (Figs. 1.24-1.27).[197] The explanation for these findings are obscure at the present time. However, one explanation could be that the ingrowth of new vessels in the pulp tissue during the revascularization period is enhanced by small movements during function.[198] Furthermore the small movements during the healing period may either prevent or eliminate small ankylosis sites.

Fig. 1.23. Effect of rigid splinting upon PDL healing of replanted mature monkey teeth. From Andreasen, 1975.[193]

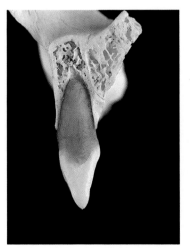
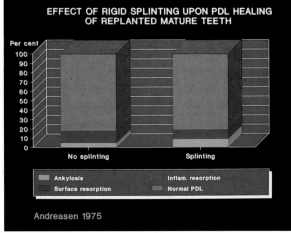
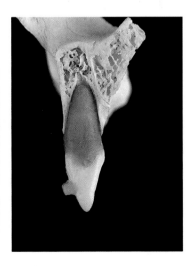

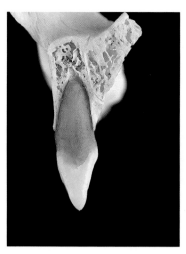
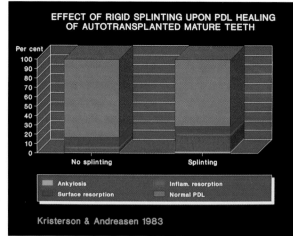
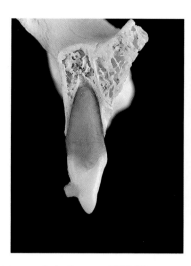

Fig. 1.24. Effect of rigid splinting upon PDL healing of autotransplanted mature monkey teeth. From Kristerson & Andreasen, 1983.[197]

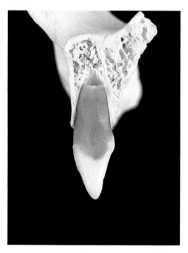
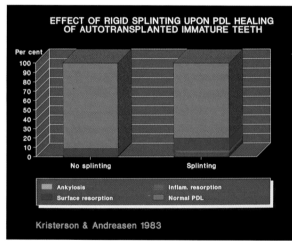
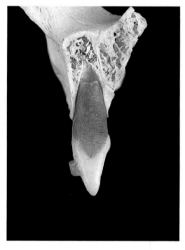

Fig. 1.25. Effect of rigid splinting upon PDL healing of autotransplanted immature monkey teeth. From Kristerson & Andreasen, 1983.[197]

Fig. 1.26. Effect of rigid splinting upon pulpal healing of autotransplanted mature monkey teeth. From Kristerson & Andreasen, 1983.[197]

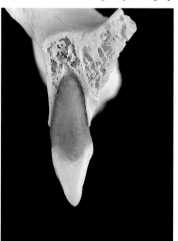
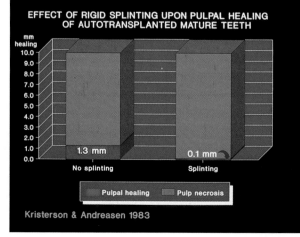
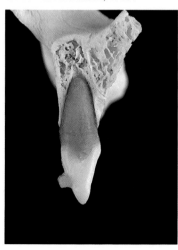

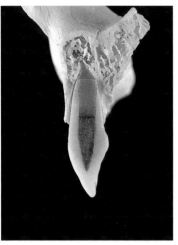
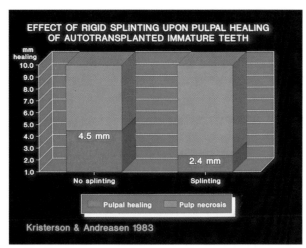
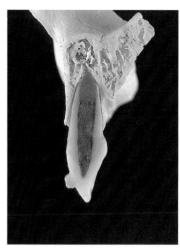

Fig. 1.27. Effect of rigid splinting upon pulpal healing of autotransplanted immature monkey teeth. From Kristerson & Andreasen, 1983,[197]

The role of antibiotics in periodontal and pulpal healing (Figs. 1.28-1.30)

Very little is known today about the value of antibiotics in periodontal and pulpal healing. In experimental studies in monkeys it has been shown that *systemic* antibiotics given in conjunction with replantation significantly reduce the extent of root resorption (Figs. 1.28 and 1.29).[199] However, when inflammatory resorption has been elicited it has been shown that the progress of resorption cannot be changed by systemic antibiotic therapy.[199] Concerning pulpal healing, no effect was found from *systemic* antibiotic therapy using doxycycline (Fig. 1.29), whereas *topical* use of the same drug (i.e., placing the teeth in a suspension of 1 mg doxycycline in 20 ml physiologic saline for 5 min) significantly increased the frequency of complete revascularization (Fig. 1.30) and at the same time reduced the frequency of ankylosis.[201]

The above-mentioned studies indicate that antibiotics should be used topically and possibly also systemically in replantation and transplantation procedures. However, the optimal type of antibiotic, dosage, and length of treatment are so far unsettled.

Fig. 1.28. Effect of systemic antibiotics upon PDL healing after replantation of mature monkey teeth. From Hammarström & al., 1986.[199']

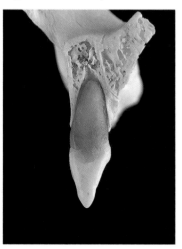
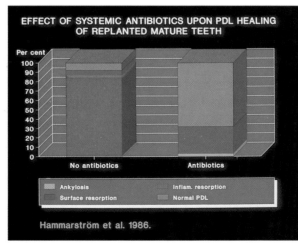
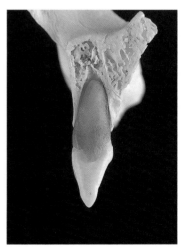

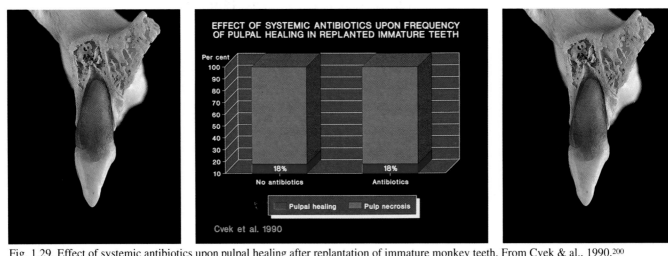

Fig. 1.29. Effect of systemic antibiotics upon pulpal healing after replantation of immature monkey teeth. From Cvek & al., 1990.[200]

Fig. 1.30. Effect of topical treatment of the root with antibiotics upon pulp healing after replantation of immature monkey teeth. From Cvek & al., 1990.[201]

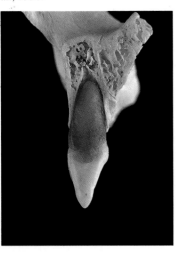
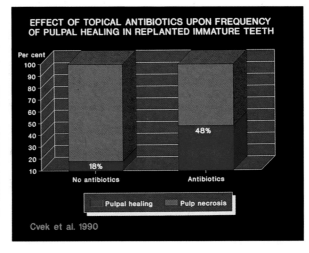
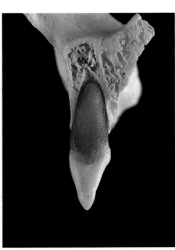

Essentials

Gingival attachment appears complete 1 week after replantation and autotransplantation.

Periodontal ligament healing is initiated after 1 week and is advanced 2 weeks after replantation; 1 or 2 weeks´ delay is found after autotransplantation.

Pulpal revascularization is initiated after 4 days and is usually complete after 4 to 5 weeks in both replanted and autotransplanted immature teeth. Revascularization is rare in mature teeth with a narrow apical foramen.

Surface resorption can develop 1 week after replantation and subsequently shows repair with newly formed cementum. This resorption type is related to damage to the innermost layers of the PDL on the root surface.

Inflammatory resorption can develop 1 week after replantation and follows a progressive course unless endodontically treated. This resorption type is related to the associated damage to the innermost layers of the PDL on the root surface and the presence of infected necrotic pulp tissue.

Replacement resorption (ankylosis) can develop 2 weeks after replantation and then appears in two forms according to the extent of damage: (1) transient replacement resorption in which a once-established ankylosis disappears, and (2) permanent replacement resorption, which gradually resorbs the entire root. Replacement resorption is related to extensive damage to the innermost layers of the PDL on the root.

Factors influencing healing

The presence of an intact and viable PDL on the root surface is the most important factor in ensuring PDL healing without root resorption.

The presence or absence of a socket wall appears to be of minor importance for healing if the PDL along the root surface is vital.

Nonphysiologic storage media (e.g., tap water, dry storage) in the extra-alveolar period result in severe cell damage and subsequent root resorption.

Too superficial repositioning of a replanted or autotransplanted immature tooth can lead to severe damage to the Hertwig´s epithelial root sheath, resulting in absent or diminutive root growth and sometimes ingrowth of bone into the pulp chamber.

Extra-alveolar root canal filling with gutta-percha and a sealer eliminates inflammatory resorption otherwise found in teeth with completed root formation; however, an ankylosis usually forms apically. Postponed endodontic treatment (i.e., 7-10 days after replantation and 3 weeks after autotransplantation) is therefore advisable.

Rigid splinting of replanted mature teeth enhances replacement resorption compared to nonsplinted teeth. In autotransplanted immature teeth, rigid splinting has a negative effect upon pulpal revascularization.

Systemic antibiotic treatment administered at the time of or before repositioning decreases the extent of root resorption but has no effect on pulpal revascularization. Topical antibiotic treatment administered before repositioning enhances pulpal revascularization.

References

1. Ten Cate AR. The development of the periodontium. In: Melcher AH, Bowen WH, eds. Biology of the periodontium. London New York: Academic Press 1969; 53-89.

2. Ten Cate AR, Mills C. The development of the periodontium: The origin of alveolar bone. Anat Rec 1972; 173: 69-78.

3. Ten Cate AR. Formation of supporting bone in association with periodontal ligament organization in the mouse. Arch Oral Biol 1975; 20: 137-38.

4. Ten Cate AR, Mills C, Solomon G. A. The development of the periodontium. A transplantation and autoradiographic study. Anat Rec 1971; 170: 365-80

5. Freeman E, Ten Cate AR. Development of the periodontium: An electron microscopic study. J Periodont 1971; 42: 387-95.

6. Hoffman RL. Formation of periodontal tissues around subcutaneously transplanted hamster molars. J Dent Res 1960; 19: 761-96.

7. Hoffman RL. Bone formation and resorption around developing teeth transplanted into the femur. Am J Anat 1960; 118: 91-102.

8. Hoffman RL. Tissue alterations in intramuscularly transplanted developing molars. Arch Oral Biol 1967; 12: 713-20.

9. Barton JM, Keenan RM. The formation of Sharpey's fibres in the hamster under nonfunctional conditions. Arch Oral Biol 1967; 12: 1331-36.

10. Freeman E, Ten Cate AR, Dickenson J. Development of a gomphosis by tooth germ implants in the parietal bone of the mouse. Arch Oral Biol 1975; 20:139-40.

11. Yoshikawa DK, Kollar EJ. Recombination experiments on the odontogenic roles of mouse dental papilla and dental sac tissues in ocular grafts. Arch Oral Biol 1981; 26: 303-07.

12. Barrett P, Reade PC. The relationship between degree of development of tooth isografts and the subsequent formation of bone and periodontal ligament. J Periodont Res 1981; 16: 456-65.

13. Cahill DR. Histological changes in the bony crypt and gubernacular canal of erupting permanent premolars during deciduous premolar exfoliation in beagles. J Dent Res 1974; 53: 786-91.

14. Cahill DR, Marks SC Jr. Tooth eruption: evidence for the central role of the dental follicle. J Oral Pathol 1980; 9: 189-200.

15. Cahill DR, Marks SC Jr. Chronology and histology of exfoliation and eruption of mandibular premolars in dogs. J Morphol 1982; 171: 213-18.

16. Marks SC Jr, Cahill DR, Wise GE. The cytology of the dental follicle and adjacent alveolar bone during tooth eruption in the dog. Am J Anat 1983; 168: 277-89.

17. Marks SC Jr, Cahill DR. Experimental study in the dog of the non-active role of the tooth in the eruptive process. Arch Oral Biol 1984; 29: 311-22.

18. Wise GE, Marks SC, Cahill DR. Ultrastructural features of the dental follicle associated with formation of the tooth eruption pathway in the dog. J Oral Pathol 1985; 14: 15-26.

19. Henry CB. Examples of reimplantation of teeth in young subjects. Proc R Soc Med 1955; 48: 1013-22.

20. Monsour FNT, Adkins KF. Aberrations involving the enamel epithelium in transplanted developing teeth. J Oral Maxillofac Surg 1983; 41: 377-84.

21. Grant D, Bernick S. Formation of the periodontal ligament. J Periodontol 1972; 43: 17-25.

22. Grant D, Bernick S, Levy BM, Dreizen S. A comparative study of periodontal ligament development in teeth with and without predecessors in marmosets. J Periodontol 1972; 43: 162-9.

23. Kristerson L, Andreasen JO. Autotransplantation and replantation of tooth germs in monkeys. Effect of damage to the dental follicle and position of transplant in the alveolus. Int J Oral Surg 1984; 13: 324-33.

24. Barfoed CP, Nielsen LH, Andreasen JO. Injury to developing canines as a complication of intranasal antrostomy. Int J Oral Surg 1984; 13: 445-47.

25. Andreasen JO, Riis I. Influence of pulp necrosis and periapical inflammation of primary teeth on their permanent successors. Combined macroscopic and histological study in monkeys. Int J Oral Surg 1978; 7: 178-87.

26. Andreasen JO. Traumatic injuries of the teeth. Second ed. Copenhagen: Munksgaard, 1981: 304.

27. Goldman HM. The topography and role of the gingival fibers. J Dent Res 1951; 30: 331-36.

28. Arnim SS, Hagerman DA.The connective tissue fibers of the marginal gingiva. J Am Dent Assoc 1953; 47: 271-81.

29. Melcher AH. The interpapillary ligament. Dent Pract 1962; 12: 461-62.

30. Smukler H, Dreyer CJ. Principal fibres of the periodontium. J Periodont Res 1969; 4: 19-25.

31. Page RC, Ammons WF, Schectman LR, Dillingham LA. Collagen fibre bundles of the normal marginal gingiva in the marmoset. Arch Oral Biol 1974; 19: 1039-43.

32. Atkinson ME. The development of transalveolar ligament fibres in the mouse. J Dent Res 1978; 57: 151 (abstract).

33. Garnick J, Walton RE. Fiber system of the facial gingiva. J Peridont Res 1984; 19: 419-23.

34. Tonna EA, Cronkite EP. The periosteum: Autoradiographic studies of cellular proliferation and transformation utilizing tritiated thymidine. Clin Orthop 1963; 30: 218-33 .

35. Tonna EA. Response of the cellular phase of the skeleton to trauma. Periodontics 1966; 4: 105-14.

36. Tonna EA. Electron microscopy of aging skeletal cells III. The periosteum. Lab Invest 1974; 31: 609-32.

37. Nasjleti CE, Caffesse RG, Castelli WA, Hoke JA. Healing after tooth reimplantation in monkeys. A radioautographic study. Oral Surg Oral Med Oral Pathol 1975; 39: 361-75.

38. Hurst RW. Regeneration of periodontal and transseptal fibres after autografts in rhesus monkeys. A qualitative approach. J Dent Res 1972; 51: 1183-92.

39. Andreasen JO. A time-related study of periodontal healing and root resorption activity after replantation of mature permanent incisors in monkeys. Swed Dent J 1980; 4: 101-10.

40. Proye MP, Polson AM. Repair in different zones of the periodontium after tooth reimplantation. J Periodontol 1982; 53: 379-89.

41. Kohler CA, Ramfjord SP. Healing of gingival mucoperiosteal flaps. Oral Surg Oral Med Oral Pathol 1960; 13: 89-103.

42. Donnenfeld OW, Hoag PM, Weissman DP. A clinical study on the effects of osteoplasty. J Periodontol 1970; 41: 131-41.

43. Wood DL, Hoag PM, Donnenfeld OW, Rosenfeld LD. Alveolar reduction following full and partial thickness flaps. J Periodontol 1972; 43: 141-45.

44. Pfeifer JS. The reaction of alveolar bone to flap procedures in man. Periodontics 1965; 3: 135-40.

45. Melcher AH, Accursi GE. Osteogenic capacity of periosteal and osteoperiosteal flaps elevated from the parietal bone of the rat. Arch Oral Biol 1971; 16: 573-80.

46. Hjørting-Hansen E, Andreasen JO. Incomplete bone healing of experimental cavities in dog mandibles. Br J Oral Surg 1971; 9: 33-40.

47. Mascres C, Marchand JF. Experimental apical scars in rats. Oral Surg Oral Med Oral Pathol 1980 ; 50 : 164-74.

48. Nwoku AL. Unusually rapid bone regeneration following mandibular resection. J Maxillofac Surg 1980; 8: 309-15.

49. Shuker S. Spontaneous regeneration of the mandible in a child. A sequel to partial avulsion as a result of a war injury. J Maxillofac Surg 1985; 13: 70-73.

50. Selvig KA. The fine structure of human cementum. Acta Odontol Scand 1965; 23: 423-41.

51. Zander HA, Hürzeler B. Continuous cementum apposition. J Dent Res 1958; 37: 1035-44 .

52. Stoot GG, Sis RF, Levy BM. Cemental annulation as an age criterion in forensic dentistry. J Dent Res 1982; 61: 814-17.

53. Roberts WE, Chamberlain JG. Scanning electron microscopy of the cellular elements of rat periodontal ligament. Arch Oral Biol 1978; 23: 587-89.

54. Beertsen W, Everts V. Junctions between fibroblasts in mouse periodontal ligament. J Peridont Res 1980; 15: 655-68.

55. Garant PR. Collagen resorption by fibroblasts. A theory of fibroblastic maintenance of the periodontal ligament. J Periodontol 1976; 47: 380-390.

56. Deporter DA, Ten Cate AR. Collagen resorption by periodontal ligament fibroblasts at the hard tissue-ligament interfaces of the mouse periodontium. J Periodontol 1980; 51: 429-32.

57. Gould TRL, Brunette DM, Dorey J. Cell turnover in health and periodontal disease. J Periodont Res 1983; 18: 353-61.

58. McCulloch CAG, Melcher AH. Continuous labelling of the periodontal ligament of mice. J Periodont Res 1983; 18: 231-41.

59. McCulloch CAG, Melcher AH. Cell density and cell generation in the periodontal ligament of mice. Am J Anat 1983; 167: 43-58.

60. McCulloch CAG, Melcher AH. Cell migration in the periodontal ligament of mice. J Periodont Res 1983; 18: 339-52.

61. Boyde A, Jones SJ. Scanning electron microscopy of cementum and Sharpey's fibre bone. Z Zellforsch 1968; 92: 536-48.

62. Shackleford JM, Zuniga MA. Scanning electron microscopic studies of calcified and noncalcified dental tissues. Proc Cambridge Stereoscan Colloquium 1970, 113-19.

63. Shackleford JM. Scanning electron microscopy of the dog periodontium. J Periodont Res 1971; 6: 45-54.

64. Shackleford JM. The indifferent fiber plexus and its relationship to principal fibers of the periodontium. Am J Anat 1971; 131: 427-42.

65. Svejda J, Krejsa O. Die Oberflächenstruktur des Alveolarknochens des extrahierten Zahnes und des Periodontiums im Rasterelektronenmikroskop (REM). Schweiz Monatsschr Zahnheilk 1972; 82: 763-76.

66. Svejda J, Skach M. The periodontium of the human tooth in the scanning electron microscope (Stereoscan). J Periodontol 1973; 44: 478-84 .

67. Kvam E. Scanning electron microsopy of organic structures on the root surface of human teeth. Scand J Dent Res 1972; 80: 297-306.

68. Kvam E. Topoprapby of principal fibers. Scand J Dent Res 1973; 81: 553-57.

69. Shackleford JM. Ultrastructural and microradiographic characteristics of Sharpey's fibers in the dog alveolar bone. Alabama J Med Sci 1973; 10: 11-20.

70. Sloan P, Shellis RP, Berkovitz BKB. Effect of specimen preparation on the appearance of the rat periodontal ligament in the scanning electron microscope. Arch Oral Biol 1976; 21: 633-35.

71. Berkovitz BKB, Holland GR, Moxham BJ. A Colour Atlas & Textbook of Oral Anatomy. London: Wolfe Medical Publications Ltd, 1978.

72. Sloan P . Scanning electron microscopy of the collagen fibre architecture of the rabbit incisor periodontium. Arch Oral Biol 1978; 23: 567-72.

73. Sloan P. Collagen fibre architecture in the periodontal ligament. J R Soc Med 1979; 72: 188-91.

74. Folke LEA, Stallard RE. Periodontal microcirculation as revealed by plastic microspheres. J Periodont Res 1967; 2: 53-63.

75. Lenz P. Zur Gefäßstruktur des Parodontiums. Untersuchungen an Korrosionspräparaten von Affenkiefern. Dtsch Zahnärztl Z 1968; 23: 357-61.

76. Edwall LGA. The vasculature of the periodontal ligament. In: Berkovitz BKB, Moxham BJ, Newman HN, eds. The periodontal ligament in health and disease. Oxford: Pergamon Press, 1982: 151-71.

77. Saunders RL de CH, Röckert HOE. Vascular supply of dental tissue including lymphatics. In Miles AEW (ed). Structural and chemical organization of teeth, vol 1 London, Academic Press, 1967; 199-245

78. Birn H. The vascular supply of the periodontal membrane. An investigation of the number and size of perforations in the alveolar wall. J Periodont Res 1966; 1: 51-68.

79. Amler MH, Johnson PL, Salman I. Histological and histochemical investigation of human alveolar socket healing in undisturbed extraction wounds. J Am Dent Assoc 1960; 61: 32-44.

80. Amler MH, Salman I, Bungener H. Reticular and collagen fiber characteristics in human bone healing. Oral Surg Oral Med Oral Pathol 1964; 17: 785-796.

81. Amler MH. The time sequence of tissue regeneration in human extraction wounds. Oral Surg Oral Med Oral Pathol 1969; 27: 309-18.

82. Amler MH. Pathogenesis of disturbed extraction wounds. J Oral Surg 1973; 31: 666-74.

83. Amler MH. The age factor in human extraction wound healing. J Oral Surg 1977; 35: 1939-99.

84. Amler MH. The interrelationship of dry socket sequelae. NY J Dent 1980; 50: 211-217.

85. Gergeley E, Bartha N. Die Rolle der Wurzelhaut bei der Heilung von Ekstraktionswunden. Dtsch Stomat 1961; 10:162-67.

86. Simpson HE. The healing of extraction wounds. Br Dent J 1969; 126: 550-57.

87. Evian CI, Rosenberg ES, Coslet JG, Corn H. The osteogenic activity of bone removed from healing extraction sockets in humans. J Periodont 1982; 53: 81-85.

88. Mandel U, Viidik A. Effect of splinting on the mechanical and histological properties of the healing periodontal ligament after experimental extrusive luxation in the vervet monkey (Cercopithecus aethiops). Arch Oral Biol 1989; 34: 209-17.

89. Andreasen JO. Rewiev of root resorption systems and models. Etiology of root resorption and the homeostatic mechanisms of the periodontal ligament. In: Davidovitch Z, ed. The biological mechanisms of tooth eruption and tooth resorption. Birmingham: EBSCO Media, 1988; 9-21.

90. Kantor M, Polson AM, Zander HA. Alveolar bone regeneration after removal of inflammatory and traumatic factors. J Periodont 1976; 47: 687-95.

91. Malooley Jr. J. Patterson S, Kafrawy A. Response of periapical pathosis to endodontic treatment in monkeys. Oral Surg Oral Med Oral Pathol 1979; 47: 545-54.

92. Moskow BS, Wasserman BH, Hirschfeld LS, Morris ML. Repair of periodontal tissues following acute localized osteomyelitis. Periodontics 1967; 5: 29-36.

93. Hammer H. Der histologische Vorgang bei der Zahnreplantation. Dtsch Kieferchir 1934; 1: 115-36.

94. Anderson AW, Sharav Y, Massler M. Periapical tissue reactions following root amputation in immediate tooth replants. Isr J Dent Med 1970; 19: 1-8.

95. Waerhaug J. Observations on replanted teeth plated with gold foil. Oral Surg Oral Med Oral Pathol 1956; 9: 780-91.

96. Hamner JE, Reed OM, Stanley HR. Reimplantation of teeth in the baboon. J Am Dent Assoc 1970; 81: 662-70.

97. Nasjleti CE, Caffesse RG, Castelli WA, Hoke JA. Healing after tooth reimplantation in monkeys. A radioautographic study. Oral Surg Oral Med Oral Pathol 1975; 39: 361-75.

98. Barbakow FH, Cleaton-Jones PE. Experimental replantation of root-canal-filled and untreated teeth in the vervet monkey. J Endod 1977; 3: 89-94.

99. Andreasen JO. A time-related study of periodontal healing and root resorption activity after replantation of mature permanent incisors in monkeys. Swed Dent J 1980; 4: 101-10.

100. Andreasen JO. Analysis of topography of surface- and inflammatory root resorption after replantation of mature permanent incisors in monkeys. Swed Dent J 1980; 4: 135-44.

101. Andreasen JO. Analysis of pathogenesis and topography of replacement root resorption (ankylosis) after replantation of mature permanent incisors in monkeys. Swed Dent J 1980; 4: 231-40.

102. Krömer H. Tannreplantasjon. Norske Tannlægeforen Tid 1952; 62: 147-57.

103. Hammer H. Der histologische Vorgang bei der Zahnreplantation nach Vernichtung der Wurzelhaut. Zahn Mund Kieferheilk 1937; 4: 179-87.

104. Löe H, Waerhaug J. Experimental replantation of teeth in dogs and monkeys. Arch Oral Biol 1961; 3: 176-84.

105. Andreasen JO. Relationship between surface and inflammatory resorption and changes in the pulp after replantation of permanent incisors in monkeys. J Endod 1981; 7: 294-301 and 1982; 8: 426-27.

106. Andreasen JO. Periodontal healing after replantation and autotransplantation of incisors in monkeys. Int J Oral Surg 1981; 10: 54-61.

107. Agnew RG, Fong CC. Transplantation of teeth - histological studies. J Dent Res 1955; 34: 669.

108. Agnew RG, Fong CC. Histologic studies on experimental transplantation of teeth. Oral Surg Oral Med Oral Pathol 1956; 9: 18-39.

109. Nordenram Å. Autotransplantation of teeth. A clinical and experimental investigation. Acta Odontol Scand 1963; 21 Suppl 33.

110. Fong C, Morris M, Grant T, Berger J. Experimental tooth transplantation in the rhesus monkey. J Dent Res 1967; 46: 492-96.

111. Shulman LO, Kalis P, Goldhaber P. Fluoride inhibition of tooth-replant root resorption in cebus monkeys. J Oral Ther Pharm 1968; 4: 331-37.

112. Andreasen JO. Periodontal healing after replantation and autotransplantation of incisors in monkeys. Int J Oral Surg 1981; 10: 54-61.

113. Kristerson L, Andreasen JO. Autotransplantation and replantation of tooth germs in monkeys. Effect of damage to the dental follicle and position of transplant in the alveolus. Int J Oral Surg 1984; 13: 324-33.

114. Schwartz O, Andreasen JO. Allotransplantation and autotransplantation of mature teeth in monkeys: The influence of endodontic treatment. J Oral Maxillofac Surg 1988; 46: 672-81.

115. Schwartz O, Andreasen JO. Allo- and autotransplantation of mature teeth in monkeys. A sequential time-related histoquantitive study. To be submitted to Endod Dent Traumatol.

116. Andreasen JO. Relationship between cell damage in the periodontal ligament after replantation and subsequent development of root resorption. A time-related study in monkeys. Acta Odontol Scand 1981; 3 9: 15-25 .

117. Andreasen JO, Kristerson L. Repair processes in the cervical region of replanted and transplanted teeth in monkeys. Int J Oral Surg 1981; 10: 128-36.

118. Andreasen JO. Effect of extra-alveolar period and storage media upon periodontal and pulpal healing after replantation of mature permanent incisors in monkeys. Int J Oral Surg 1981; 10: 43-53.

119. Andreasen JO, Kristerson L. The effect of limited drying or removal of the periodontal ligament. Periodontal healing after replantation of mature permanent incisors in monkeys. Acta Odontol Scand 1981; 39: 1-13.

120. Andreasen JO, Hjørting-Hansen E. Replantation of teeth. I. Radiographic and clinical study of 110 human teeth replanted after accidental loss. Acta Odontol Scand 1966; 24: 263-86.

121. Kristerson L, Andreasen JO. Influence of root development on periodontal and pulpal healing after replantation of incisors in monkeys. Int J Oral Surg 1984; 13: 313-23.

122. Frost HM. Tetracycline-based histological analysis of bone remodelling. Calcif Tissue Res 1969; 3: 211-37.

123. Andreasen JO. Periodontal healing after replantation of traumatically avulsed human teeth. Assessment by mobility testing and radiography. Acta Odontol Scand 1975; 33: 325-335.

124. Baume LJ. The biology of pulp and dentine. A historic, terminologic-taxonomic, histologic biochemical, embryonic and clinical survey. Monographs in Oral Science l980; 5: 1-220.

125. Ruch JV. Odontoblast differentation and the formation of the odontoblast layer. J Dent Res 1945 ; 64: 489-98.

126. Holland GR. The odontoblast process: Form and function. J Dent Res 1985; 64: 499-514.

127. Couve E. Ultrastructural changes during the life cycle of human odontoblasts. Arch Oral Biol 1986; 31: 643-51.

128. Melsen B, Melsen F, Rölling I. Dentin formation rate in human teeth. Calcif Tissue Res 1977; 24: Suppl: Abstr no 62.

129. Kramer IRH, Russel LH. Observations on the vascular architecture of the dental pulp. J Dent Res 1956; 35: 957.

130. Kramer IRH. The vascular architecture of the human dental pulp. Arch Oral Biol 1960; 2: 177-89.

131. Saunders RL de CH. X-ray microscopy of the periodontal and dental pulp vessels in the monkey and in man. Oral Surg Oral Med Oral Pathol 1966; 22: 503-18.

132. Takahashi K, Kishi Y, Kim S. Scanning electron microscope study of the blood vessels of dog pulp using corrosion resin casts. J Endod 1982; 8: 131-35.

133. Bernick S. Differences in nerve distribution between erupted and non-erupted human teeth. J Dent Res 1964; 43: 406-11.

134. Fulling H-J, Andreasen JO. Influence of maturation status and tooth type of permanent teeth upon electrometric and thermal pulp testing. Scand J Dent Res 1976; 84: 286-90.

135. Johnsen DC, Harshbarger J, Rymer HD. Quantitative assessment of neural development in human premolars. Anat Rec 1983; 205: 421-29.

136. Johnsen DC. Innervation of teeth: Qualitative, quantitative, and developmental assessment. J Dent Res 1985; 64 (Spec. Iss.): 555-63.

137. Andreasen JO, Paulsen HU, Yu Z, Ahlquist R, Bayer T, Schwartz O. A long-term study of 370 autotransplanted premolars. Part 1. Surgical procedures and standardized techniques for monitoring healing. Eur J Orthod 1990; 12: 3-13.

138. Öhman A. Healing and sensitivity to pain in young replanted human teeth. Odontologisk Tidskrift (Göteborg) 1965; 73: 165-228.

139. Anderson AW, Sharav Y, Massler M. Reparative dentine formation and pulp morphology. Oral Surg Oral Med Oral Pathol 1968; 26: 837-47.

140. Johnson DS, Burich RL. Revascularization of reimplanted teeth in dogs. J Dent Res 1979; 58: 671.

141. Sheppard PR, Burich RL. Effects of extra-oral exposure and multiple avulsions on revascularization of reimplanted teeth in dogs. J Dent Res 1980; 59: 140.

142. Skoglund A, Tronstad L, Wallenius K. A microangiographic study of vascular changes in replanted and autotransplanted teeth of young dogs. Oral Surg Oral Med Oral Pathol 1978; 45: 17-28.

143. Scheibe B, Düker J. Umbauvorgänge nach Re- und Transplantationen von Zähnen im Tierversuch. Dtsch Zahnärztl Z 1980; 35: 784-88.

144. Skoglund A. Vascular changes in replanted and autotransplanted apicoectomized mature teeth of dogs. Int J Oral Surg 1981; 10: 100-10.

145. Skoglund A. Pulpal changes in replanted and autotransplanted apicectomized mature teeth of dogs. Int J Oral Surg 1981; 10: 11-21.

146. Skoglund A, Hasselgren G, Tronstad L. Oxidoreductase activity in the pulp of replanted and autotransplanted teeth in young dogs. Oral Surg Oral Med Oral Pathol; 1981; 52: 205-09

147. Heyeraas KJ, Myking AM. Pulpal blood flow in immature permanent dog teeth after replantation. Scand J Dent Res 1985; 93: 227-38.

148. Vidair RV, Butcher EO. Regeneration of tissue into the pulp canal of monkeys' teeth. J Dent Med 1955; 10: 163-67.

149. Skoglund A. Vascular changes in replanted and autotransplanted apicoectomized mature teeth of dogs. Int J Oral Surg 1981; 10: 100-10.

150. Noble HW, Carmichael AF, Rankine DM. Electron microscopy of human developing dentine. Arch Oral Biol 1962; 7: 395-99.

151. Diamond M, Applebaum E. The epithelial sheath: histogenesis and function. J Dent Res 1942; 21: 403-11.

152. Grant D, Bernick S. Morphodifferentiation and structure of Hertwig's root sheath in the cat. J Dent Res 1971; 50: 1580-88.

153. Owens PDA. A light microscopic study of the development of the roots of premolar teeth in dogs. Arch Oral Biol 1974; 20: 525-38.

154. Owens PDA. Ultrastructure of Hertwig's epithelial root sheath during early root development in premolar teeth in dogs. Arch Oral Biol 1978; 23: 91-104.

155. Andreasen FM, Andreasen JO. The relationship in monkeys between the functional, histological and radiographic diameter of the apical foramen and blood supply to the pulp. In preparation 1990.

156. Diab MA, Stallard RE. A study of the relationship between epithelial root sheath and root development. Periodontics 1965; 3: 10-17.

157. Shibata F, Stern IB. Hertwig's sheath in the rat incisors. II Autoradiographic study. J Periodont Res 1968; 2: 111-20.

158. Andreasen JO, Kristerson L, Andreasen FM. Damage of the Hertwig's epithelial root sheath: effect upon root growth after autotransplantation in monkeys. Endod Dent Traumatol 1988; 4: 145-51.

159. Anderson AW, Massler M. Periapical tissue reactions following root amputation in immediate tooth replants. Isr J Dent Med 1970; 19: 01-08.

160. Stewart DJ. Traumatised incisors. An unusual type of response. Br Dent J 1960; 108: 396- 99.

161. Rule DC, Winter GB. Root growth and apical repair subsequent to pulpal necrosis in children. Br Dent J 1966; 120: 586-90.

162. Barker BCW, Mayne JR. Some unusual cases of apexification subsequent to trauma. Oral Surg Oral Med Oral Pathol 1975; 39: 144-50.

163. Torneck CD, Smith J. Biologic effects of endodontic procedures on developing incisor teeth. Effect of partial and total pulp removal. Oral Surg Oral Med Oral Pathol 1970; 30: 258-66.

164. Lieberman J, Trowbridge H. Apical closure of nonvital permanent incisor teeth where no treatment was performed: case report. J Endod 1983; 9: 257-60.

165. Holland R, de Souza V. Ability of a new calcium hydroxide root canal filling material to induce hard tissue formation. J Endod 1985; 11: 535-43.

166. Van Hassel HJ, Oswald RJ, Harrington GW. Replantation 2. The role of the periodontal ligament. Endod 1980; 6: 506-08.

167. Oswald RJ, Harrington GW, Van Hassel HJ. A postreplantation evaluation of air-dried and saliva-stored avulsed teeth. J Endod 1980; 6: 546-51.

168. Blomlöf L, Lindskog S, Hedström K-G, Hammarström L. Vitality of periodontal ligament cells after storage of monkey teeth in milk or saliva. Scand J Dent Res 1980; 88: 441-45.

169. Nyman S, Karring T, Lindhe J, Plantén S. Healing following implantation of periodontitis-affected roots into gingival connective tissue. J Clin Periodontol 1980; 7: 394-401.

170. Andreasen JO. Delayed replantation after submucosal storage in order to prevent root resorption after replantation. An experimental study in monkeys. Int J Oral Surg 1980; 9: 394-403 .

171. Oswald RJ, Harrington GW, Van Hassel HJ. Replantation 1. The role of the socket. J Endod 1980; 6: 479-84.

172. Andreasen JO. Interrelation between alveolar bone and periodontal ligament repair after replantation of mature permanent incisors in monkeys. J. Periodont Res 1981; 16: 228-35.

173. Hoffman RL. Formation of periodontal tissues around subcutaneously transplanted hamster molars. J Dent Res 1960; 39: 71-98.

55

174. Hoffman RL. Tissue alterations in intramuscularly transplanted developing molars. Arch Oral Biol 1967; 12: 713-20.

175. Barton JM, Keenan RM. The formation of Sharpey´s fibres in the hamster under nonfunctional conditions. Arch Oral Biol 1967; 12: 1331-36.

176. Ten Cate AR. Mills C, Solomon G. The development of the periodontium. A transplantation and autoradiographic study. Anat Rec 1971; 170: 365-78.

177. Ten Cate AR, Mills C. The development of the periodontium. The origin of alveolar bone. Anat Rec 1972; 173: 69-78.

178. Barret AP, Reade PC. The relationship between degree of development of tooth isografts and subsequent formation of bone and periodontal ligament. J Periodont Res 1981; 16: 456-65.

179. Borring-Møller G, Frandsen A. Autologous tooth transplantation to replace molars lost in patients with juvenile periodontitis. J Clin Periodontol 1978; 5: 152-58.

180. Andreasen JO. The effect of pulp extirpation or root canal treatment on periodontal healing after replantation of permanent incisors in monkeys. J Endod 1981; 7: 245-52 and 1982; 8: 426-27.

181. Andreasen JO, Kristerson L. The effect of extra-alveolar root filling with calcium hydroxide on periodontal healing after replantation of permanent incisors in monkeys. J Endod 1981; 7: 349-54 and 1982; 8: 426-27.

182. Andreasen JO. Treatment of fractured and avulsed teeth. J Dent Child 1971; 38: 29-48.

183. Cvek M, Granath L-E, Hollender L. Treatment of non-vital permanent incisors with calcium hydroxide. III. Variation of occurrence of ankylosis of reimplanted teeth with duration of extra-alveolar period and storage environment. Odont Revy 1974; 25: 43-56.

184. Tronstad L, Andreasen JO, Hasselgren G, Kristerson L, Riis I. Changes in dental tissues after root canal filling with calcium hydroxide. J Endod 1981; 7: 17-22.

185. Edwards TSF. Treatment of pulpal and periapical disease by replantation. Br Dent J 1966; 121: 159-66.

186. Anderson AW, Sharav Y, Massler M. Periodontal reattachment after tooth replantation. Periodontics 1968; 6: 161-67.

187. Groper JN, Bernick S. Histological study of the periodontium following replantation of teeth in the dog. J Dent Child 1970; 37: 25-35.

188. Blomlöf L, Lindskog S, Andersson L, Hedström K-G, Hammarström L. Storage of experimentally avulsed teeth in milk prior to replantation. J Dent Res 1983; 62: 912-16.

189. Blomlöf L, Andersson L, Lindskog S, Hedström K-G, Hammarström L. Periodontal healing of replanted monkey teeth prevented from drying. Acta Odontol Scand 1983; 41: 117-23.

190. Hörster W, Altfeld F, Planko D. Behandlungsergebnisse nach Replantation total luxierter Frontzähne. Fortschr Kiefer Gesichtschir 176; 20: 127-29.

191. Coccia CT. A clinical investigation of root resorption rates in reimplanted young permanent incisors: a five-year study. J Endod 1980; 6: 413-20.

192. Morris ML, Moreinis A, Patel R, Prestrup A. Factors affecting healing after experimentally delayed tooth transplantation. J Endod 1981; 7: 80-84.

193. Andreasen JO. The effect of splinting upon periodontal healing after replantation of permanent incisors in monkeys. Acta Odontol Scand 1975; 33: 313-23.

194. Morley RS, Malloy R, Hurst RVV, James R. Analysis of functional splinting upon autologously reimplanted teeth. J Dent Res 1978; 57: IADR Abstract no. 593.

195. Nasjleti CE, Castelli WA, Caffesse RG. The effects of different splinting times on replantation of teeth in monkeys. Oral Surg Oral Med Oral Pathol 1982; 53: 557-66.

196. Andreasen JO. The effect of excessive occlusal trauma upon periodontal healing after replantation of mature permanent incisors in monkeys. Swed Dent J 1981; 5: 115-22.

197. Kristerson L, Andreasen JO. The effect of splinting upon periodontal and pulpal healing after autotransplantation of mature and immature permanent incisors in monkeys. Int J Oral Surg 1983; 12: 239-49.

198. Andersson L, Lindskog S, Blomlöf L, Hedström K-G, Hammarström L. Effect of masticatory stimulation on dentoalveolar ankylosis after experimental tooth replantation. Endod Dent Traumatol 1985; 1: 13-16.

199. Hammarström L, Blomlöf L, Feiglin B, Andersson L, Lindskog S. Replantation of teeth and antibiotic treatment. Endod Dent Traumatol 1986; 2: 51-57.

200. Cvek M, Cleaton-Jones P, Austin J, Lownie J, Kling M, Fatti P. Pulp revascularization in reimplanted immature monkey incisors - predictability and the effect of antibiotic systemic prophylaxis. Endod Dent Traumatol 1990; 6: 157-69.

201. Cvek M, Cleaton-Jones P, Austin J, Kling M, Lownie J, Fatti P. Effect of topical application of doxycycline on pulp revascularization and periodontal healing in reimplanted monkey incisors. Endod Dent Traumatol 1990; 6: 170-76.

202. Monsour FNT, Adkins KF. Aberrations in pulpal histology and dentinogenesis in transplanted erupting teeth. J Oral Maxillofac Surg 1985; 43: 8-13.

203. Monsour FNT, Adkins KF. Histological changes following transplantation of developing teeth to more advanced functional positions. Aust Dent J 1987; 32: 104-09.

204. Möller Å, Fabricius L, Dahlén G, Öhman A, Heyden G. Influence on periapical tissues of indigenous oral bacteria and necrotic pulp tissue in monkeys. Scand J Dent Res 1981; 89: 475-84.

205. Berude JA, Lamar H, Sauber JJ, Li S-H. Resorption after physiological and rigid splinting of replanted permanent incisors in monkeys. J Endod 1988; 14: 592-600.

206. Schendel KU, Schwartz O, Andreasen JO, Hoffmeister B. Reinnervation of autotransplanted teeth. A histological investigation in monkeys. Int J Oral Maxillofac Surg 1990; 19: 247-249.

207. Öhman A. Healing and sensitivity to pain in young replanted human teeth. An experimental and histological study. Odontol Tidskr 1965; 73: 168-227.

Chapter 2
Replantation of avulsed teeth

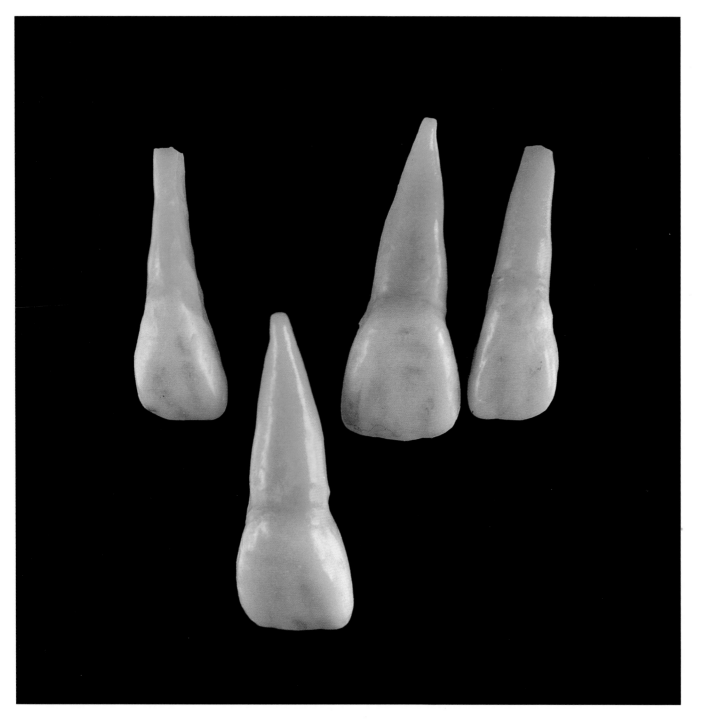

Indications and treatment planning

Avulsion of anterior teeth is a rather frequent event in children (Fig. 2.1). The success of a replantation procedure is very dependent upon when and how this procedure is performed. This has been the subject of numerous survey articles[2-13,180-182] and case reports dealing with replantation of immature[14-30,184] and mature teeth.[31-118,174-179,193] In the following, treatment procedures for avulsed teeth will be described which are based primarily on results from animal experiments and clinical studies (see Chapter 1, p. 45).[119-141,183-192]

Case reports of replantation of primary incisors have been published.[142-146] However, the risk of injury to the permanent successor is so great due to either the replantation procedure or subsequent pulp necrosis of the replanted primary tooth that this procedure should not be carried out.[147]

Examination of the avulsed tooth

The apical area should be inspected for possible fracture. The presence of an intact apex should be noted. However, the presence of a fracture is not a contraindication for replantation. In these cases, the replanted coronal fragment is considered the replant and endodontic intervention is limited to that part of the tooth.

The level of the attachment apparatus on the root should be recorded. The presence of a ring of calculus or discoloration is usually a good marker (Fig. 2.2). In teeth with immature root formation, the integrity of the apical third of the pulp should be noted. Severance of the pulp in this location can occur with avulsion, implying that the apical pulp stump and Hertwig's epithelial root sheath have been left behind in the socket, which could complicate healing (see p. 91). Finally, the tooth is examined for the presence of macroscopic contamination.

Fig. 2.1. Avulsed central incisor in a 7-year-old boy. The tooth has been wrapped in paper for 60 minutes.

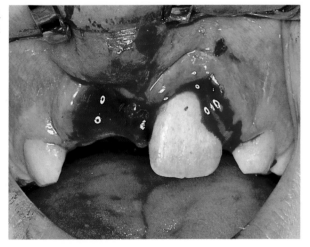

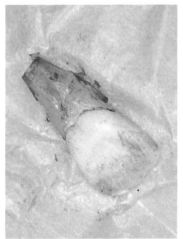

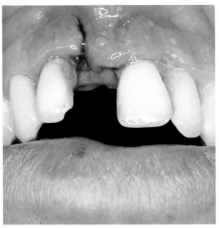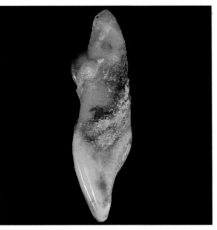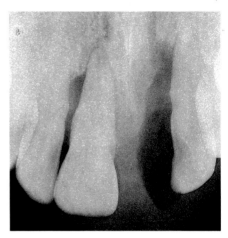

Fig. 2.2. A ring of calculus on the root surface indicates the level of PDL attachment.

Any treatment procedure for avulsed teeth starts immediately after avulsion, where the patient, relatives, or others can do several things to minimize the otherwise serious consequences of such a traumatic event. The most effective information to the public is that avulsed teeth can be saved and that a necessary initial step towards successful treatment is, immediate replantation by the patient, parents, or relatives. This will significantly improve healing. If this is not possible the avulsed tooth should be placed in the oral cavity between the lips and the gingiva (Fig. 2.3). This, however, implies that the patient is conscious so that accidental swallowing or aspiration of the tooth does not occur. If storage of the tooth in the patient's own mouth is not possible, storage in another's will do. By placing the tooth in saliva, the periodontal ligament (PDL) is immediately protected from the harmful effect of drying. The tooth can be kept in this location for several hours before a noticeable effect on pulpal and periodontal healing can be observed (see p. 76). However, if physiological saline is immediately available, storage in this medium is to be preferred, as it has been shown to result in slightly better periodontal healing (see p. 76).

When the patient arrives at the treatment center (e.g., hospital emergency service, dental office), the next problem is replantation: when and how. Replantation in itself is a relatively simple procedure. However, certain procedures are essential in order to minimize damage to the PDL and pulp. These procedures include adequate cleansing of the tooth and the socket and atraumatic replantation. In most cases, this implies replantation by an experienced dentist - even at the expense of a longer extraoral period - on the condition that the avulsed tooth is kept in a suitable storage medium until replantation. If stored dry or in the oral cavity until arrival at the treatment center, it should be transferred immediately to physiologic saline. Placed in this medium, several hours can elapse before any significant effect on periodontal or pulpal healing can be demonstrated (see p. 73).

The initial patient examination should include the following:

Visual inspection of the socket area

Notice should be paid to evidence of contusion or fracture of the alveolar socket walls (Figs. 2.4 and 2.5). Laceration of the gingiva should be recorded.

Fig. 2.3. An avulsed central incisor is kept moist in saliva.

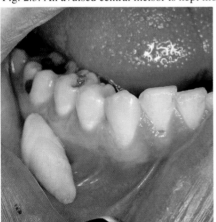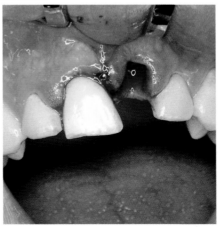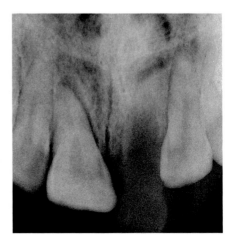

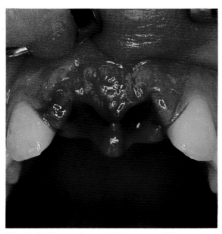 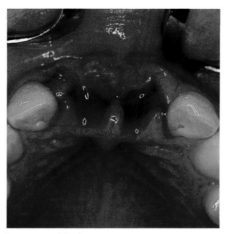 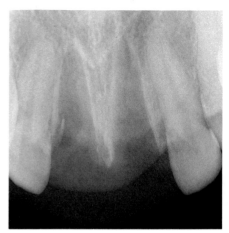

Fig. 2.4. Contusion and fracture of the sockets of two central incisors.

When clinical examination of the socket area and the avulsed tooth is complete, the patient history should be recorded to reveal circumstances related to injury and storage conditions (including storage media and sequence of these). In this context, it should be mentioned that replantation in adults is possible even after prolonged extra-alveolar storage, such as where several days have elapsed. In these cases, a total ankylosis can be expected; a protracted resorption process can be anticipated. To further prolong the resorptive process in these cases, chemical treatment of the root surface should be considered (see p. 69).

Finally, a treatment plan is made for the avulsed tooth. In some cases replantation is not indicated. This is generally true if the tooth has been broken down by caries or the PDL has been severely reduced due to marginal periodontitis. Severe crowding in the area coupled with an estimated poor prognosis of the replanted tooth could lead to a decision not to replant the avulsed tooth.

Fig. 2.5. An avulsed central incisor with heavy macroscopic contamination and fracture of labial bone plate.

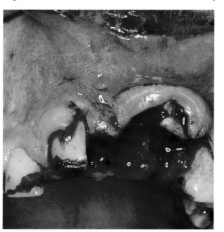 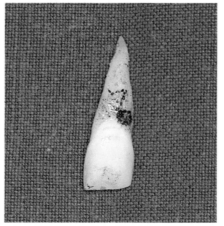 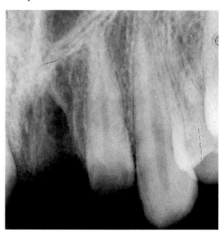

Surgical procedure

If replantation is indicated, it is necessary to consider whether it represents a permanent treatment solution or whether the replanted tooth will merely serve as a space maintainer until the time when final treatment is deemed appropriate. In the latter case, special treatment of the root surface might be indicated to prolong the life expectancy of the replant (see p. 69). In the following, replantation, including preservation of an intact PDL as a permanent treatment solution will be described (Fig. 2.6).

If inspection of the alveolus reveals fracture or contusion of bone, usually confined to the labial socket wall, the first step in treatment will be the recontouring of the socket with an amalgam carver or straight elevator. It should be noted that loss of the labial socket wall is usually not a contraindication for replantation, as long as the rest of the socket is intact (see Chapter 1, p. 45). When the socket area has been found suitable for replantation, the next step is the preparation of the root surface. This implies adequate cleansing of the PDL and pulp entering the apical foramen for the elimination of bacterial contaminants and foreign bodies. Cleansing is best accomplished by grasping the tooth by the crown with a forceps and thereafter rinsing with a continuous flow of saline along the root surface and apex for several minutes until the root is macroscopically clean.

The coagulum must also be removed from the socket with a jet of saline or evacuated with suction. When the root surface appears clean, the tooth can be replanted. If several teeth are avulsed, it is necessary to identify all teeth with respect to anatomy and location in the dental arch. Thereafter, the tooth is placed three-quarters up into the socket. At this time, slight, continuous finger pressure incisally is used to reposition the tooth.

If resistance is met during the replantation procedure, it is necessary to remove the tooth, place it again in physiologic saline, and reexamine the alveolus for loose, unrepositioned bone fragments. If the obstacle to complete repositioning cannot be located, it is better to accept incomplete repositioning than to forcefully reposition the tooth completely. Forceful repositioning can damage large areas of PDL on the root surface and lead to root resorption. Furthermore, incomplete repositioning not only does not impede periodontal healing, but in cases of PDL damage might actually improve healing. In such situations, it would appear that distance from the alveolar wall might favor PDL repair from adjacent intact PDL areas over bony healing from the socket.

Splinting

In a replantation situation, the purpose of the splint is to provide stability during the initial stages of healing, where the tooth might be very loose. However, it should also be noted that at least rigid splinting seems to result in more ankylosis and possibly impedes pulpal revascularization (see Chapter 1, p. 47). These findings imply that a minimal fixation period should generally be used (i.e., 1 week) in order to allow initial PDL healing to take place and at the same time to prevent ankylosis sites from becoming permanent. However, in cases with extensive bone damage, a fixation period of 3-4 weeks or longer may be necessary. The same applies to teeth where the PDL has been removed and the root surface chemically treated, where a fixation period of 6 weeks is recommended.

An acid-etch/acrylic splint is easy to apply and reliable (Fig. 2.6). The incisal half of the facial surface of the replanted and the two adjacent teeth are etched with phosphoric acid, avoiding the interproximal surfaces. The acid is removed thoroughly and the surfaces air dried, with the air stream directed axially towards the gingiva. Thereafter, the splinting material is applied to the etched enamel surface, avoiding the gingiva and proximal surfaces. These precautions facilitate oral hygiene and later removal respectively.

Regarding the choice of splinting material, temporary crown and bridge materials have been found quite suitable in that they are slightly elastic, allowing some mobility, and are easy to remove. If these materials are not available, ordinary composite material can be used. If adjacent supporting teeth are not available, as can be the case in the mixed dentition, acid-etch/acrylic supplemented with an arch bar can be used.

After replantation of immature, incompletely erupted incisors, a suture "splint" can be applied, using a single suture extending from the oral to the facial gingiva or a nylon fishing line or Kevlar thread bonded to the replant and adjacent teeth (Fig. 2.7).

Radiographic examination

Once replantation and fixation are complete, a final radiograph is taken to document the degree of repositioning achieved and to serve as a reference for the diagnosis of possible healing complications. This radiograph should be taken using a reproducible technique in order to optimize the chance of detecting complications in periodontal and pulpal healing.

Antibiotic therapy

An essential part of the immediate treatment of avulsed teeth is to provide the patient with antibiotic coverage in order to prevent periodontal healing complications and to assist pulpal revascularization (see Chapter 1, p. 49).

It should be mentioned that the value of antibiotic coverage has only been demonstrated experimentally. However, it seems reasonable to assume that some of these benefits might also be anticipated clinically. The optimal choice and dosage of antibiotics for a replantation situation have not yet been determined. It is, therefore, recommended that usual therapeutic doses of penicillin are used in the period immediately after replantation (i.e., 4-7 days).

Tetanus prophylaxis

Finally, tetanus prophylaxis should be considered if the patient is not already adequately covered. Although no cases of tetanus related to replantation of teeth have been reported, such an event is certainly possible.

Post-trauma follow-up

The patient is now scheduled for follow-up (see Appendix 1, p. 289). The first appointment is usually 1 week after injury. At this time, the gingival or mucosal sutures are removed. It should also be considered whether pulpal revascularization can be anticipated. The decisive factors in this matter are the stage of root development and extra-alveolar storage conditions. Minimal requirements for pulpal revascularization are a wide open apical foramen and an extra-alveolar period of less than 2 hours, with a moist storage environment in the greater part of that period. If these conditions have been met, there is a chance (although limited) for pulpal revascularization. In all other cases, pulpal revascularization is not likely to occur. In these instances, in order to prevent periapical inflammation and inflammatory root resorption, the pulp should be extirpated and root canal treatment initiated.

Timing of endodontic therapy

The optimal time for initiating endodontic therapy is not known. Theoretically, it would seem best to wait until apical periodontal healing has begun in order to prevent the seepage of cytotoxic medicaments (e.g., calcium hydroxide, camphorated paramonophenol) through the apical foramen, which would further damage the already injured PDL.[148-149] *PDL healing* thus dictates a *delay* of several weeks prior to endodontic treatment. However, the onset of inflammatory root resorption is another important factor to consider. Attack on the root surface usually begins (at least experimentally) with a few initial resorption cavities 1 week after injury and becomes very prominent after 2 weeks. These initial resorption cavities can be the prelude to either surface resorption, replacement resorption, or inflammatory resorption. The last event will only take place when the initial resorption attack penetrates dentinal tubules that are in direct contact with infected, necrotic pulp tissue (see Chapter 1, p. 28). Development of *root resorption* thus dictates *early* endodontic therapy. Data presently available from clinical studies indicate that endodontic treatment carried out at the time of replantation leads to apical ankylosis (see p. 46).[123,137] Postponement of treatment for 2 weeks at which time PDL healing is advanced, but inflammatory resorption is marked, is undesirable. A compromise between these two treatment periods appears to be 7-10 days after replantation. The endodontic treatment can then be combined with splint removal. At this time, pulp extirpation and endodontic therapy can be initiated with the replanted tooth still stabilized by the splint. This procedure will limit trauma to the periodontium by the various endodontic procedures. After completion of initial endodontic therapy at this appointment, the splint can be removed.

Endodontic treatment

Endodontic therapy after replantation or transplantation differs in some respects from endodontic therapy due to caries. For the first, pulp necrosis after replantation or transplantation is not usually accompanied by painful clinical symptoms. For this reason, endodontic treatment, including pulp extirpation, can easily be performed without the use of local anesthetics. That the patient can respond to stimuli in the apical area means that helpful information regarding the amputation level can be gained directly from patient response.

A second difference concerns the requirements for successful treatment. In the caries/necrosis situation, presumably only the apical periodontium has been involved in the disease process. This implies that a tight root filling apically will usually result in successful healing. However, after replantation or transplantation, one can anticipate that areas of traumatized PDL along the entire root surface will be potential sites for external root resorption. Thus, endodontic therapy after replantation or transplantation requires a tight root filling along the entire root length.

Fig. 2.6. Replanting an avulsed central incisor

The patient is an 8-year-old girl who had an incisor knocked out during a fall. The tooth was immediately picked up, and stored in the oral cavity. After admission to the emergency service the tooth was transferred to saline. The total extra-alveolar time before treatment was 60 minutes.

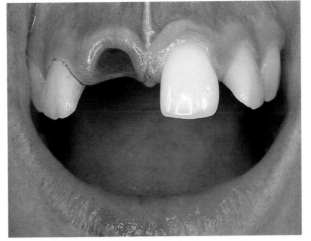
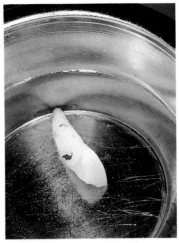

Clinical and radiographic examination

If the labial bone plate is lost it is no contraindication to replantation as long as the remaining socket is intact. In this case there is no sign of contusion or fracture of the socket wall.

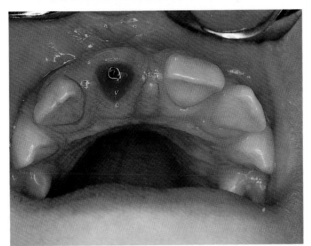
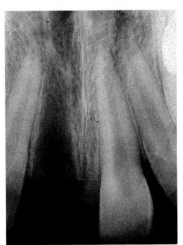

Cleansing the tooth and the socket

The tooth is grasped with forceps by the crown and the root surface is inspected for the PDL attachment level and obvious contamination. Thereafter the root surface and especially the apical area is cleansed with a flow of saline. Finally the socket is evacuated of the coagulum by saline rinsing.

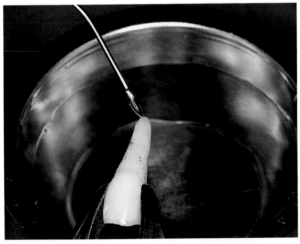
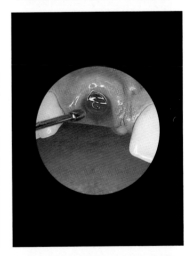

Replanting the tooth

The tooth is partly repositioned. The final part of the repositioning procedure is completed with gentle finger pressure. If any resistance is felt the most obvious reason is a fracture of the socket wall; in this instance the replanted tooth should be removed again and the socket wall repositioned with an amalgam carver or a straight elevator.

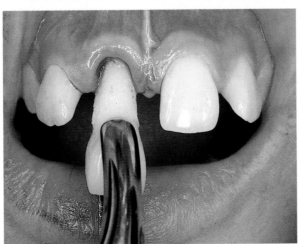
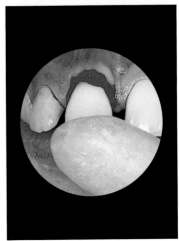

Fig. 2.6. Continued

Etching the labial surface

The labial surfaces of the replanted tooth and the two adjacent teeth are etched with a conditioner. The conditioner is removed with a flow of water and compressed air. The stream of air should be directed axially to remove blood and saliva from the interproximal areas.

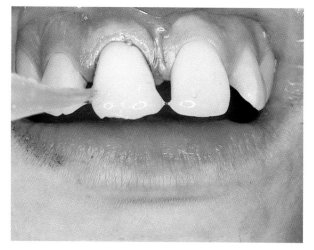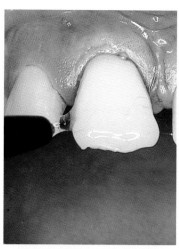

Applying the splinting material

A temporary bridge material is placed incisally (Protemp, Espe, GmbH, D-8031, Seefeld, Germany) and the tooth is kept repositioned with gentle pressure during setting. After setting the splint is smoothened with a fissure bur.

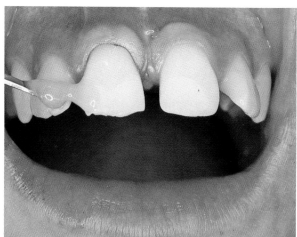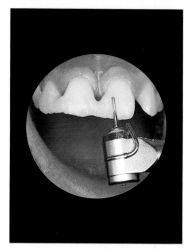

Radiographic control

A radiograph serves as a control for proper repositioning and as a reference for later controls.

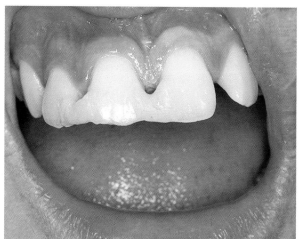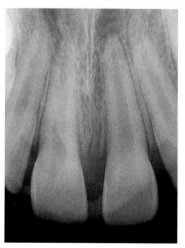

Endodontic treatment

7 days has elapsed since replantation. A rubber dam is prepared; because of the splint the rubber dam has to span over three teeth and three connecting holes are punched out. The rubber dam is placed over the splinted teeth.

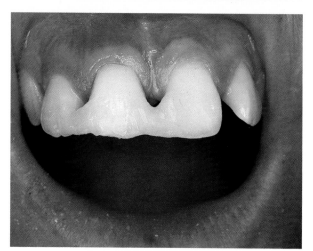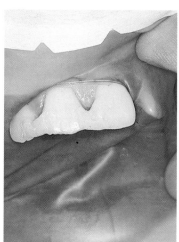

Fig. 2.6. Continued

Opening to the root canal

A fold of the rubber dam mesially and distally ensures the stability. The palatal surface of the replanted incisor is cleansed, first with 3 % hydrogen peroxide followed by a disinfectant. Thereafter an access cavity is made to the pulp chamber which corresponds to the axial projection of the root canal upon the palatal surface.

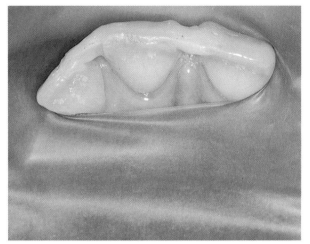 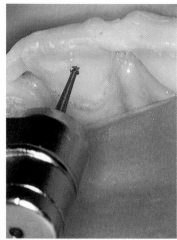

Extirpating the pulp

The extirpation needle is inserted half the distance to the apical foramen, and the pulp is extirpated. It is noted whether the entire pulp has been extirpated. If this is not the case the extirpation is repeated.

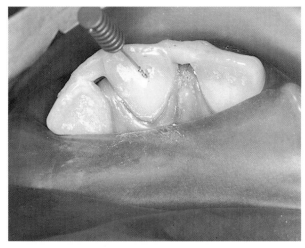 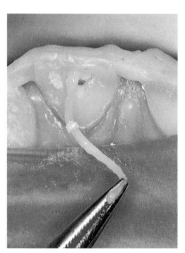

Locating the amputating site

The coronal access cavity is cleansed for pulp remnants with a small excavator. Thereafter a reamer is slowly inserted in the root canal and the patient is asked to indicate the level of sensation in the tooth. That level serves as the pulp amputation level and the root canal should not be instrumented beyond that limit.

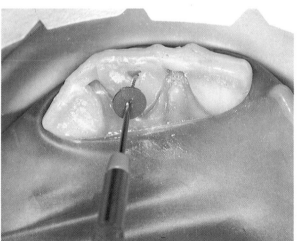 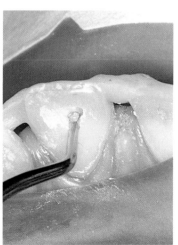

Instrumenting the root canal

The root canal is enlarged with reamers and files. During this procedure the root canal is rinsed repeatedly with a 2% sodium hypochlorite solution, finally followed by a rinse with saline.

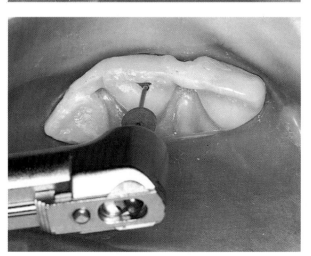 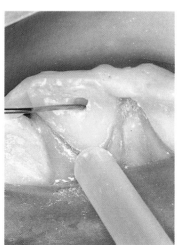

Fig. 2.6. Continued

Filling the root canal with calcium hydroxide

The root canal is filled with a calcium hydroxide compound using a syringe (e.g., Calasept, Scania Dental AB, S-74100 Knivsta, Sweden). Calcium hydroxide is carried to the amputation level using a mechanically driven spiral.

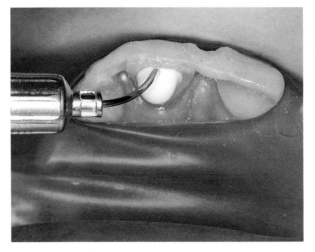
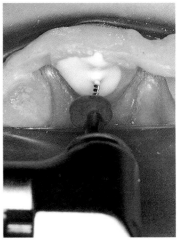

Condensing the calcium hydroxide

The calcium hydroxide is condensed using paper points inserted with their cut end first in the root canal. This procedure is repeated 2-3 times. Finally the calcium hydroxide content in the root canal is compressed with a small cotton pellet. This serves to further condense the calcium hydroxide and extract moisture and the cotton pellet is left in place approximately 3 mm below the access opening.

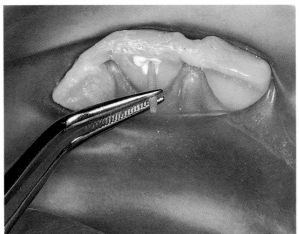
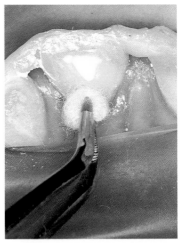

Sealing the access cavity

A water rinsing is performed, followed by a prolonged compressed air drying in order to make a tight seal possible. A temporary seal is placed in the entrance opening (e.g., Cavit, Espe GmbH, D-8031 Seefeld, Germany or I.R.M, de Trey Dentsply, GmbH, D-6072 Dreieich, Germany). Finally a radiograph verifies the level and standard of the root filling.

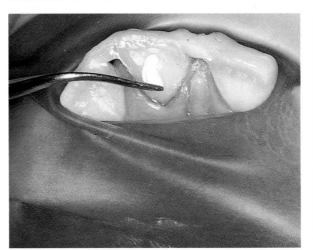
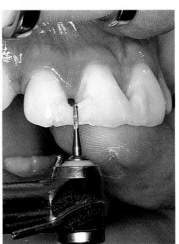

Removing the splint

When the radiographic examination has revealed a satisfactory root filling, the splint is removed with a fissure bur. During the final phase of removal the incisal edge is supported with a finger as the tooth at this time is quite loose in its socket.

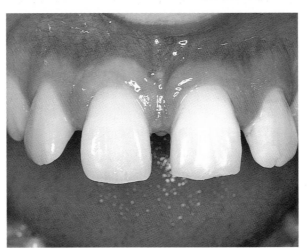
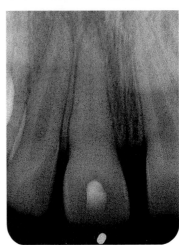

Fig. 2.7. Kevlar thread (Wingen Prod HB, S-59600 Skeninge, Sweden) bonded to the replanted tooth and two adjacent teeth with an acid-etch technique acts as a functional splint. If more stability is needed Protemp, can be added to the Kevlar thread.

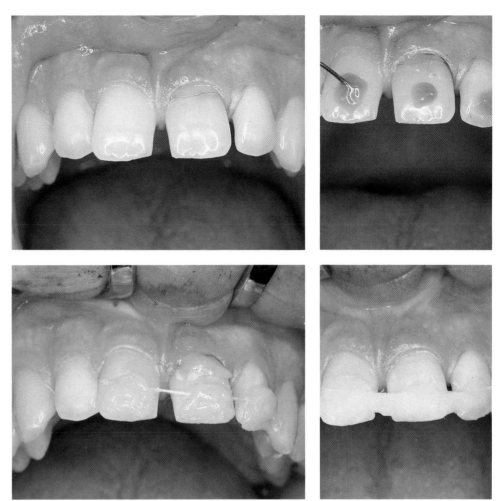

If at all possible, a rubber dam is applied. It is normally possible to include the replanted tooth and the splinted adjacent teeth in the dam. This can be done by punching adjacent connecting holes in the dam to accommodate all splinted teeth. A piece of rubber dam material is then wedged between the last tooth in the splint on either side and the non splinted adjacent tooth (Fig. 2.6). It is essential not to place any clamps or ligatures upon the replanted tooth in order not to disturb the healing processes in the cervical region.

After sterilization of the oral surface, an entrance is made into the pulp chamber which will ensure maximum access to the pulp canal. A barbed broach is then placed approximately halfway down the canal. With extirpation, separation of the pulp will usually occur at the narrow leukocyte zone found between the vital pulp stump apically and the necrotic and infected pulp coronally. After extirpation, a reamer is introduced into the canal and advanced apically until the patient feels slight pressure. This will be the amputation zone and is normally found approximately 2 mm from the apical foramen. However, in teeth with immature root formation, this zone can be found at varying distances, sometimes even at the mid-root level. When the amputation level has been determined, it is essential that this structure be protected from further damage during the chemomechanical preparation of the canal, as this part of the pulp is essential for hard tissue closure of the root canal. In the case of immature teeth, this vital tissue may even ensure continued root formation.

Adequate chemomechanical preparation of the root canal in a replanted tooth is very critical for successful treatment, as infected tissue remnants in the canal can sustain an inflammatory root resorption process already present on the root surface. The mechanical preparation of the canal can be carried out using sodium hypochlorite at a concentration of 2% as a tissue solvent. Thereafter, the canal is cleared of sodium hypochlorite with a copious flow of physiologic saline.

A dressing should then be used which ensures a sterile canal and arrest of osteoclastic activity on the root surface. Calcium hydroxide has been shown to be effective for this purpose.[152] More recently, antibiotic solutions have also been found to be effective in animal experiments.[153]

Once the canal has been rinsed thoroughly and there is no sign of hemorrhage, calcium hydroxide paste (e.g., Calasept Scania Dental AB, S-74100 Knivsta, Sweden) can be introduced into the canal. Interposition of a coagulum or secretion between the calcium hydroxide paste and amputation site seems to neutralize the effect of calcium hydroxide.[152] Calcium hydroxide is injected into the moist canal and then distributed throughout the length of the canal using a lentulo spiral and thereafter compressed with paper points. A canal which is moist with saline allows the calcium hydroxide paste to flow to the apex, whereas injection of the paste into a dry canal could entrap air bubbles apically and impede complete filling. Injection, spiraling, and compression of the paste should be repeated several times to ensure complete filling of the canal and intimate contact between the calcium hydroxide and the amputation site (Fig. 2.6).

Fig. 2.8. Replantation of two avulsed incisors after fluoride treatment of the root surfaces

This is an 18-year-old patient who had had two central incisors knocked out four hours previously. The teeth were recovered on the ground and then placed in a pocket until admission to the emergency service. The PDL is completely dried out and the root surface heavily contaminated.

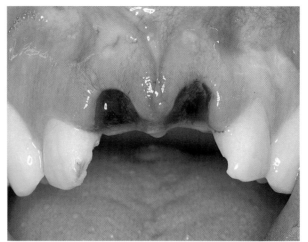

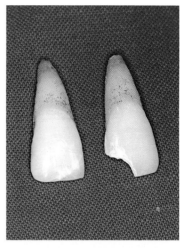

Endodontic treatment

The tooth is grasped proximally with forceps, whereafter an entrance cavity is made to the pulp chamber. The pulp is extirpated and the root canal enlarged with reamers and files. The PDL is removed with a surgical blade until the root surface appears completely devoid of any soft tissue. The teeth are then placed for 20 min in a 2.4% sodium fluoride solution acidulated to a pH of 6.5. Before replantation the teeth are rinsed with saline to remove surplus toxic fluoride solution.

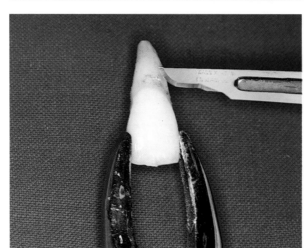

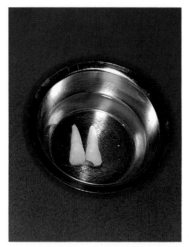

Fluoride treatment and filling the root canal

After drying the canal it is obturated with gutta-percha and a sealer using lateral condensation. Finally surplus root filling is removed after setting of the sealer.

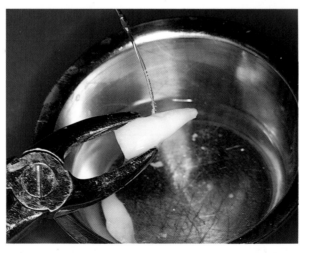

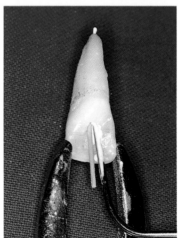

Preparing the sockets and replantation

Before replantation the coagulum already formed is removed with a curette and a saline rinse. The incisors are then repositioned in their respective sockets and the occlusion is checked.

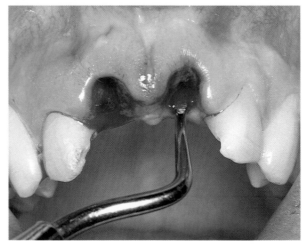

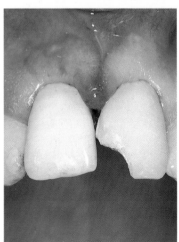

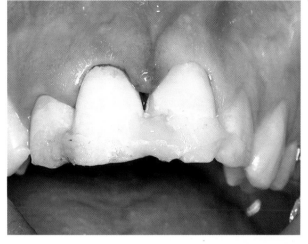

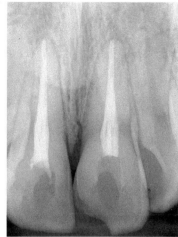

Follow-up
The percussion test shows an ankylosis. Radiographic appearance at 1 year follow-up. There is very little progression of the ankylotic process.

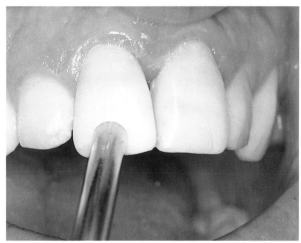

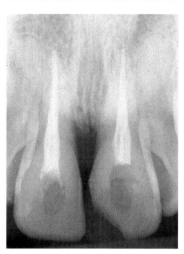

Filling complete, the entrance to the root canal is sealed with a temporary sealing material (e.g., IRM cement). However, placement of the temporary sealer is done only after the margins of the coronal entrance are carefully cleaned of all excess calcium hydroxide. As calcium hydroxide is water soluble, paste around the margins can wash out, leaving an insufficient seal which is vulnerable to bacterial contamination from the oral cavity and leakage of calcium hydroxide.

Treatment of the root surface

In cases where total loss of cell viability is likely, chemical treatment of the root surface may be indicated to make it resistant to osteoclastic activity.[135,150-151] Such cases would include teeth which have been kept dry 60 minutes or more as well teeth kept in non physiologic media, such as sterilizing solutions (e.g., alcohol, chloramine, and hydrogen peroxide). Nonphysiologic preservation of avulsed teeth will ultimately lead to total ankylosis of the root surface.

Treatment with fluoride solutions has been used clinically to achieve this result.[135,150,151] In the following, this treatment modality will be described (Fig. 2.8).

Fluoride treatment

Before treatment of the root surface, the pulp should be extirpated. The tooth is held by the crown with a forceps during the endodontic procedure. Adequate mechanical preparation and obturation of the root canal are essential, as pulp tissue remnants can lead to inflammatory resorption.[148] After pulp extirpation, the root canal is filled with a well-condensed gutta-percha filling and sealer. The tooth is then immersed for 20 min in a 2.4% sodium fluoride solution, acidulated at pH 5.5. The tooth is then rinsed thoroughly with saline, replanted, and splinted for 6 weeks.

In one clinical study of 125 fluoride-treated replanted incisors, the resorption process was found to be significantly protracted when evaluated over a 5-year period.[135] This protraction of the resorptive process was seen irrespective of the length of the extra-alveolar period (Fig. 2.9).

Completion of endodontic treatment

Upon completion of initial calcium hydroxide root filling, a radiograph is taken to serve as a reference for later follow-up visits. Radiographically, a tooth with an adequate calcium hydroxide root filling resembles a tooth with no root canal. That is, calcium hydroxide has the same radiopacity as dentin.

Fig. 2.9a. Comparison of root resorption after 1 year of replanted permanent incisors with and without fluoride treatment. The vertical bars indicate the reduction in mm. in the length due to root resorption. From Coccia, 1980.[135]

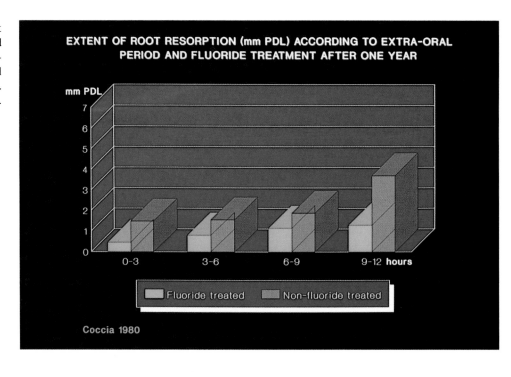

Fig. 2.9b. Comparison of root resorption after 3 years of replanted permanent incisors with and without fluoride treatment. The vertical bars indicate the reduction in mm in the length due to root resorption. From Coccia, 1980.[135]

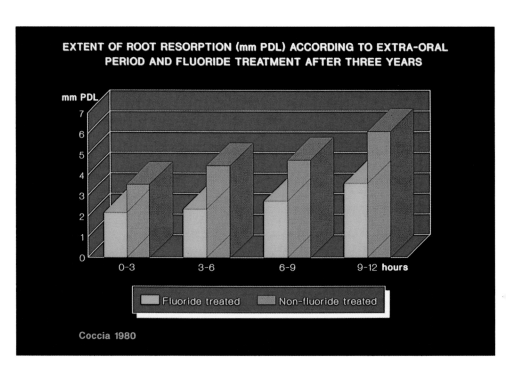

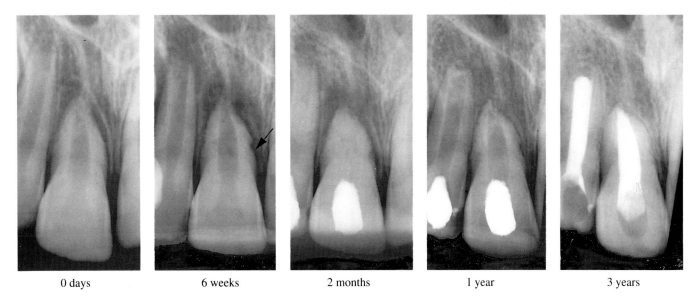

| 0 days | 6 weeks | 2 months | 1 year | 3 years |

Fig. 2.10. Formation of an apical hard tissue barrier and arrest of inflammatory root resorption (arrow) in a replanted central incisor after initial endodontic treatment with calcium hydroxide. From Andreasen & al., 1991.[191]

The patient is scheduled for revision of the calcium hydroxide dressing material 1 month after initial filling. Experimentally, this has been shown to result in a more complete apical bridge than a one appointment procedure.[154] The root filling is controlled radiographically after 2-3 months (i.e., 3-4 months after initial filling). At this time, there should be evidence of arrest of any root resorption and/or apical rarefaction. If the radiographic examination demonstrates a loss of calcium hydroxide from the canal, the root canal is refilled. Such a radiographic loss of calcium hydroxide has been shown to be accompanied by a similar drop in pH, from a pH of approximately 12.5 towards a more neutral level.[155]

The next visit should be 6 months after replantation, at which time another radiographic examination is made. In accordance with the above-mentioned guidelines, the dressing is either maintained or renewed. At this time, most cases will show reestablishment of a PDL space adjacent to previous resorption sites as well as apical repair. In teeth with completed root formation, an apical barrier is normally found. However, in teeth with open apices, a period of 12-18 months is necessary before a solid apical hard tissue barrier can be demonstrated, at which time final endodontic therapy can be carried out (Fig. 2.10).[156,157]

Table 2.1. Long-term results of replantation of avulsed permanent teeth

	Observation period, years (mean)	Age of patients, years (mean)	Number of teeth	Tooth survival %	PDL healing %	Pulp healing %	Gingival healing %
Lenstrup & Skieller, 1957, 1959 [120,121]	0.2-5	5-18	47	57	9	4	
Andreasen & Hjörting-Hansen, 1966 [123]	0.2-15	6-24	110	54	20	4	95
Ravn & Helbo, 1966 [125]		5-15	28		4	4	
Gröndahl & al., 1974 [130]	2-5		45	69	23	7	67
Cvek & al., 1974 [129]	2-6.5	6-17 (11)	38		50		
Hörster & al., 1976 [132]			38		26		
Kemp & Phillips, 1977 [134]	0.1-10	10-15	71	61	30		
Ravn, 1977 [133]		7-16	20		20	5	
Kock & Ullbro, 1982 [137]	1-9	7-17	55	65	27	4	
Herforth, 1982 [136]	1-8 (4.5)	7-15	79	51	11	4	
Jacobsen, 1986 [183]	1-14 (5)		59	39	29	15	
Gonda & al., 1990 [192]	0.6-6.5	(16)	27	70	41	15	
Andreasen & al., 1991 [187-191]	0.2-20 (5.1)	5-52 (13.4)	400	70	36	8	93

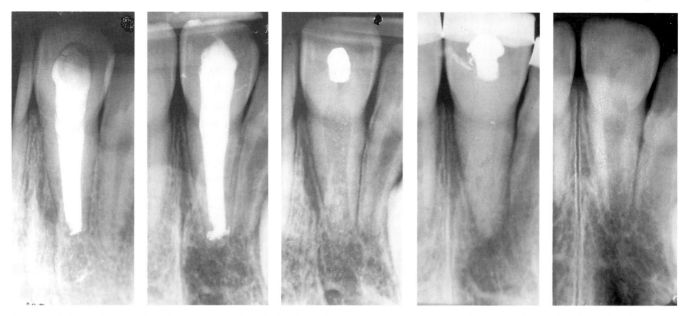

Fig. 2.11. Initial calcium hydroxide treatment followed after 1 year by a gutta-percha root filling of a replanted central incisor. There is no root resorption. From Andreasen et & al., 1991.[191]

Final endodontic treatment, consisting of a gutta-percha root filling and sealer, can be performed after 6 months in teeth with completed root formation. However, in some cases, a flare-up of resorption activity might be seen. This could be due to a rather thin cementum layer covering the repaired resorption cavity, which is not able to shield the PDL from the toxic effect of bacteria in the root canal. For this reason, final root filling should normally be postponed until 1 year after replantation in teeth with completed root formation.

The permanent root filling should aim at three-dimensional obturation of the root canal, as insufficient filling could reactivate resorption processes (Fig. 2.11).

Prognosis

Today there are relatively few studies based on larger patient materials which can give information about the long-term prognosis of replanted avulsed permanent teeth. In Table 2.1 the results are listed from clinical studies where adequate documentation is given for pulp and periodontal healing complications.

Tooth survival

It appears from Fig. 2.12 that tooth survival is strongly related to tooth development at time of injury.

Fig. 2.12. Tooth survival related to stage of root development at time of injury. From Andreasen & al., 1991.[187]

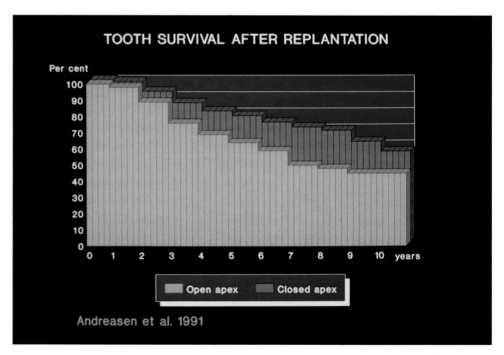

Fig. 2.13a. Relation between pulpal healing of teeth with incomplete root formation and type and length of extra-alveolar dry storage. From Andreasen & al, 1991.[188]

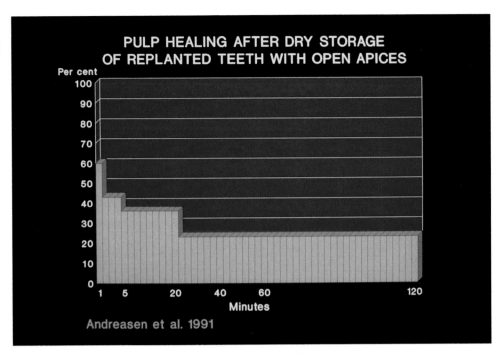

Pulpal healing and pulp necrosis

As an avulsion injury implies a severed vascular supply, pulp necrosis is inevitable unless revascularization of the pulp can occur. Clinically, this has only been found to take place in teeth with open apices.[140,188] Therefore, instead of awaiting radiographic or clinical signs of pulp necrosis in teeth with completed root formation, pulp extirpation is justified on the assumption that revascularization cannot be anticipated. However, in cases of incomplete root formation, pulpal revascularization is possible. This has been found to be related to the type and length of extra-alveolar storage.[140,184,188] Thus, immediate replantation favors the chance of revascularization,[188] whereas dry and wet storage limits the possibility of revascularization. The relationship between extra-alveolar period and pulp survival in humans is illustrated in Fig. 2.13a and b.

Fig. 2.13b. Relation between pulpal healing of teeth with incomplete root formation and length of extra-alveolar wet storage. From Andreasen & al., 1991.[188]

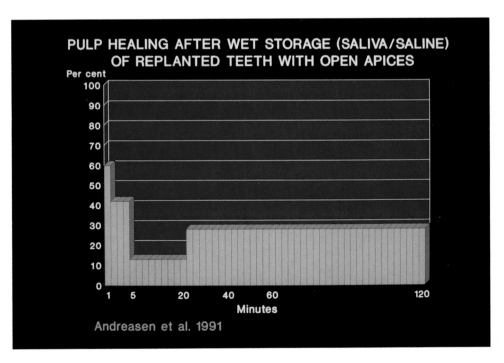

It appears from this study that pulpal revascularization is dependent upon storage conditions. If the avulsed teeth are kept *wet* (ie in saline or saliva), revascularization takes place in approximately one-third of the cases stored up to 3 hours (Figs. 2.13 and 2.14).

Fig. 2.14. Pulpal healing in three replanted incisors with an extra-alveolar period of 2 minutes dry and 88 minutes in saline in an 8-year-old boy. From Andreasen & al., 1991.[188]

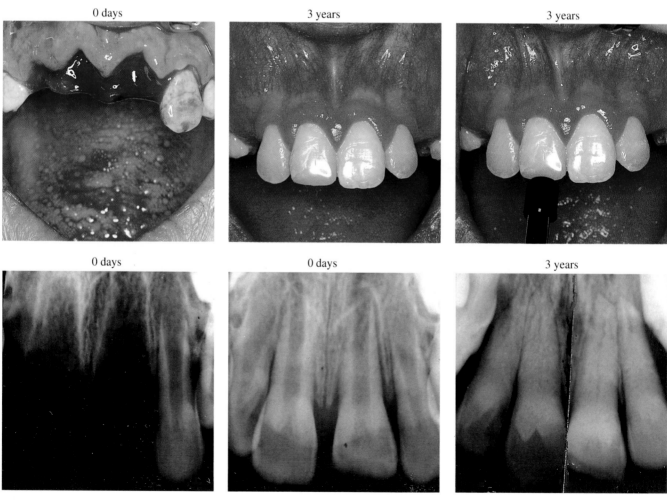

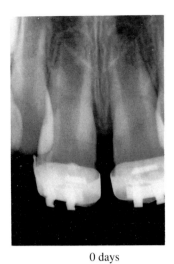

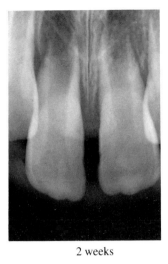

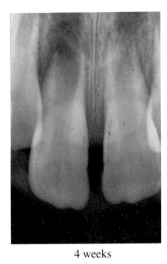

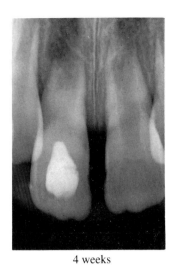

| 0 days | 2 weeks | 4 weeks | 4 weeks |

Fig. 2.15. Pulp necrosis seen as periapical radiolucency 4 weeks after replantation in a replanted right central incisor. From Andreasen & al., 1991.[188]

Revascularization after *dry* storage usually occurs in about half of the cases when the storage period is less than 5 min. Then, the frequency of revascularization drops to about one third in the period from 6 to 20 min, and then continues to decrease with increasing drying periods. Furthermore, it has been found that revascularization took place only in teeth with an apical diameter which exceeded 1 mm.[140]

Finally pulpal length has been found to be a very important factor with increasing risk of pulp necrosis with increasing pulp lengths.[188]

Radiographic controls should be carried out after 2, 3 and 4 weeks in order to demonstrate signs of pulp necrosis, such as periapical radiolucency (Fig. 2.15) and inflammatory root resorption (Fig. 2.16).

0 days

0 days

Fig. 2.16. Pulp healing in a replanted right central incisor in a 6-year-old boy where the apical foramen was protected by the blood clot in the socket. The left central incisor, which was completely dislodged from the socket and was stored in alveolar sulcus for 170 min, has developed pulp necrosis and inflammatory resorption. From Andreasen & al., 1991.[188]

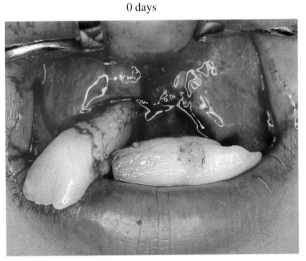

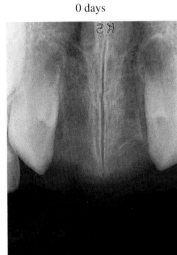

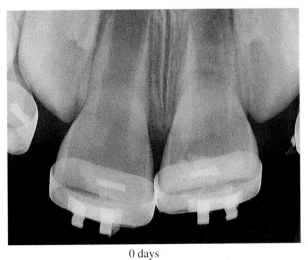

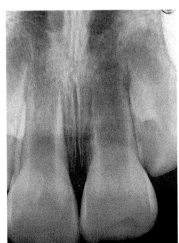

| 0 days | 3 weeks |

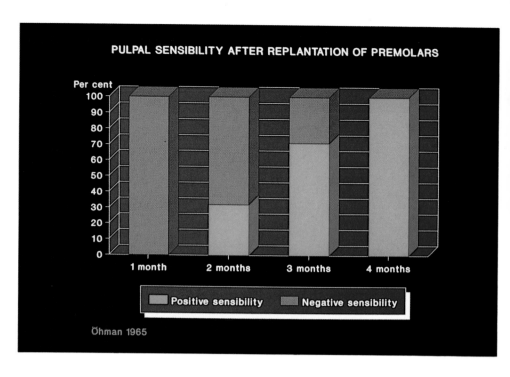

Fig. 2.17. Return of pulpal sensibility related to observation period in 86 intentionally extracted and immediately replanted premolars with open apices. From Öhman, 1965.[158]

In cases of pulp survival, the earliest sensibility reaction can be expected approximately 36 days after replantation. The frequency of positive pulpal response increases up to 100 days postreplantation (Fig. 2.17).[158]

In the few cases where pulp revascularization has taken place, *pulp canal obliteration* normally follows, the first signs of which can be detected 3 months after replantation, accompanied by a normal sensibility response (Fig. 2.18).

An alternative healing modality following pulpal revascularization is ingrowth of bone and PDL into the pulpal chamber, creating an internal PDL (Fig. 2.19). This is presumably due to damage to the Hertwig's epithelial root sheath, either at the time of avulsion or at the time of replantation (see Chapter 1, p. 43).

PDL healing and root resorption

Root resorption has been found to be closely related to the stage of root development, the extra-alveolar storage media, and the storage period (Figs. 2.20 and 2.21). In the following the typical characteristics of surface inflammatory and replacement resorption will be described.

Fig. 2.18. Pulp canal obliteration after replantation of a left central incisor. The canal obliteration becomes apparent after 6 months. From Andreasen & al., 1991.[188]

0 days	2 months	6 months	1 years	5 years	10 years

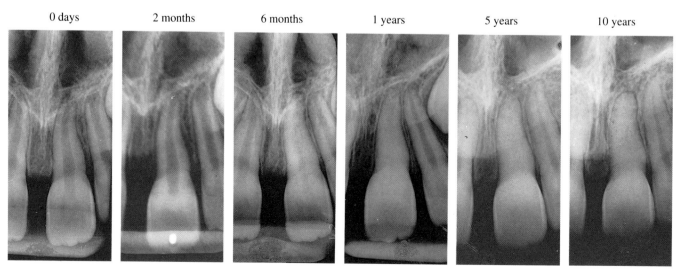

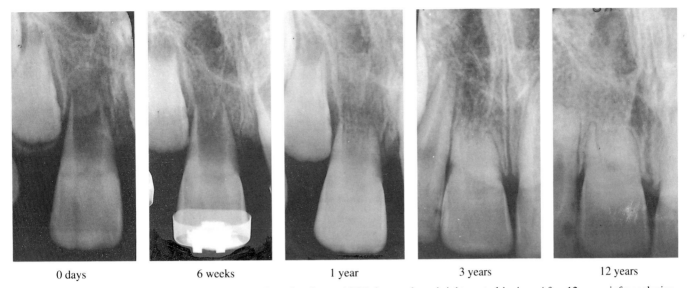

| 0 days | 6 weeks | 1 year | 3 years | 12 years |

Fig. 2.19. Bone invasion in the pulp canal and formation of an internal PDL in a replanted right central incisor. After 12 years infraocclusion was found apparently due to an internal ankylosis process. From Andreasen & al., 1991.[189]

Fig. 2.20a. Relation between PDL healing and length of extra-alveolar dry storage. From Andreasen & al., 1991.[190]

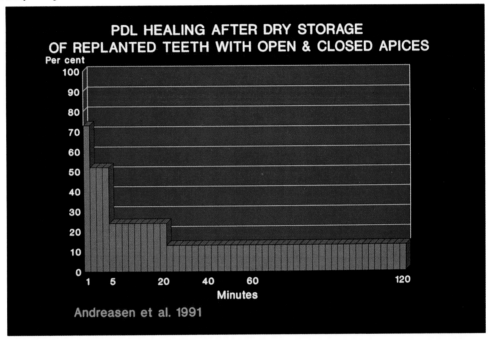

Fig. 2.20b. Relation between PDL healing and length of extra-alveolar wet storage. From Andreasen & al., 1991.[190]

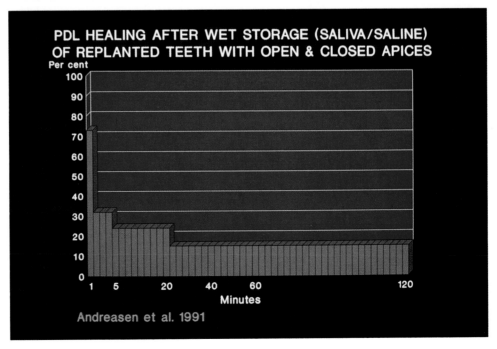

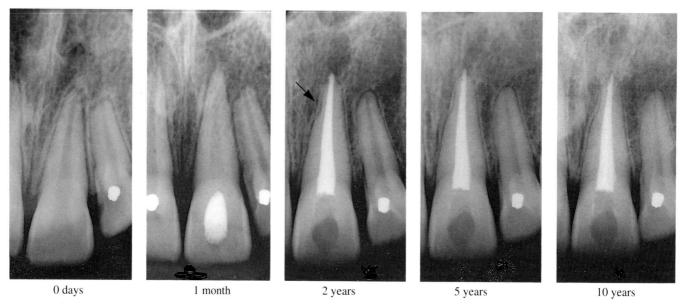

| 0 days | 1 month | 2 years | 5 years | 10 years |

Fig. 2.21. Surface resorption (arrow) of a replanted right central incisor. Note the superficial appearance on the root and sparse involvement of the lamina dura. The resorption cavity is stationary during the entire observation period. From Andreasen & al., 1991.[190]

Surface resorption

Surface resorption is the response to a limited injury to the PDL or root surface which subsequently heals from adjacent intact PDL (see Chapter 1, p. 27). These resorption cavities are always present on the root surface after replantation, but cannot normally be demonstrated radiographically because of their small dimensions. In rare instances, however, these resorption cavities can be seen, initially as shallow cavities on the root surface and the socket wall which later heal with a normal PDL space and intact lamina dura which follows the outline of the residual defect along the root surface.

A characteristic finding which usually makes it possible to distinguish between surface and inflammatory resorption (see later) is the more shallow nature of bone and root involvement with surface resorption than with inflammatory resorption. Another distinguishing feature, as mentioned earlier, is the self-limiting nature of the resorption process (Fig. 2.21). It is important to remember that surface resorption sites become stationary and can be seen many years after replantation. Most important, this resorption process requires no treatment.

Inflammatory resorption

This type of resorption is a response to a combined injury to the PDL and the pulp. When a resorption cavity on the root surface exposes dentinal tubules and these tubules communicate with infected necrotic pulp tissue, inflammation in the PDL can ensue and stimulate resorption activity (see Chapter 1, p. 28).

Inflammatory resorption is a very frequent complication after replantation and has been found to be significantly related to the stage of root development (i.e., being more prominent in teeth with incomplete root development than in teeth with completed root development).[123] Furthermore, this resorption type has also been found to be related to the type of storage medium and the length of the extraalveolar period (Fig. 2.20).[190] Thus, dry storage leads to extensive inflammatory resorption, whereas even prolonged storage in saline or saliva is followed by only a moderate increase in the extent of inflammatory resorption compared to immediate replantation.

Bowl-shaped inflammatory resorption cavities on the proximal root surfaces and in the adjacent bone can be demonstrated radiographically as early as 2-3 weeks after replantation and are usually first visible in the cervical or middle thirds of the root (Fig. 2.22).

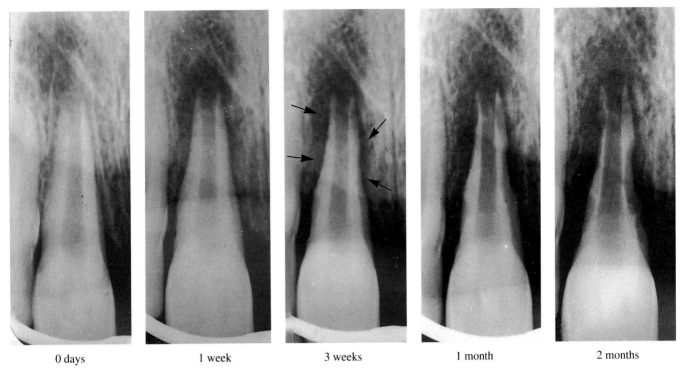

0 days	1 week	3 weeks	1 month	2 months

Fig. 2.22. Inflammatory resorption of a replanted right central incisor. Note the excavating nature of the resorption process on the root (arrows) and a corresponding marked resorption of the lamina dura. From Andreasen & Hjörting-Hansen, 1966 [123].

When placed facially or orally, inflammatory resorption cavities are seen as circular radiolucent zones within the root mass (Fig. 2.23).

Combined radiographic and histologic studies have shown that inflammatory resorption cavities are usually quite extensive before they can be diagnosed radiographically. Furthermore, it could be shown that artificial root resorption cavities made in human premolars in autopsy material are first visible when they reach a depth of 0.6 mm and a width of 1.2 mm.[161] Other factors which appear to be of importance for the visualization of resorption cavities are the viewing conditions and the radiographic technique used. The essential requirement for viewing conditions appears to be that extraneous light be eliminated, as this markedly limits the chance of

detecting minor variations in radiolucency in the radiographs. The most effective means of eliminating extraneous light is the use of an enclosed viewer, which not only eliminates light around the radiographs, but also slightly magnifies the image.[160]

Another important feature is that the contrast of the radiograph is optimal. It was found that the exposure time influenced the possibility of detecting artificial resorption cavities. Thus, an underexposed radiograph hid many resorption cavities, while a darker radiograph revealed more.[161]

Finally, the use of "identical" exposures is necessary in determining change from one examination to another. This can only be achieved by using a filmholder and a fixed film-focus distance.[160]

Fig. 2.23. Inflammatory resorption of a right central incisor. The resorption cavities appear as circular radiolucent zones within the root mass (arrows). Courtesy of Dr. AJ Ragne, Uppsala, Sweden.

0 days	4 weeks	4 months	5 months

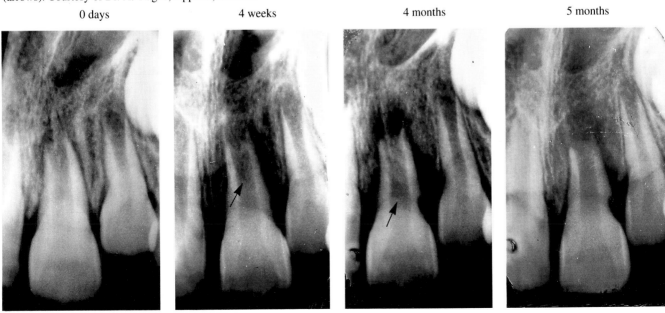

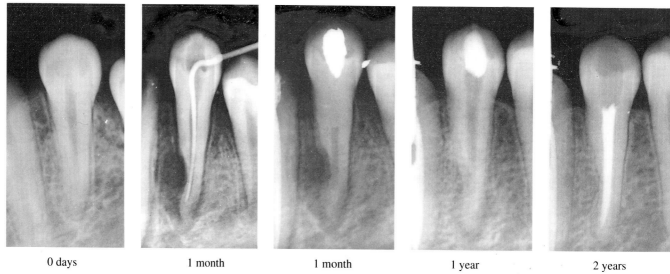

| 0 days | 1 month | 1 month | 1 year | 2 years |

Fig. 2.24. Arrest of inflammatory resorption using endodontic treatment with gutta-percha and a sealer; however, replacement resorption developed. From Andreasen & al., 1991.[191]

Treatment of inflammatory resorption

As soon as inflammatory resorption is diagnosed, endodontic treatment must be initiated, as the resorption process has been found to proceed with a speed of up to 0.1 mm per day. This speed implies rapid perforation to the root canal if treatment is not begun immediately.

Treatment of inflammatory resorption depends on endodontic intervention to combat effectively the bacteria present in the root canal and dentinal tubules.

In most cases it is possible to arrest even severely resorbed teeth if appropriate endodontic procedures are instituted (Figs. 2.10 and 2.11). However, it should be noted that in cases where large areas of the root have been resorbed, the healing which takes place can be in the form of an ankylosis (Figs. 2.24 and 2.25). This type of healing might be explained by a size factor. There is experimental evidence to suggest that the extent of injury to the root surface is decisive for the development of ankylosis (see Chapter 1, p. 30).

Delay in treating inflammatory resorption thus increases the risk of both perforation to the root canal and subsequent ankylosis.

Fig. 2.25. Endodontic treatment using calcium hydroxide has changed inflammatory resorption into replacement resorption evident as an obliteration of the PDL space 8 months after replantation. From Andreasen & al., 1991.[191]

| 0 days | 6 weeks | 8 months | 1 year | 3 years |

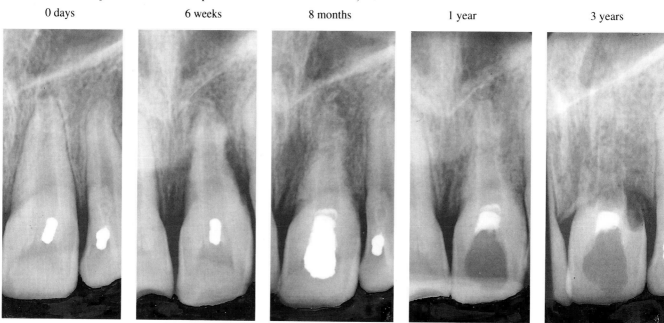

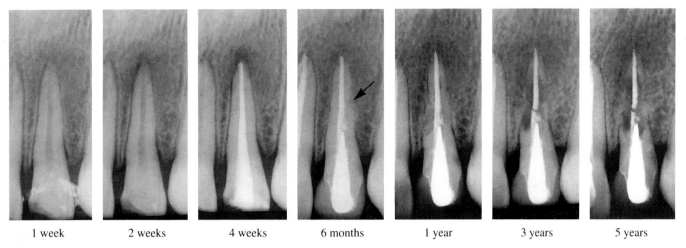

| 1 week | 2 weeks | 4 weeks | 6 months | 1 year | 3 years | 5 years |

Fig. 2.26. Ankylosis is evident as an obliteration of the PDL space 6 months after replantation (arrow). Note later development of inflammatory resorption. From Andreasen & al., 1991.[190]

Replacement resorption (ankylosis)

This type of resorption results from extensive injury to the innermost layer of the PDL and possibly also to the cemental surface.[163] In these cases healing processes are initiated from bone on the alveolar side of the PDL or from the adjacent bone marrow and result in an ankylosis between the socket wall and the root surface (Fig. 2.26).[124] The development of ankylosis is strongly related to the extent of damage to the PDL on the root surface of the avulsed tooth during the extra-alveolar period (Figs. 2.20 a and b).[185,186,190] Already after 5 min *dry* storage, the first signs of ankylosis become manifest; and after 20 min dry storage, ankylosis will affect almost all replanted teeth with complete root formation (Fig. 2.20a). In teeth with open apices the critical drying period appears to be 40 min. If teeth are stored *wet* (i.e. saliva or saline) extended storage has only a moderate effect upon periodontal ligament healing (Fig. 2. 20b). Also extended storage in nonphysiologic media, such as tap water, will lead to extensive ankylosis (see Chapter 1, p. 30).

Another factor known to lead to ankylosis is a fracture of the socket wall or alveolar process adjacent to the replantation site.[123] In these instances, the repair processes initiated in the alveolar bone apparently invade the root surface of the replanted tooth (Fig. 2.27)

Finally, it should be mentioned that extra-alveolar root filling procedures have been associated with a high frequency of replacement resorption.[123,137]

Fig. 2.27. The socket of the lateral incisor is involved in an alveolar fracture, leading to subsequent replacement resorption of the replanted incisor.

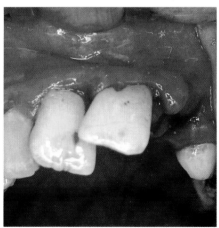
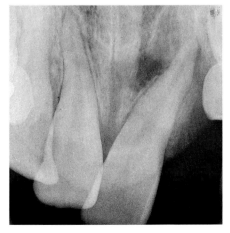
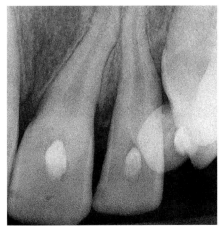

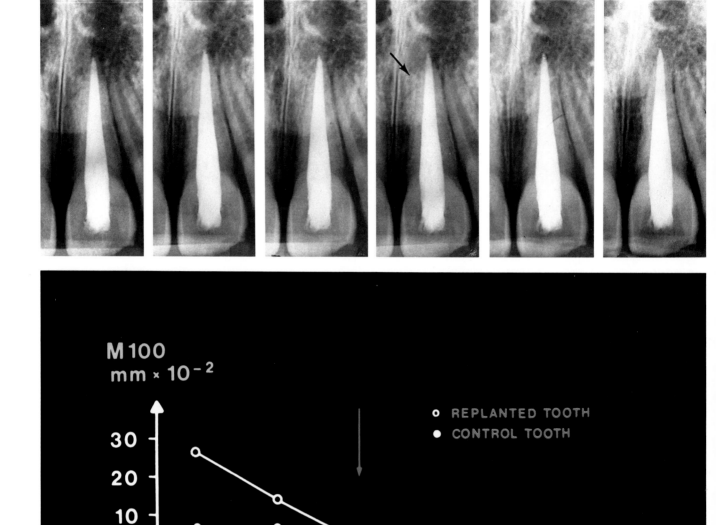

Fig. 2.28. Mobility testing a.m. Mühlemann shows restricted and later absent labiolingual excursion when ankylosis is established. Radiographically ankylosis can be demonstrated 6 weeks after replantation. From Andreasen, 1975.[141]

Diagnosis of replacement resorption

Early diagnosis of replacement resorption relies entirely upon clinical findings. The first clinical sign of ankylosis is a change in the percussion sound to a high metallic sound when the tooth is percussed on the facial aspect. Also, if the percussed tooth is supported by the examiner's finger, ankylosis can often be felt, in that vibration from percussion will not be felt through an ankylosed tooth. If mobility testing is performed (e.g., ad modum *Mühlemann*), a marked decrease in the normal labiolingual excursion can be demonstrated, indicating either transient or permanent ankylosis if repeated tests are made (Figs. 2.28 and 2.29).[141]

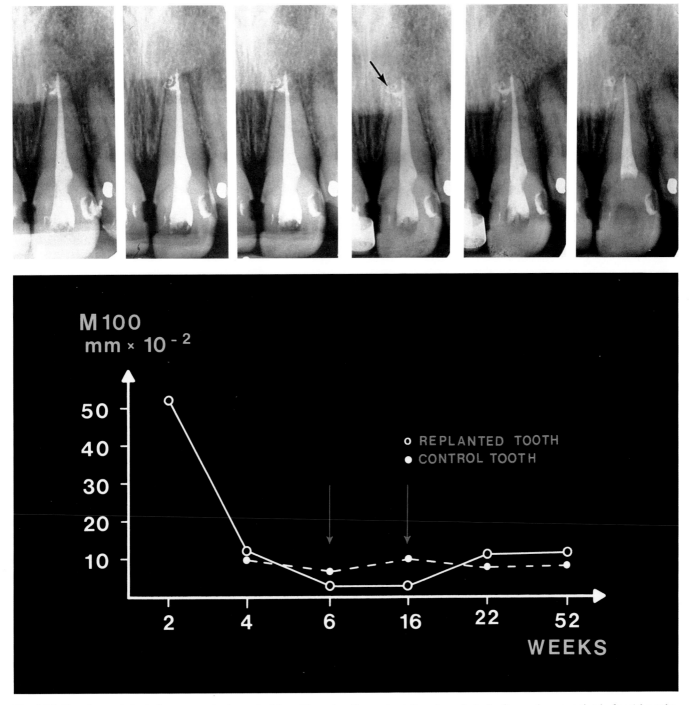

Fig. 2.29. Transient ankylosis is apparent in the period 6 to 16 weeks after replantation. An ankylosis site can be recognized after 16 weeks using mobility testing. From Andreasen, 1975.[141]

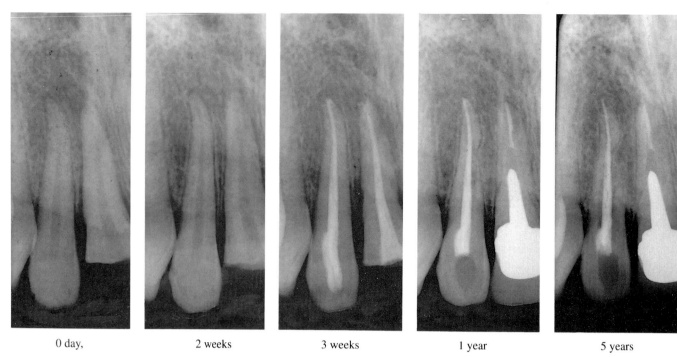

| 0 day, | 2 weeks | 3 weeks | 1 year | 5 years |

Fig. 2.30. Progression of replacement resorption is followed by tunneling inflammatory resorption along the root filling. From Andreasen & al., 1991.[191]

After 6 weeks, ankylosis is sometimes visible radiographically as an obliteration of the PDL space (Fig. 2.28). However, experimental studies have shown that the radiographic visualization of ankylosis requires involvement of at least 40% of the proximal root surface; and ankylosis sites located labially or lingually cannot be detected.[162]

In conclusion, early diagnosis of ankylosis depends very much on the percussion test or mobility testing; radiographic examination is less sensitive. The lower limit for diagnosing ankylosis by changes in mobility or percussion testing appears to be about 20% involvement of the root surface. Apparently small ankylosis sites can create bridging between the root surface and the socket wall, while still allowing tooth mobility.[162,163]

Factors influencing replacement resorption

The rate of the replacement resorption process is age dependent, progressing at the normal remodeling rate of the skeleton.[186] It has thus been found that the remodeling of bone in young individuals can be at the rate of 50% annually compared to a 2% annual turnover in older individuals.[164]

Apart from the remodeling factor, another phenomenon could exacerbate the resorption process, namely the superimposition of inflammatory resorption. If replacement resorption or surface resorption exposes dentinal tubules which communicate with bacteria present either in the proximal part of the dentinal tubules or in the root canal, inflammatory resorption may take over (Figs. 2.30 and 2.31).

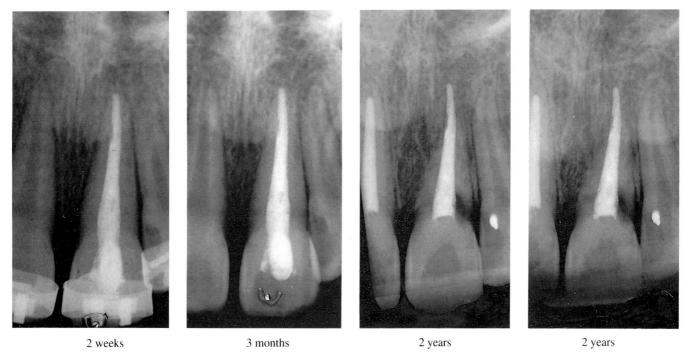

| 2 weeks | 3 months | 2 years | 2 years |

Fig. 2.31. Change of replacement resorption into inflammatory resorption presumably under the influence of infected necrotic tissue remnants in the root canal. From Andreasen & al., 1991.[191]

In this situation, instead of osteoclasts functioning at a pace corresponding to bone remodeling, their functional speed is accelerated to that for combating infection, implying an enormous intensification of the resorption process (see also Chapter 1, p. 28). This process becomes manifest when ankylosis has penetrated cementum and is stimulated by either bacteria in infected necrotic pulp tissue or bacteria present along an insufficient root filling.

It should be considered that ankylosis can occur even with pulp survival, as the pulp is less sensitive to external damage (Fig. 2.32).

Treatment of replacement resorption

If the initial ankylosis site is limited (i.e., an extra-alveolar period of less than 60 min), the ankylotic process can be temporary, being eliminated by healing events in the PDL within the first year after injury.[131] This process is apparently dependent upon normal function of the tooth (i.e. absence of rigid splinting). During normal function in the healing period, forces are transmitted to the PDL; stress created at the ankylosis sites apparently favoring their resorption (see Chapter 1, p. 47). Thus the first treatment principle for the prevention of permanent ankylosis appears to be the omission of rigid fixation after replantation.[131,165]

Fig. 2.32. Development of replacement resorption in spite of pulp revascularization. The extraoral period was 10 minutes dry storage and 155 minutes storage in tap water. From Andreasen & al., 1991.[190]

| 0 days | 1 month | 1 month | 1 year | 2 years |

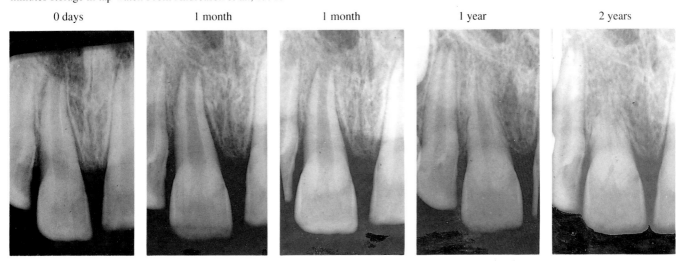

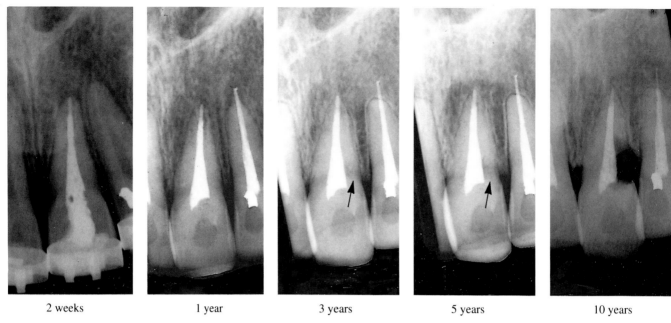

2 weeks	1 year	3 years	5 years	10 years

Fig. 2.33. Late appearance of ankylosis. Resorption activity is suspected after 3 and 5 years (arrows) and becomes manifest after 10 years. From Andreasen & al., 1991.[191]

Prognosis for replanted teeth with respect to replacement resorption cannot usually be determined earlier than the first year after injury because of the possibility of temporary replacement resorption, unless the extra-alveolar period is so extreme as to exclude any possibility of normal PDL healing. In some cases, ankylosis first becomes apparent several years after injury (Fig. 2.33).[190]

When ankylosis has been diagnosed, several factors must be determined, i.e., the probable extent of the ankylotic process and the probable remodeling rate of the skeleton.[191] In older individuals with replanted teeth and extreme extra-alveolar periods, an extended life expectancy of the replant still can be anticipated (Fig. 2.34).

In younger individuals, the effects of extreme extra-alveolar periods must be considered. Ankylosis will impede growth of that portion of the alveolar process containing the replanted tooth, ultimately resulting in infraocclusion (Fig. 2.35). Once the tooth is 1 - 2 mm in infraocclusion, two treatment alternatives exist: (1) extraction or (2) luxation and orthodontic extrusion.

Fig. 2.34. Long-term survival in spite of ankylosis of a replanted right central incisor in a 22-year-old individual. From Andreasen & al., 1991.[191]

0 days	6 weeks	6 weeks	1 year	3 years	5 years

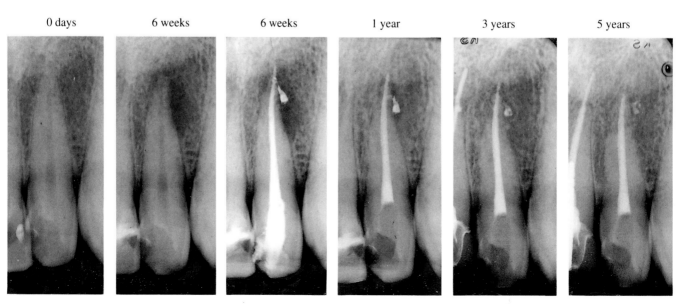

Fig. 2.35. Infraocclusion after replantation and subsequent ankylosis of a right central incisor

The replantation was carried out at the age of 7.

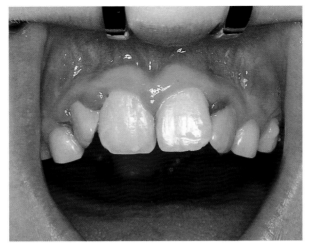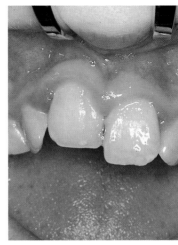

In cases where only limited ankylosis is suspected (i.e., with extra-alveolar periods of less than 1 hour), it might be worthwhile to break up the ankylosis sites by luxation. A local anesthetic is administered and the tooth grasped with a forceps. Using slight rotating movements, the tooth is then loosened. The patient is then instructed to keep the tooth in function and to rock the tooth back and forth with finger pressure, e.g., for 1 minute three times daily for a month to prevent reestablishment of the ankylosis. Clinical experience has shown that this procedure can in some cases result in a normally functioning PDL (Fig. 2.36).

If extraction is decided upon, future treatment must be considered. If orthodontic movement of the adjacent teeth into the extraction site is not planned, partial tooth removal (i.e., removal of only the supra-alveolar part of the tooth) can be performed (Fig. 2.37). The crown is fractured off and root substance is removed 1 mm below the cervical margin of the socket, whereafter the root filling is removed. By leaving the root in the alveolus, which is ultimately replaced by bone, the height of the alveolar process will be maintained and sometimes even slightly increased.[166]

Fig. 2.36. Ankylosis treated by luxation

Ankylosis is manifest by a percussion test 2 months after replantation.

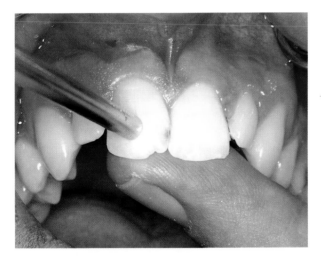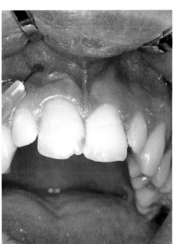

Loosening the incisor

After administration of a local analgesic the tooth is loosened with forceps using rotation movements. The tooth should be completely mobile in the socket. The patient should then undertake rocking movements for several minutes a day over a 1-month period.

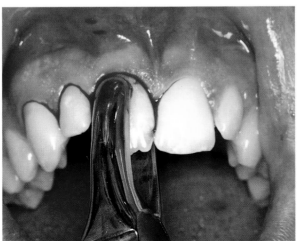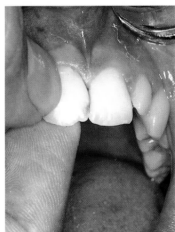

Fig. 2.37. Removal of an ankylosed tooth

5 years after replantation in a 9-year-old individual at the time of trauma, severe ankylosis and infra-occlusion are present.

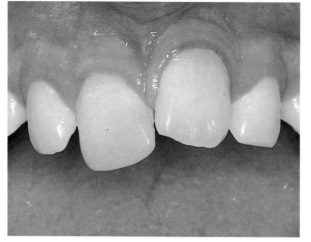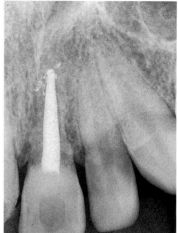

Extraction of the crown

The crown portion is removed with forceps.

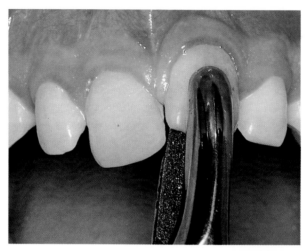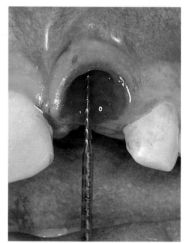

Removing the root filling

The gutta-percha root filling is removed with thumb forceps or a root canal file.

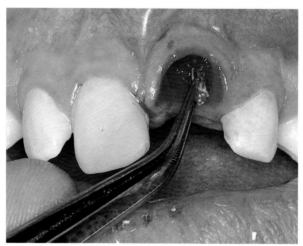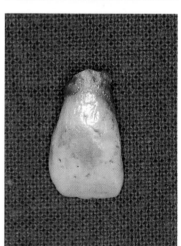

Removal of gutta-percha fragments

If gutta-percha fragments are present in the bone, a canal can be burred into the alveolus following the path of the root filling. Thereafter gutta-percha fragments can be washed out with saline. Finally a radiograph is taken to verify complete removal.

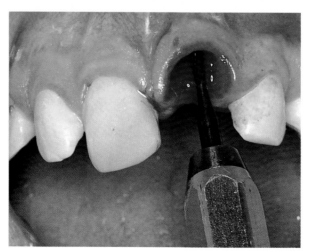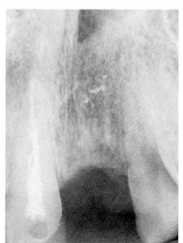

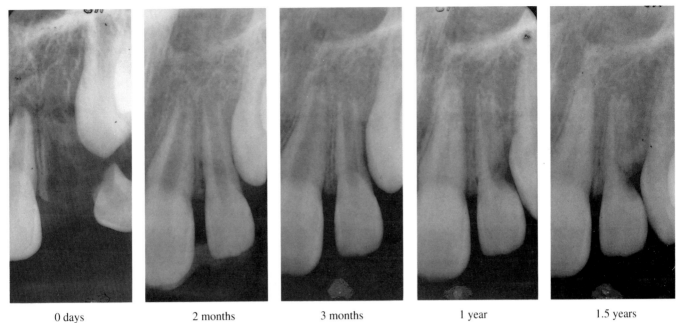

| 0 days | 2 months | 3 months | 1 year | 1.5 years |

Fig. 2.38. Resorption of a replanted lateral incisor by an erupting canine. From Andreasen & al., 1991.[190]

Erupting teeth causing resorption

In the case of replanted lateral incisors, erupting cuspids may cause resorption of the root of the replanted tooth (Fig. 2.38).[190] In these cases, extraction of the primary cuspid is recommended in order to alter the path of eruption of the permanent cuspid and avoid resorption.

Root development and developmental disturbances

In most cases where teeth with incomplete root formation are replanted, a total or partial arrest of root formation will result, the decisive factor for further root development being the integrity of Hertwig's epithelial root sheath.[189] In cases where this structure can be kept vital, complete root formation can occur (Fig. 2.39). In the event of partial damage, partial root formation is possible (Fig. 2.40). In this context, it should be remembered that completed root formation by no means implies pulp survival. Thus, root development can take place even where a partial pulp necrosis is present (Fig. 2.41). In most cases, however, the Hertwig epithelial root sheath is apparently so damaged that total arrest of root formation is the result. Subsequent pulpal repair will then result in the ingrowth of bone and PDL through the apical foramen, filling the canal with bone separated from the dentinal wall by an internal PDL (Fig. 2.42) (see also Chapter 1, p. 43).

Fig. 2.39. Completed root formation after replantation of a right central incisor. From Andreasen & al., 1991.[189]

| 0 days | 6 months | 1 year | 2 years | 5 years | 10 years |

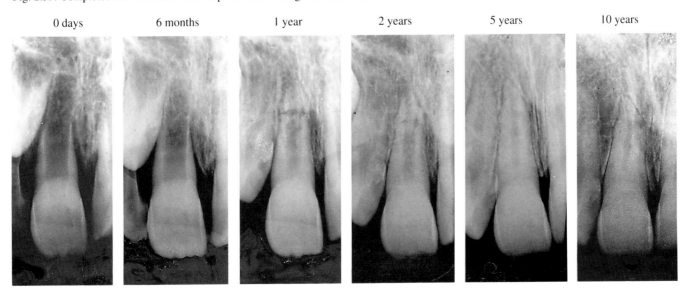

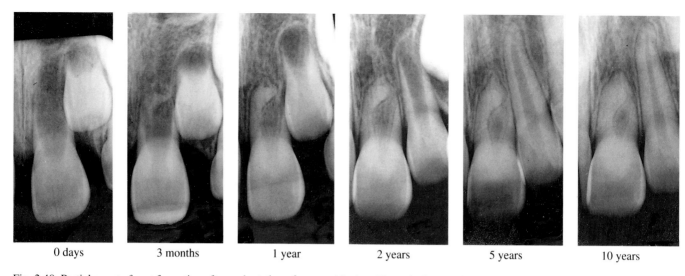

| 0 days | 3 months | 1 year | 2 years | 5 years | 10 years |

Fig. 2.40. Partial arrest of root formation after replantation of a central incisor. From Andreasen & al., 1991.[189]

Fig. 2.41. Completion of root formation in spite of partial pulp necrosis. From Andreasen & al., 1991.[189]

| 0 days | 3 weeks | 6 months | 1 year |

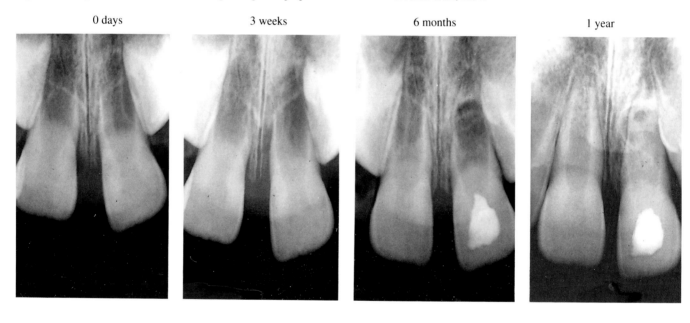

Fig. 2.42. Arrested root formation and ingrowth of apical bone and PDL after replantation of a right central incisor. From Andreasen & al., 1991.[189]

| 0 days | 6 months | 2 years | 10 years | 10 years |

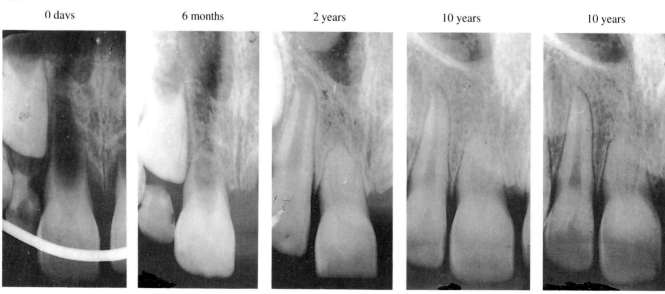

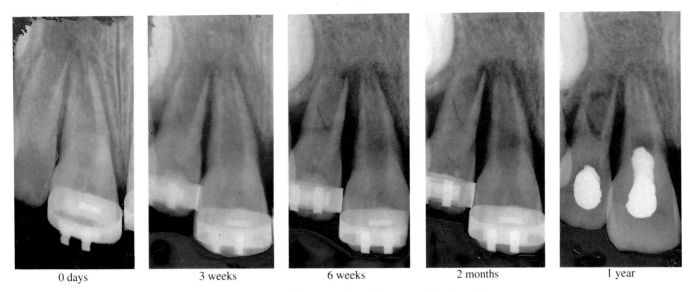

| 0 days | 3 weeks | 6 weeks | 2 months | 1 year |

Fig. 2.43. Loss of marginal bone support due to contusion of the alveolar socket at time of replantation.

Gingival healing and marginal attachment loss

Loss of marginal periodontal support is not a typical complication after replantation. The few cases where this complication occurs are usually in older individuals where the socket wall is crushed at the time of injury (Fig. 2.43).

Phantom root formation

In cases where teeth with immature root formation have been avulsed and replantation is not indicated, the tooth should be examined for the presence of the pulp in the root canal. If the pulp is missing, it has been left behind in the alveolus. If such a pulp is allowed to remain, a root fragment will develop from this tissue which could indicate later surgical removal (Fig. 2.44).[167-173] The explanation for this is that the pulp tissue is able to continue to form dentin even when all hard tissue has been removed (see Chapter 1, p. 43). Furthermore, the Hertwig's epithelial root sheath can continue to initiate root development, even in its "disembodied" state.

Fig. 2.44. Phantom root development subsequent to avulsion of a tooth with incomplete root formation. The pulp has remained in the socket and formed the new root. From Ravn, 1970.[169]

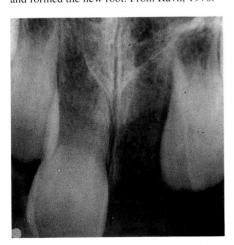
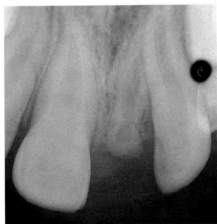
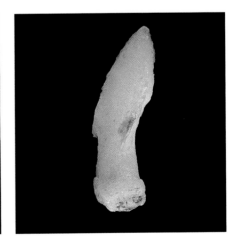

Essentials

Indications

Before replantation consider the following:

1. Only permanent teeth should be replanted.

2. Caries and periodontal status. Serious neglect may contra-indicate replantation.

3. Length of the extra-alveolar period. Dry periods of more than 60 min usually result in ankylosis. In these cases, special replantation procedures using chemical treatment of the root may be indicated (see p. 68).

4. Condition of the socket. Associated bone fractures result in ankylosis.

Surgical procedure (Fig. 2.6).

1. Examine the avulsed tooth for the presence of PDL, and in immature teeth, for the condition of the apical pulp.

2. Place the avulsed tooth in physiologic saline.

3. Examine the socket area for signs of fracture or contusion and the presence of foreign bodies. If the socket area appears damaged, take a radiograph.

4. If replantation is decided upon, cleanse the root surface and apical part of the pulp with a copious flow of saline until the tooth appears clean.

5. Reposition the tooth in the socket. It is usually not necessary to remove the coagulum.

6. Splint the tooth with an acid-etch/ acrylic splint, a Kevlar or nylon fish line/acid-etch splint, or in cases of incompletely erupted teeth, with a suture across the incisal edge.

7. Administer antibiotic coverage (e.g., penicillin, 0.5 million IU x 4 daily for 4-7 days).

8. Consider tetanus prophylaxis.

9. Reschedule the patient 1 week later for splint removal. In cases of completed root formation, the pulp is extirpated before splint removal. A calcium hydroxide dressing is placed and the access cavity is sealed with a fortified zinc oxide eugenol cement (e.g., IRM). The dressing is renewed 4 weeks later.

In cases with incomplete root formation, the splint is removed and the patient is rescheduled 2, 3, and 4 weeks after replantation for diagnosis of signs of pulp necrosis and inflammatory resorption. At all controls, radiographs are taken. If signs of healing complications are detected, the pulp is extirpated immediately and the root canal filled with calcium hydroxide, as in teeth with completed root formation.

10. In the event of pulp extirpation, the tooth should be examined radiographically 3 months after replantation. If the radiograph shows persistent calcium hydroxide in the canal, arrest of the inflammatory resorption process, and/or diminished apical rarefaction, the patient is rescheduled for the next control 6 months after replantation. Otherwise, the calcium hydroxide dressing is renewed.

11. In teeth with complete root formation, a final root filling using a gutta-percha technique is possible 6 months after replantation. In teeth with incomplete root formation, the final endodontic treatment must await apexification, which normally takes 12-18 months.

Follow up

See Appendix 1, p. 289

Tooth survival (5 years)
Incomplete root formation:	66%
Complete root formation:	82%

Pulp healing (5 years)
Incomplete root formation:	30%
Complete root formation:	0%

PDL healing (5 years)
Incomplete root formation:	39%
Complete root formation:	17%

References

1. Andreasen JO. Traumatic injuries of the teeth. 2nd ed. Copenhagen: Munksgaard, 1981; 203-42.

2. Axhausen G. Die histologischen Gesetze der Wiedereinheilung replantierter Zähne. Dtsch-Zahn-Mund Kieferheilk 1937; 4: 169-78.

3. Öhman A. Behandling av olycksfallsskadade incisiver på barn. Replantation av utslagna eller accidentellt extraherade tänder och tandanlag. Odontol Tidskr 1957; 65: 150-59.

4. Jachno R. Present state of immediate replantation of teeth. Cesk Stomatol 1962; 62: 203-08.

5. Hammer H. Il reimpianto biologico dei denti. Mondo Odontostomatol 1967; 9: 291-302.

6. Natiella JR, Armitage JE, Greene GW. The replantation and transplantation of teeth. A review. Oral Surg Oral Med Oral Pathol 1970; 29: 397-419.

7. Spreter von Kreudenstein T. Indikation und Erfolg der Frontzähneimplantation. Zahnärztl Prax 1972; 23: 345-47.

8. Massler M. Tooth replantation. Dent Clin North Am 1974; 18: 445-52.

9. Grasser H. Reimplantation im Milch- und Wechselgebiss. Zahnärztl Prax 1975; 26: 5.

10. Barbakow F, Imfeld T. Principles in the replantation of permanent teeth (I). Oral Surg 1982; 3: 289-94.

11. Barbakow F, Imfeld T. Principles in the replantation of permanent teeth (II). Oral Surg 1982; 13: 401-05.

12. Essade J. La réimplantation dentaire chez l'enfant apres un traumatisme accidentel. Présentation de cas cliniques. Schweiz Monatsschr Zahnheilk 1979; 89: 1134-35.

13. Scott JN, Zelikow R. Replantation - a clinical philosophy. J Am Dent Assoc 1980; 101: 17-19.

14. Hess W. Zur Frage der Replantation von Zahnkeimen. Schweiz Monatschr Zahnheilk 1943; 53: 672-77.

15. Pålsson F. Zur Frage der Replantation von Zahnkeimen. Acta Odontol Scand 1944; 5: 63-78 .

16. Herbert WE. Three successful cases of replacement of teeth immediately following dislocation. Br Dent J 1953; 94: 182-84.

17. Edlan A. Can the pulp preserve its vitality following replantation of the totally displaced tooth? Cesk Stomatol 1955; 55: 165-67.

18. Ljungdahl L, Mårtensson K. Ett fall av multipla tandreplantationer. Odontol Rev 1955; 55: 222-232.

19. Lindahl B, Mårtensson K. Replantation of a tooth. A case report. Odontol Rev 1960; 11: 325-30.

20. Henning FR. Reimplantation of luxated teeth. Aust Dent J 1965; 10: 306-12.

21. Adatia AK. Odontogenesis following replantation of erupted maxillary central incisor. Dent Pract 1971; 21: 153-55.

22. Porteous JR. Vital reimplantation of a maxillary central incisor tooth: Report of a case. J Dent Child 1972; 39: 429-31.

23. Barry GN. Replanted teeth still functioning after 42 years: Report of case. J Am Dent Assoc 1976; 92: 412-13.

24. Eckstein A. Replantation bleibender Frontzähne mit nicht abgeschlossenem Wurzelwachstum. Fortschr Kiefer Gesichtschir 1976; 20: 125-27.

25. Meyer-Bardowicks J. Eine Zahnreplantation mit Erhaltung der Pulpavitalität. Quintessenz 1977; 28: 39-42.

26. Kemp WB, Mourino A. Accidental extraction and replantation of an immature permanent tooth. J Endod 1977; 3: 240-41.

27. Todaro CJ. Fuss Z. Successful self-replantation of avulsed tooth with 42-year follow-up. Endod Dent Traumatol 1985; 1: 120-22.

28. Kildebo H. Eksartikulation av fronttenner. En Kasusbeskrivelse. Nor Tannlægeforen Tid 1983; 93: 463-64.

29. Fuss Z. Successful self-replantation of avulsed tooth with 42-year follow-up. Endod Dent Traumatol 1985; 1: 120-22.

30. Johnson WT, James GA. Replantation of avulsed teeth with immature root development. Oral Surg Oral Med Oral Pathol 1985; 60: 420-27.

31. Pleasant SA. Tooth replantation. Br Dent J 1942; 73: 308-10.

32. Axhausen G. Ein Beitrag zur Zahnreplantation ZWR 1948; 3: 130-32.

33. Krömer H. An auxiliary device for the performance of replantation. Br Dent J 1948; 84: 210-13.

34. Krepil H. Für die Praxis: Ist der von der Alveole getrennte Zahn ein totes Hartgebilde? Dtsch Zahnärztl Z 1949; 4: 638-39.

35. Pindborg JJ, Hansen J. A case of replantation of an upper lateral incisor: A histological study. Oral Surg Oral Med Oral Pathol 1951; 4: 661-67.

36. Ciriello G. Alcune considerazioni sulla tecnica del reimpianto dentario. Riv Ital Stomatol 1953; 8: 764-99.

37. Ciriello G. Impianti acrilici ed innesti dentarii nei tessuti mascellari a sostegno de protesi. Riv Ital Stomatol 1954; 9: 1088-1143.

38. Ciriello G. Considerazioni critiche sugli impianti a sostegno di protesi. Riv Ital Stomatol 1956; 11: 464-75.

39. Healey HJ. Replantation: A brief review and a report of a case sequel. Oral Surg Oral Med Oral Pathol 1953; 6: 775-79.

40. Ingle JI, Dow P. Replantation following total luxation. Dent Digest 1953; 59: 386-90.

41. Kupfer IJ, Kupfer SR. Tooth replantation following traumatic avulsion. NY State Dent J 1953; 19: 80-84.

42. Miller HM. Reimplanting human teeth. Dent Survey 1953; 29: 1439-43.

43. Carmichael AF, Nixon GS. Two interesting cases of root resorption. Dent Record 1954; 74: 258-60.

44. Douglas BL, Douglas W. Clinical observations on replantation of upper anterior teeth. Oral Surg Oral Med Oral Oral Pathol 1954; 7: 29-31.

45. Lovel RW, Hopper FE. Tooth replantation: A case report with serial radiographs and histological examination. Br Dent J 1954; 97: 205-08.

46. Ogus WI Research report on the replant-implant of individual teeth. Dent Dig 1954; 60: 358-61.

47. Keresztesi K. Die Reimplantation von Zähnen in der modernen Zahnheilkunde. Öster Z Stomatol 1955; 52: 16-22.

48. Olech E. Replanted upper central incisor. Oral Surg Oral Med Oral Pathol 1956; 9: 106-09.

49. Thonner KE. Vitalliumstift vid reimplantation av totalluxerade tänder. Sven Tandläkarförb Tidn 1956; 48: 216-17.

50. Drahonovsky V. Otazka vitality replantovanych zubu. Prakt Zubn Lek 1957; 5: 148-51.

51. Kluge R. Indikation und Erfolgsaussichten bei Zahnrückpflanzung. Zahnärztl Prax 1957; 23: 3-10.

52. Walter KL. Beitrag zur Replantation einwurzeliger Zähne. Zahnärztl Rundsch 1957; 66: 315-18.

53. Herbert WE. A case of complete dislocation of a tooth. Br Dent J 1958; 94: 137-38.

54. McCagie JNW. A case of re-implantation of teeth after five days. Dent Pract 1958; 8: 320-21.

55. Best EJ, Olsen NH. The management of traumatic injuries by replantation. Dent Dig 1959; 65: 298-301.

56. Bataille R. Reimplantation de 3 dents dans un foyer de fracture, utilisees ensuite comme piliers de prothese fixe. Rev Stomatol 1959; 60: 339-42.

57. Bataille R. Reimplantation - transplantation - implantation. Acta Stomatol Belg 1963; 60: 455-64.

58. Kilian J. Replantace zubu Prakt Zubn Lek 1959; 7: 68-75.

59. Burley MA, Crabb HSM. Replantation of teeth. Br Dent J 1960; 108: 190-93.

60. Friedman JW. Replantation of evulsed teeth: A case report. Dent Dig 1961; 67: 568-69.

61. Kustaloglu O. Replantation of an upper central incisor in a pretraumatized area. Oral Surg Oral Med Oral Pathol 1961; 14: 270-75.

62. Mathieu P. Aspect chirurgical des traumatismes des dents anterieures chez les jeunes sujets. Deux cas de réimplantation de dent fracturée. Rev Belg Soc Dent 1961; 16: 485-98.

63. Bodecker CF. Tooth replantation registry. NY State Dent J 1962; 28: 78-79.

64. Hirsch S. Travaux originaux. Réimplantations post-traumatiques la contention. Inf Dent 1962; 7: 2589-95.

65. Rabinowitch BZ. Replantation of teeth and management of root fractures. Dent Clin North Am 1962; July: 555-68.

66. Recant BS, Kaufman PS. Reimplantation of an avulsed maxillary lateral incisor tooth. NY State Dent J 1962; 28: 401-03.

67. Traiger J. Replantation of teeth. Dent Radiogr Photogr 1964; 37: 44-45.

68. Lange D. Untersuchungen zur enossalen "biologischen Implantation" bei therapeutischen und posttraumatischen replantationen. Dtsch Zahnärztl Z 1965; 20: 1157-64.

69. Moginier C. Über das Schicksal eines angeblich reponierten Zahnes. Schweiz Monatschr Zahnheilk 1966; 75: 1222-23.

70. Edwards TSF. Treatment of pulpal and periapical disease by replantation. Br Dent J 1966; 121: 159-66.

71. Mangiante P, Mantero F. Alcune variazione sul reimpianto dentale nella traumatolgia maxillo-facciale. Minerva Stomatol 1966; 15: 47-52.

72. de Rysky S, Nidoli G, Caprioglio D. Trapianti e reimpianti dentali. Contributo personale. Riv Ital Stomatol 1966; 21: 3-15.

73. Talim ST, Antia FE. A roentgenographic evaluation of reimplanted teeth. Oral Surg Oral Med Oral Pathol 1966; 21: 602-08.

74. Broglia ML, Guasta G. Il problema, terapeutico della lussazione totale traumatica degli incisivi permaneneti pazienti di eta pediatrica. Minerva Stomatol 1968; 6: 549-56.

75. Benqué E-P. Réimplantations et auto-transplantation par transfixation - Methode personnelle. Inf Dent 1968; 50: 125-38.

76. Hovinga J. Replantantie en transplantantie van tanden. Een experimenteel en klinisch onderzoek (Thesis). Amsterdam: Oosterbaan & Le Cointre, 1968.

77. Marzola C. Reimplante dental. Consideraçoes cirurgicas, clinicas e radiograficas. Rev Bras Odontol 1968; 25: 254-69.

78. Messing JJ. Reimplantation of teeth. Dent Pract 1968; 18: 241-48.

79. LeCavalier L. Reimplantation of maxillary anterior teeth: Report of case. J Am Dent Assoc 1969; 79: 1427-30.

80. Bertoft H. Replanterad tand med lång observationstid. Sven Tandläkarförb Tidn 1969; 61: 1289

81. Elsey HJ. An interesting case of reimplantation. Dent Pract 1969; 20: 18-20.

82. Florence M. Replantation of a luxated incisor. Can Dent Assoc J 1969; 35: 23-25.

83. Di Giulio PJ. Reimplantation of three permanent anterior teeth accidentally evulsed. NY State Dent J 1969; 35: 219-22.

84. Holmes LW. Case report. Replantation of right central incisor. J NJ Dent Assoc 1969; 41: 9-16.

85. Pfeifer H. Erhaltung traumatisch geschädigter Zähne? Dtsch Zahnärztl Z 1969; 24: 263-67.

86. Severineanu V, Pasevschi-Colesnic A. Replantation as an emergency therapeutic method. Stomatologia (Romania) 1969; 14: 307-12.

87. Bell JG. Reimplantation and post-operative observation of a traumatically extracted upper central incisor. Dent J 1970; 66: 175-76.

88. Monsour FNT. The reimplantation of displaced teeth. Aust Dent J 1970; 21: 361-64.

89. Pongraez P. Die Frage der Replantation, mit besonderer Hinsicht auf die Verletzungen im Frontzahnbereich. Fogorv Sz 1970; 63: 151-56.

90. Tosti A. Reimplantation: Report of a case. Dent Dig 1970; 76: 98-100.

91. Matthews RW. Successful replantation of an anterior tooth with an apical third fracture. Br Dent J 1971; 130: 117-18.

92. Colletti GDN. A new technique for replants and transplants: Clinical report of 229 cases. J Oral Med 1971; 26: 82-84.

93. Barbakow FH. Reimplantation of teeth: A review of the literature and a case report. J Dent Assoc S Afr 1971; 26: 177-81.

94. Harndt R, Hoefig W. Replantation of traumatically avulsed teeth. Quintessence Int 1972; 3: 19-23.

95. Spreter von Kreudenstein T. Indikation und Erfolg der Frontzahnreimplantation. Zahnärztl Prax 1972; 23: 345.

96. Nosonowitz DM. On intentional replantation. NY J Dent 1272; 42: 44-64.

97. Gomes GR, Gomes JMR. Evaluacion de la vitalidad del tejido periodontal en los reimplantes y transplantes. Rev Asoc Odontol Argent 1973; 61: 168-173.

98. Milton LU. Replantation of avulsed anterior teeth in patients with jaw fractures. Plast Reconstr Surg 1973; 51: 377-83.

99. Richardson MB. Replantation of avulsed teeth. NC Dent J 1973; 56: 24-25.

100. Bellizzi R. Replantation of avulsed anterior teeth: An unusual technique. Oral Surg Oral Med Oral Pathol 1974; 38: 614-17.

101. Dind E. A propos de la duree des reimplantations. Schweiz Monatschr Zahnheilk 1974; 84: 770-71.

102. White E. Delayed replantation of avulsed teeth. J Endod 1975; 1: 247-48.

103. Matusow RJ. Clinical observations regarding the treatment of traumatically avulsed mature teeth. Part 2. Oral Surg Oral Med Oral Pathol 1985; 60: 428-35.

104. Pullinger PC, Craig GG. Loss of upper permanent incisor teeth. Case report. Aust Dent J 1976; 21: 395-96.

105. Rodriguez CLN. Contribucion al estudio de los reimplantes dentarios. (Thesis). Barcelona: Universidad de Barcelona,1976.

106. Shusterman S, Meller SM, Kane J. Reimplantation of traumatically avulsed immature incisor: Report of case. J Dent Child 1976 ; 43 : 49-52.

107. Wepner F. Die Replantation der Frontzähne nach traumatischen Zahnverlust. Öster Z Stomatol 1976; 73: 275-82.

108. Gombos F. Su di una particolare tecnica di reimpianto e trapianto dentario. Studio sperimentale. Arch Stomatol (Napoli) 1978; 19: 153-208.

l09. Marosky JE. Treating the avulsed tooth. Ill Dent J 1978; 47 : 58-61.

110. Valletta G. Reimpianti e trapianti dentari. Arch Stomatol (Napoli) 1978; 19: 209-17.

111. Gombos F, Caruso F, Preteroti AM. Gli insuccessi negli autotrapianti e nei reimpianti dentari. Arch Stomatol (Napoli) 1979; 20: 21-35.

112. Holthaus V. Reimplantation von total luxierten Frontzähnen bei einer Patientin mit genuiner Epilipsie, Fallbericht: Behandlung und Verlauf. ZWR 1979; 88: 312-14.

113. Chamberlin JH, Goerig AC. Rationale for treatment and management of avulsed teeth. J Am Dent Assoc 1980; 101: 471-75.

114. Järvinen S, Ojala E. Replantation of young permanent incisors. A long term follow-up study of seven cases with eleven replanted teeth. Acta Odontol Pediatr 1980; 2: 83-87.

115. Melczer K. Felsö frontfogak reimplantaciója. Fogorv Sz 1980; 73: 150-52.

116. O'Riordan MW, Ralstrom CS, Doerr SE. Treatment of avulsed permanent teeth: an update. J Am Dent Assoc 1982; 105: 1028-30.

117. Cameron JA. The endodontic management of a replanted avulsed tooth with severe root resorption - a case report. Int Endod J 1984; 17: 76-79.

118. Matusow RJ. Clinical observations regarding the treatment of traumatically avulsed mature teeth. Part 1. Oral Surg Oral Med Oral Pathol 1985; 60: 94-99.

119. Stålhane I, Hedegård B. Traumatized permanent teeth in children aged 7-15 years. Part II. Swed Dent J 1975; 68: 157-69.

120. Lenstrup K, Skieller V. Efterundersögelse af tænder replanteret efter exartikulation. Tandlægebladet 1957; 61: 570-83.

121. Lenstrup K, Skieller V. A follow-up study of teeth replanted after accidental loss. Acta Odontol Scand 1959; 17: 503-09.

122. Deeb E, Prietto PP, McKenna RC. Reimplantation of luxated teeth in humans. South Cal State Dent Assoc 1965; 33: 194-206.

123. Andreasen JO, Hjörting-Hansen E. Replantation of teeth I. Radiographic and clinical study of 110 human teeth replanted after accidental loss. Acta Odontol Scand 1966; 24: 264-286.

124. Andreasen JO, Hjörting-Hansen E. Replantation of teeth II. Histological study of 22 replanted anterior teeth in humans. Acta Odontol Scand 1966; 24: 287-306.

125. Ravn JJ, Helbo M. Replantation af akcidentelt eksartikulerede tænder. Tandlægebladet 1966; 70: 805-15.

126. Rivas LA. Ergebnisse der Replantation nach Trauma im Frontzahnbereich bei Jugendlichen. Dtsch Zahnärztl Z 1968; 23: 484-89.

127. Grossman LI, Ship II. Survival rate of replanted teeth. Oral Surg Oral Med Oral Pathol 1970; 29: 899-906.

128. Andreasen JO. Treatment of fractured and avulsed teeth. J Dent Child 1971; 38: 29-48

129. Cvek M, Granath L-E, Hollender L. Treatment of non vital permanent incisors with calcium hydroxide. III. Variation of occurrence of ankylosis of reimplanted teeth with duration of extra-alveolar period and storage environment. Odontol Rev 1974; 25: 43-56.

130. Gröndahl H-G, Kahnberg K-E, Olsson G. Traumatiserade tänder. En klinisk efterundersökning. Göteborgs Tandläkar-Sällskaps Artikelserie 1974; No 384:37-50.

131. Andreasen JO. Periodontal healing after replantation of traumatically avulsed human teeth. Assessment by mobility testing and radiography. Acta Odontol Scand 1975; 33: 325-35.

132. Hörster W, Altfeld F, Planko D. Behandlungsergebnisse nach Replantation total luxierter Frontzahne. Fortschr Kiefer Gesichtschir 1976; 20: 127-29.

133. Ravn JJ. En redegørelse for behandlingen efter eksartikulation af permanente incisiver i en skolebarnspopulation. Tandlægebladet 1977; 81: 563-69.

134. Kemp WB, Phillips J. Evaluation of 71 replanted teeth. J Endod 1977; 3: 30-35.

135. Coccia CT. A clinical investigation of root resorption rates in reimplanted young permanent incisors: A five-year study. J Endod 1980; 6: 413-20.

136. Herforth A. Traumatische Schädigungen der Frontzähne bei Kindern und Jugendlichen im Alter von 7 bis 15 Jahren. Berlin: Quintessenz Verlag GmbH, 1982.

137. Koch G, Ullbro C. Klinisk funktionstid hos 55 exartikulerade och replanterade tänder. Tandläkartidningen 1982; 74: 18-25.

138. Heimdal A, von Konow L. Lundquist G. Replantation of avulsed teeth after long extra-alveolar periods. Int J Oral Surg 1983; 12: 413-17.

139. Wettensshwiler H. Unfallbedingte Totalluxation von bleibenden Frontzähnen. Befund, Sofortbehandlung und Langzeitprognose. Inaugural Dissertation. Zürich 1984.

140. Kling M, Cvek M, Mejare I. Rate and predictability of pulp revascularization in therapeuticially reimplanted permanent incisors. Endod Dent Traumatol 1986; 2: 83-89.

141. Andreasen JO. Periodontal healing after replantation of traumatically avulsed human teeth. Assessment by mobility testing and radiography. Acta Odont Scand 1975; 33: 325-35.

142. Smelhaus S. Über die Replantation der Milchzähne. Z Stomatol 1925; 23: 52-57.

143. Sakellariou PL. Replantation of infected deciduous teeth: A contribution to the problem of their preservation until normal shedding. Preliminary report. Oral Surg Oral Med Oral Pathol 1963; 16: 645-53.

144. Eisenberg MD. Reimplantation of a deciduous tooth. Oral Surg Oral Med Oral Pathol 1965; 19: 588-90.

145. Crabb JJ, Crabb VP. Reimplantation of a primary central incisor: A case report. Dent Pract 1971; 21: 353-54.

146. Mueller BH, Whitsett BD. Management of an avulsed deciduous incisor. Oral Surg Oral Med Oral Pathol 1978; 46: 442-46.

147. Andreasen JO. Ravn JJ. The effect of traumatic injuries to primary teeth on their permanent successors. II. A clinical and radiographic follow-up study of 213 teeth. Scand J Dent Res 1971; 79: 284-94.

148. Andreasen JO. The effect of pulp extirpation or root canal treatment on periodontal healing after replantation of permanent incisors in monkeys. J Endod 1981; 7: 245-51 and 8: 426-27.

149. Andreasen JO. A time-related study of periodontal healing root resorption activity after replantation of mature permanent incisors in monkeys. Swed Dent J 1980; 4: 101-10.

150. Shulman LB. Allogenic tooth transplantation. J Oral Surg 1972; 30: 395-409.

151. Shulman LB, Gedalia I, Feingold RM. Fluoride concentration in the root surfaces and alveolar bone of fluoride-immersed monkey incisors three weeks after replantation. J Dent Res 1973;52:1314-16.

152. Tronstad L, Andreasen JO, Hasselgren G, Kristerson L, Riis I. pH changes in dental tissues after root canal filling with calcium hydroxide. J Endod 1981; 7: 17-21.

153. Hammarström L, Blomlöf L Feiglin B, Andersson L, Lindskog S. Replantation of teeth and antibiotic treatment. Endod Dent Traumatol 1986; 2: 51-57.

154. Holland R, Nery MJ, de Mello W, de Souza V, Bernabe PFE, Otoboni Filho JA. Root canal treatment with calcium hydroxide. Effect of overfilling and refilling. Oral Surg Oral Med Oral Pathol 1979; 47: 87-92.

155. Jensen L, Andreasen FM, Andreasen JO. Long-term pH changes in the root canal subsequent to placement of calcium hydroxide. 1990; In preparation.

156. Cvek M. Treatment of non-vital permanent incisors with calcium hydroxide. I. Follow-up of periapical repair and apical closure of immature roots. Odont Rev 1972; 23: 27-44.

157. Vernieks AA, Messer LB. Calcium hydroxide induced healing of periapical lesions: a study of 78 non-vital teeth. J Br Endod Soc 1978; 11: 61-69.

158. Öhman A. Healing and sensitivity to pain in young replanted human teeth. An experimental and histological study. Odontol Tidskr 1965; 73: 168-227.

159. Andreasen JO. Effect on extra-alveolar period and storage media upon periodontal and pulpal healing after replantation of mature permanent incisors in monkeys. Int J Oral Surg 1981; 10: 43-53.

160. Andreasen FM, Andreasen JO. Diagnosis of luxation injuries: The importance of standardized clinical, radiographic and photographic techniques in clinical investigations. Endod Dent Traumatol 1985; 1: 160-69.

161. Andreasen FM, Sewerin I, Mandel U, Andreasen JO. Radiographic assessment of simulated root resorption cavities. Endod Dent Traumatol 1986; 2: 21-27.

162. Andersson L, Blomlöf L, Lindskog S, Feiglin B, Hammarström L. Tooth ankylosis. Clinical, radiographic and histological assessments. Int J Oral Surg 1984; 13: 423-31.

163. Andreasen JO. Analysis of pathogenesis and topography of replacement root resorption (ankylosis) after replantation of mature permanent incisors in monkeys. Swed Dent J 1980; 4: 231-40.

164. Frost HM. Tetracycline-based histological analysis of bone remodelling. Calcif Tissue Res 1969; 3: 211-37.

165. Kristerson L, Andreasen JO. The effect of splinting upon periodontal and pulpal healing after autotransplantation of mature and immature permanent incisors in monkeys. Int J Oral Surg 1983; 12: 239-49.

166. Malmgren B, Cvek M, Lundberg M, Frykholm A. Surgical treatment of ankylosed and infrapositioned reimplanted incisors in adolescents. Scand J Dent Res 1984; 92: 391-99.

167. Gibson ACL. Continued root development after traumatic avulsion of partly formed permanent incisor. Br Dent J 1969; 126: 356-57.

168. Lysell G, Lysell L. A unique case of dilaceration. Odontol Rev 1969; 20: 43-46.

169. Ravn JJ. Partiel roddannelse efter eksartikulation af permanent incisiv hos en 7-årig dreng. Tandlægebladet 1970; 74: 906-10.

170. Oliet S. Apexogenesis associated with replantation. Dent Clin North Am 1974; 18: 457-64.

171. Barker BCW, Mayne JR. Some unusual cases of apexification subsequent to trauma. Oral Surg Oral Med Oral Pathol 1975; 39: 144-50.

172. Burley MA, Reece RD. Root formation following traumatic loss of an immature incisor. Br Dent J 1976; 141: 315-16.

173. Hill FJ, Lee KW. Continued development of the dental papilla after removal of premaxillary supernumerary teeth. Br Dent J 1983; 154: 333.

174. Levine BC, Sadowsky D. Management of an avulsed central incisor: an unusual approach. Gen Dent 1982; 30: 62-63.

175. O'Donnel D, Cooke MS, Wei SHY. Esthetic treatment of an avulsed maxillary central incisor: report of a case. J Am Dent Assoc 1989; 119: 629-31.

176. Vijayan L. Avulsed teeth. Sing Dent J 1985; 10: 9-12.

177. Bockisch H. Replantation total luxierter Frontzähne - ein kasuistischer Bereicht. Stomatol DDR 1980; 30: 499- 503.

178. Symons AL. Root resorption: a complication following traumatic avulsion. ASDC J Dent Child 1986; 53: 271-74.

179. Harris WE. Unusual cervical resorption after reinjury. J Am Dent Assoc 1982; 105: 240-42.

180. Johnson R. The treatment of traumatized incisor in the child patient. In: Cohen DW, ed. Continuing dental education. Chicago: Quintessence Publishing Co., Inc. 1980; vol 10.

181. Petrin P. Kriterien des autogenetischen Replantationerfolges nach Luxationstraumen bei Jugendlichen. ZWR 1982; 91: 54-55.

182. Jacobsen I. Clinical problems in the mixed dentition: traumatized teeth - evaluation, treatment and prognosis. Int Dent J 1981; 31: 99-104.

183. Jacobsen I. Long term evaluation, prognosis and subsequent management of traumatic tooth injuries. In: Gutmann JL, Harrison JW, eds. Proceedings of the International Conference on Oral Trauma. Chicago: American Association of Endodontists Endowment & Memorial Foundation, 1986; 129-34.

184. Krenkel C, Grunert I. Replantierte nicht endodontisch behandelte Frontzahne mit offenem Foramen Apicale. Zahnärtzl Prax 1986; 8: 290-98.

185. Andersson L, Bodin I. Avulsed human teeth replanted within 15 minutes - a long-term clinical follow-up study. Endod Dent Traumatol 1990; 6: 37-42.

186. Andersson L, Bodin I, Sörensen S. Progression of root resorption following replantation of human teeth after extended extraoral storage. Endod Dent Traumatol 1989; 5: 38-47.

187. Andreasen JO, Borum M, Jacobsen HL, Andreasen FM. Replantation of 400 traumatically avulsed permanent incisors. I. Diagnosis of healing complications. Endod Dent Traumatol 1991, To be submitted.

188. Andreasen JO, Borum M, Jacobsen HL, Andreasen FM. Replantation of 400 avulsed permanent incisors. II. Factors related to pulp healing. Endod Dent Traumatol 1991, To be submitted.

189. Andreasen JO, Borum M, Andreasen FM. Replantation of 400 avulsed permanent incisors. III. Factors related to root growth after replantation. Endod Dent Traumatol 1991, To be submitted.

190. Andreasen JO, Borum M, Jacobsen HL, Andreasen FM. Replantation of 400 avulsed permanent incisors. IV. Factors related to periodontal ligament healing. Endod Dent Traumatol 1991; To be submitted.

191. Andreasen JO, Borum M, Jacobsen HL, Andreasen FM. Replantation of 400 avulsed permanent incisors. V. Factors related to the progression of root resorption. Endod Dent Traumatol 1991; To be submitted.

192. Gonda F, Nagase M, Chen R-B, Yakata H, Nakajima T. Replantation: An analysis of 29 teeth. Oral Surg Oral Med Oral Pathol; 70: 650-5.

193. Abrams RA. Tooth replantation: 11-year follow-up. Aust Dent J 1987; 32: 417-19.

Chapter 3
Intentional replantation

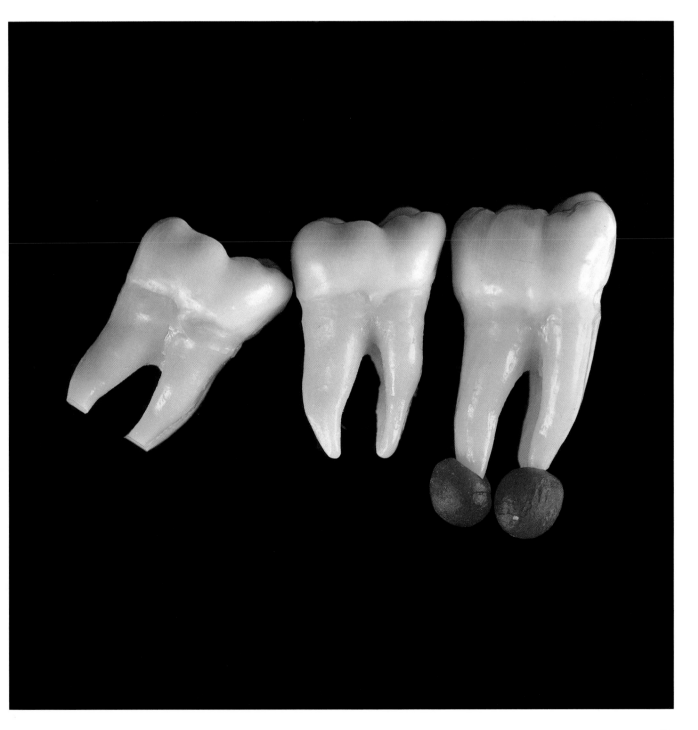

Indications

Extraction and extraoral endodontic therapy followed by replantation has been developed as a supplementary endodontic treatment modality, primarily for molars because of their complicated root canal anatomy (Fig. 3.1). However, before the indication for this procedure is described, it might be useful to consider the general healing results after conventional and surgical endodontic treatment of molars.

Conventional endodontic therapy is usually a successful procedure, with reported success rates for molars ranging from 61% to 93% of the reexamined cases.[1-5] Similarly, surgical endodontic therapy has been found to have a favorable prognosis, with reported healing rates of 71% to 90%.[6-14] However, in both conservative and surgical endodontic procedures, the root filling procedure is often compromised because of the complicated anatomy of the molar root canals.[15-17] Furthermore, problems in obtaining surgical access to the apices due to associated structures such as the maxillary sinus or the mandibular canal, or the density of bone covering the root, could contraindicate surgical intervention.[18] In these cases, extraction and extraoral root filling under direct visual inspection (i.e., intentional replantation) can be the treatment of choice, as demonstrated by several case reports[14-59,85,86] and clinical studies.[60-69]

Although this procedure can ease endodontic treatment considerably, the technique is also accompanied by the risk of root resorption, which is rarely encountered after either conservative or surgical endodontics.[44,62,70] This risk is most likely due to the combined effect of the extraction trauma to the root surface and faulty root canal obturation, which can result in the presence of infected pulpal remnants in the root canal.[71]

Intentional replantation of primary molars in order to avoid problems of space loss has also been reported.[72-74] However, a follow-up study of 94 intentionally replanted primary molars revealed that only 53 of those teeth were in place 1 year after treatment. Moreover, most of the remaining teeth showed radiographic signs of ankylosis[75]. Based on these findings and the unknown risk of damaging the permanent successor due to either the extraction or the replantation procedure, it does not seem justified at present to use this method in the primary dentition.

Finally, it should be mentioned that intentional replantation of roots with subsequent mucosal coverage has been advocated in order to maintain the alveolar process in denture cases.[76-79,87] However, the long-term effect of root preservation appears to be questionable, as atrophy of the alveolar ridge is apparently not prevented.[80]

0 days   9 years   11 years

Fig. 3.1. Healing after intentional replantation of a first mandibular molar. From Emmertsen & Andreasen, 1966.[62]

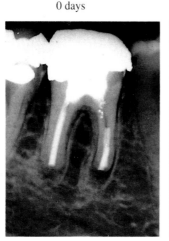 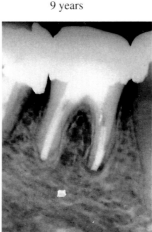 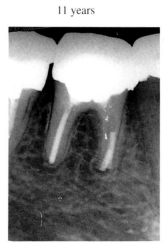

Treatment planning

Regarding intentional replantation as a treatment alternative to either surgical or conservative endodontics, it must be remembered that the primary treatment of choice should always be conservative endodontics. If this treatment procedure fails and it is not possible or desirable to progress with a surgical endodontic procedure, intentional replantation could be considered as a final resort. Before this procedure is carried out, however, it is necessary to determine whether the tooth can be extracted atraumatically and whether a sufficient root filling can be made to ensure that the entire root canal, or at least the majority of the canal, is obturated. Only if both of these requirements can be met should intentional replantation be decided upon.

Prior to extraction, an adequate radiographic survey, including the marginal and periapical periodontium, should be made in order to determine whether the tooth can be extracted without risk of fracture of the crown and/or root. This normally implies that intentional replantation is not indicated in teeth with divergent roots and where the strength of the crown or root has been markedly compromised due to caries, extensive crown restorations, or posts placed in the root canals. If intentional replantation, is decided upon, it is advisable to fill the root canals optimally using a coronal approach prior to the surgical procedure. This will improve the quality of the final root filling.

Surgical procedure

The clinical procedure is shown in Fig. 3.2. Preparation of the canals should aim at reaching the cervical region or at least the level of the previously attempted root filling. Thereafter, a retrograde gutta-percha root filling is made. If the gutta-percha root filling does not completely obliterate the prepared apical foramen, a cavity is prepared apically and heat-adapted gutta-percha cemented with a fortified zinc oxide-eugenol sealer (e.g. IRM) is used as a retrograde filling. The depth of the cavity should be at least 3 mm in order to minimize the chance of leakage.[81] The canal walls should diverge apically in order to allow trial and heat adaptation of the gutta-percha point prior to cementation with a zink oxide-eugenol based sealer. During the entire endodontic procedure the root surface should be kept moist with saline.

The tooth is then replanted in the socket; no efforts should be made to remove the coagulum prior to replantation. If the roots are divergent, it is sometimes necessary to perform a minor oblique resection of the mesial or distal aspect of the root complex in order to facilitate replantation with a minimum of trauma. Splinting is normally not indicated if there is adequate bony support around the tooth. However, occlusion should be relieved by slight grinding of the antagonist.

Postoperative follow-up

This follows the guidelines for replanted avulsed teeth with the exception that pulp healing can be disregarded (see Appendix 1, p. 289). The tooth is usually firm in its socket after 2-3 weeks and gingival healing established.

Fig. 3.2. Intentional replantation of a second mandibular molar

After administration of penicillin given 1 hour prior to surgery and a local anesthesia the marginal gingiva is incised with a scalpel or a gingivectomy knife. The tooth is then extracted with gentle luxating movements. Immediately after extraction, the socket should be covered with a gauze sponge in order to prevent saliva from contaminating the blood clot.

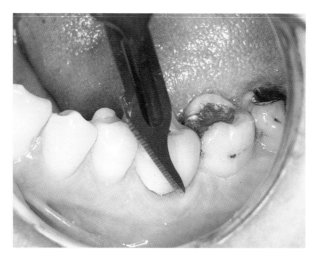 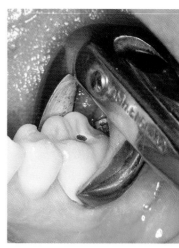

Apicoectomy

While out of its socket, the tooth is held by the crown with forceps and the periodontal ligament left untouched. If the apex is obliterated or curved, it is resected with a diamond or fissure bur under a copious flow of saline.

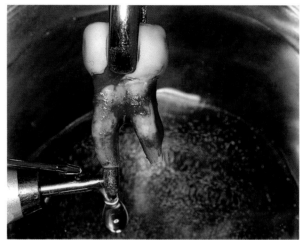 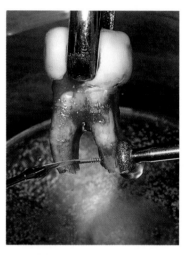

Preparation of the root canals

The root canals are enlarged with reamers and files. The preparation of the canals should aim at reaching the cervical region or at least the level of the previously attempted root filling. Thereafter, gutta-percha points are fitted into the root canal and cemented with a root canal sealer. Because of the oval cross-section of the apical portion of most root canals, a lateral condensation technique should be used.

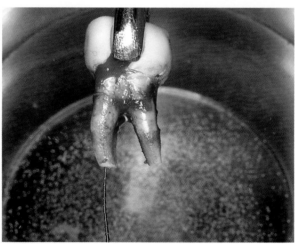 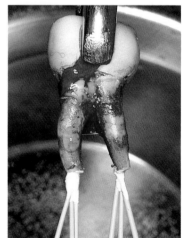

Removing surplus root filling material

Excess root filling material is removed with a scalpel. In the case of a divergent root, it is necessary to perform a minor oblique resection of the mesial or distal aspect of the root complex in order to facilitate replantation. The tooth is then replanted in its socket. Splinting is normally not indicated if there is adequate bony support around the tooth. However, occlusion should be relieved by slight grinding of the antagonist.

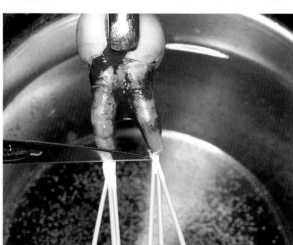 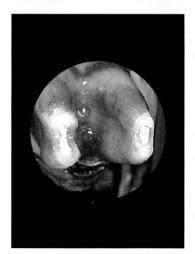

Prognosis

Only a few studies have been published where there is adequate documentation for postoperative healing.[60-63,68,70] In this context, it must be considered that the healing criteria should include both the periodontal healing with respect to periapical inflammation (Figs. 3.3 and 3.4) and progressive inflammatory and replacement resorption (Figs. 3.5 and 3.6). Only if the replanted tooth shows no sign of these complications can treatment be considered successful (Figs. 3.3 and 3.4).[62]

Fig. 3.3. Periapical healing and no root resorption after intentional replantation of a second mandibular molar. An extra oral retrograde root filling was made with gutta-percha. From Emmertsen & Andreasen, 1966.[62]

0 days	0 days	4 years

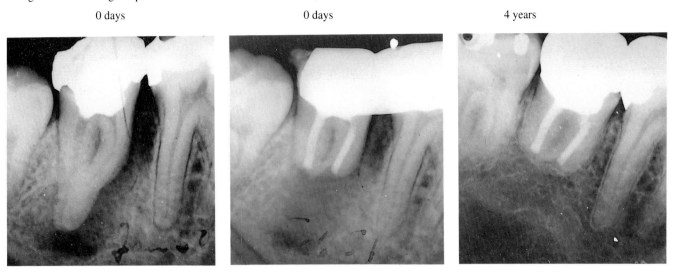

Fig. 3.4. Periapical healing and no root resorption after intentional replantation of a mandibular first molar. The tooth was root filled retrograde with both gutta-percha and amalgam. From Emmertsen & Andreasen, 1966.[62]

0 days	2 years	10 years

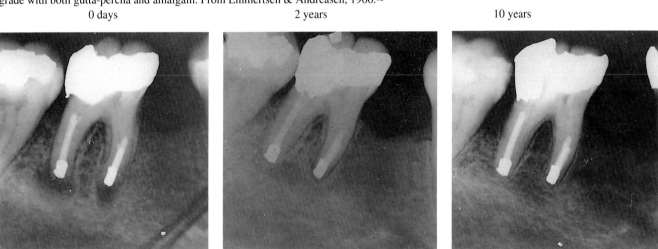

Fig. 3.5. Marked inflammatory resorption after intentional replantation of mandibular first molar. From Emmertsen & Andreasen, 1966.[62]

0 days	6 months	1.5 years

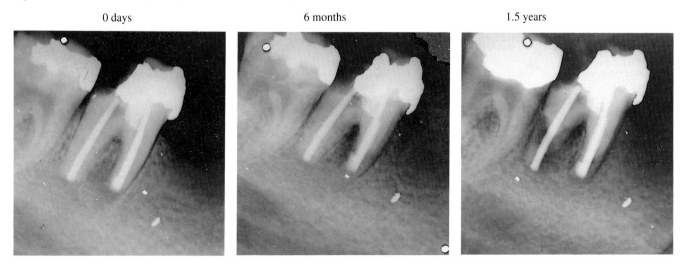

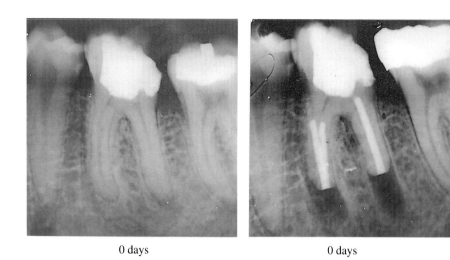
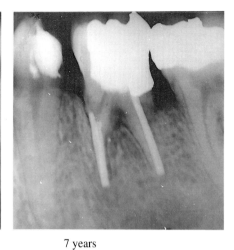

| 0 days | 0 days | 7 years |

Fig. 3.6. Replacement resorption after intentional replantation of a mandibular first molar. From Emmertsen & Andreasen, 1966.[62]

In Table 3.1, the results of four studies are listed, where healing of both periapical inflammation and progressive root resorption is documented. It appears that successful healing was found in 39% to 62% of the intentionally replanted teeth. In these studies long-term success covering observation periods of up to 10-20 years could be documented[62,68] (Figs. 3.3 and 3.4). When a time relationship between surgery and failure is analyzed, it is possible to estimate "survival" curves for intentional replantations based on one large study (Fig. 3.7). It appears from this study that a 5-year tooth survival rate of 85% can be expected after intentional replantation.[68] In one large clinical study of 1692 intentionally replanted teeth a median "survival" time was 10 years.[89]

So far, only a few factors have been found to influence periodontal healing. These are: choice of root filling, age of the patient, and presence of a preoperative radiolucency.

Choice of root filling

In two clinical studies, it was found that a retrograde amalgam filling resulted in more root resorption than a retrograde gutta-percha filling.[61,62] A possible explanation could be that when a retrograde amalgam technique was used, the infected necrotic pulp remnants remaining in the root canal caused periapical inflammation due to leakage around the root filling and possibly by lateral root resorption initiated by the extraction trauma. Trauma from extraction exposes dentinal tubules which are in contact with the infected root canal and initiates the resorption process (Fig. 3.8).[61,62] In one clinical study no difference in healing was found between gutta-percha or cones of aluminium oxide, titanium or hydroxylapatite.[88]

Fig. 3.7. Prognosis of successful healing of intentionally replanted permanent premolars and molars. From Grossmann,1980.[68]

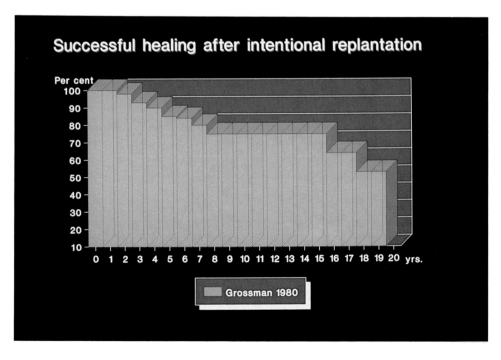

Fig. 3.8. Normal periodontal ligament healing after intentional replantation of a mandibular molar
There is periapical healing and no progressive root resorption. The tooth was removed 10 years after replantation because of extensive caries. Periodondal ligament healing has taken place in a few areas with initial surface resorption (arrow). In most places, however, there is a normally structured periodontal ligament without any sign of root resorption. From Emmertsen & Andreasen, 1966.[62]

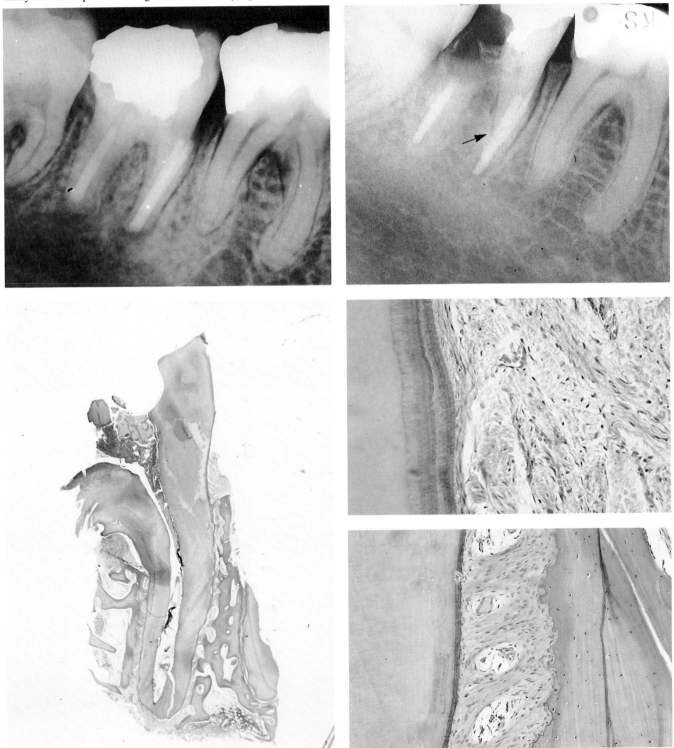

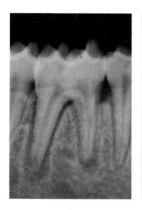 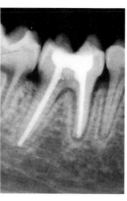 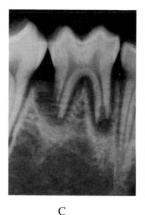 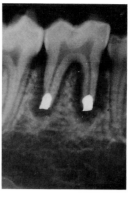 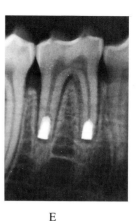

A	B	C	D	E

Fig. 3.9. Experimental intentional replantation of permanent molars in monkeys. Observation period 8 weeks. A. Replantation without endodontic treatment. A periapical radiolucency has developed. B. Periapical healing has occurred when the entire root canal is filled with gutta-percha and Kerr sealer using an extraoral coronal approach. C. Replantation after apicoectomy and preparation of a retrograde cavity. D. Same procedure but supplemented with a retrograde amalgam. E. Same procedure supplemented with a retrograde gutta-percha root filling and Kerr sealer. From Andreasen, 1990[82].

If a bacteria-tight root filling is made, periapical healing can take place, including repair of the previous trauma-induced resorption cavities (Fig. 3.8). This explanation is supported by recent experiments in monkeys where various endodontic procedures were carried out in intentionally replanted molars. It was shown that a retrograde amalgam restoration alone was not able to prevent periapical inflammation and inflammatory root resorption, whereas a root filling of the entire canal or a partial root filling with gutta-percha and a sealer was able to control both complications (Fig. 3.9).[82,83] In vitro experiments have further shown that retrograde amalgam as the only filling material was not able to prevent bacteria placed in the root canal from reaching the root surface.[83,84]

Age

In one clinical study, it was found that in the age group 10-30 years, inflammatory root resorption and periapical inflammation were significantly more frequent than in older age groups, a finding possibly related to the wider root canals and/or dentinal tubules in younger individuals which allow passage of bacterial toxins to the periodontium (see Chapter 1, p. 28).[62, 82]

Preoperative radiolucency

Preoperative radiolucency has been found to be related to healing without root resorption (Fig. 3.3).[62] This finding could be related to the fact that the extraction procedure in teeth with apical radiolucencies is considerably easier and results in less damage to the root surface (see Chapter 1, p. 30).

In conclusion, intentional replantation has a limited application in modern endodontics. Due to the risk of progressive root resorption, this procedure should only be considered in those cases where neither conservative nor surgical endodontics is feasible. Teeth where the extraction trauma can be kept to a minimum due to periapical inflammation are especially good candidates for this procedure. In those selected cases in which intentional replantation is attempted, pre- and peroperative endodontics should aim at obturating the entire root canal system as completely as possible.

Table 3.1. Long -term results of intentional replantation of teeth

	Observation period, years (mean)	Age of patients, years (mean)	Number of teeth	Tooth survival %	PDL healing %	Periapical healing %	Succesful healing %
Bielas & al., 1959[60]	1-6 (3.3)		610				59
Deeb & al., 1965[61] *	5		55		44		
**	5		165		74		
Emmertsen & Andreasen, 1966[62]	1-13 (4.3)	14-58 (30.1)	100	80	69	50	39
Grossman, 1966[63]	2-11 (5.6)	10-50 (27.5)	45	80			62
Grossman, 1980[68]	2-19 (6.5)				77		
Raasch, 1984[69]	0.7 (0.7)	11-53 (27.0)	18	83	83	78	56

* Retrograde root filling with amalgam
** Ortograde root filling

Essentials

Indication
Where conservative or surgical endodontics cannot be performed.

Treatment planning
Preoperative radiographs to evaluate the possibility of atraumatic extraction without crown and/or root fracture and the possibility of effective obturation through a combined orthograde and retrograde procedure.

Preoperative endodontic procedures
An attempt is made via a coronal approach to fill the root as far as possible in the apical direction.

Surgical endodontic procedure (Fig. 3.2).
1. Administer a local anesthetic.
2. Incise the marginal gingiva with a scalpel as far apically as possible in the periodontal ligament space.
3. The tooth is extracted.
4. The socket is covered with a gauze sponge in order to prevent salivary contamination of the blood clot.
5. The apex is resected with a diamond or fissure bur while the root surface is kept moist with saline.
6. The root canal is cleansed and enlarged from the apical end to the level of the coronally placed root filling.
7. The root canal is filled with gutta-percha and a sealer using lateral condensation.
8. The tooth is then replanted. If there is resistance to replantation, it may be necessary to grind the proximal aspects of the roots in order to ensure atraumatic replantation.
9. The occlusion is relieved by grinding the antagonist.
10. A postoperative radiograph is taken.

Follow-up
See Appendix 1, p. 289

Prognosis
Periapical healing without progressive root resorption (10 years): 75%

Risk factors
Younger individuals (younger than 30 years)
Teeth without periapical inflammation
Teeth where the entire root canal system cannot be filled using a combined orthograde-retrograde technique

References

1. Selden HS. Pulpoperiapical disease: Diagnosis and healing. Oral Surg Oral Med Oral Pathol 1974; 37: 271-83.

2. Ingle JI, Beveridge EE. Endodontics. 2nd ed. Philadelphia : Lea & Febiger,1976: 34-57.

3. Jokinen MA, Kotilainen R, Poikkeus P, Poikkeus R, Sarkki L. Clinical and radiographic study of pulpectomy and root canal therapy. Scand J Dent Res 1978; 86: 366-73.

4. Kerekes K, Tronstad L. Long-term results of endodontic treatment performed with a standardized technique. J Endod 1979; 5: 83-90.

5. Nelson IA. Endodontics in general practice - a retrospective survey. Int Endod J 1982; 15: 168-72.

6. Peter K. Die Wurzelspitzenresektion der Molaren. Leipzig: Hermann Meusser; 1936.

7. Kristen K. Ergebnisse der apikalen Radikaloperation im Seitenzahnbereich. Dtsch Zahn Mund Kieferheilk 1963; 39: 1-07.

8. Tolmeijer JA. Apicoectomy on molars. Ned Tijdschr Tandheelkd 1972; 79: 137-42.

9. Altonen M, Mattila K. Follow-up study of apicoectomized molars. Int J Oral Surg 1976; 5: 33-40.

l0. Wörle M, Wirsching R. Die Wurzelspitzenresektion im Seitenzahnbereich als Alternative zum Implantat. Dtsch Zahnärztl Z 1977; 32: 340-42.

11. Bull HG, Neugebauer W. Die Wurzelspitzenresektion an Molaren des Ober- und Unterkiefers. Indikation, Technik und Fehlerquellen sowie Langzeitergebnisse. Dtsch Zahn-Mund-Kiefer Gesichtschir 1979; 3: 229-32.

12. Harris MH. Apicoectomy and retrograde amalgam in mandibular molar teeth. Oral Surg Oral Med Oral Pathol 1979; 48: 405-07.

13. Persson G. Periapical surgery of molars. Int J Oral Surg 1982; 11: 96-100.

14. Ioannides C, Borstlap WA. Apicoectomy on molars: a clinical and radiographical study. Int J Oral Surg 1983; 12: 73-79.

15. Pomeranz HH, Eidelman DL, Goldberg MG. Treatment considerations of the middle mesial canal of mandibular first and second molar. J Endod 1981; 7: 565-68.

16. Block RM, Bushell A. Retrograde amalgam procedures for mandibular posterior teeth. J Endod 1982; 8: 107-12.

17. Hartwell G, Bellizzi R. Clinical investigation of in vivo endodontically treated mandibular and maxillary molars. J Endod 1982; 8: 555-57.

18. Lin L, Skribner J, Shovlin F, Langeland K. Periapical surgery of mandibular posterior teeth: Anatomical and surgical considerations. J Endod 1983; 9: 496-501.

19. Ilg VK. Die Zahnreplantation und ihre besondere Bedeutung für den "Kriegs-Zahnärzt". Zahnarzt Rundsch 1940; 48: 588-89.

20. Ilg VK. Ein Beitrag zur Replantation. Zahnärztl Welt 1949; 4: 605.

21. Ilg VK. Zur Theorie und Praxis der Replantation I. Dtsch Zahnärztl Z 1951; 6: 585-94.

22. Ilg VK. Zur Theorie und Praxis der Replantation. II. Dtsch Zahnärztl Z 1951; 6: 653-63.

23. Perint EJ. Results of reimplantation of posterior teeth after root filling. Oral Surg Oral Med Oral Path 1951; 4: 573-77.

24. Keresztesi K. Die Reimplantation von Zähnen in der modernen Zahnheilkunde. Öster Z Stomatol 1955; 52: 16-22.

25. Tracksdorf H. Erfolge bei Replantationen. ZWR 1957; 58: 153-54.

26. Kadankov D. Implantation, Transplantation oder Replantation Dtsch Stomatol 1960; 10: 699-702.

27. Nosonowitz DM. Planned replantation of permanent molars to correct endodontic failure. Preliminary report of four cases. Oral Surg Oral Med Oral Pathol 1962; 15: 1131-35.

28. Jachno R. Present state of immediate replantation of teeth. Cesk Stomatol 1962; 62: 203-08.

29. Bataille R. Reimplantation - Transplantation - Implantation. Acta Stomatol Belg 1963; 60: 455-64.

30. Counsell LA. Intentional reimplantation of teeth. Report of two cases. Oral Surg Oral Med Oral Pathol 1964; 18: 681-85.

31. Bhat KS. Intentional replantation. (A report of two cases). J Indian Dent Assoc 1965; 37: 291-92.

32. Friez P, Laroche J-F, Lesage C-L. Les implants naturels et leurs resultats. Leur utilisation possible comme pilier de bridge. Revue de Stomatologie 1967; 5: 406-19.

33. Lautenbach E. Die Zahnplantationen - Methodik und Wertung. Dtsch Stomatol 1967; 17: 526-34.

34. Guasta G. Studio clinico sul "reimpianto dentario". Minerva Stomatol 1968; 17: 765-73.

35. Mitsis F. Reimplantation de dents extraites a dessein. Rev Fr Odontostomatol 1969; 16: 1377-82.

36. Messing JJ. Planned re-implantation. J Br Endod Soc 1970; 4: 02-05.

37. Cagidiaco M. Nota pratica sul reimpianto dentario. Mondo Odontostomatol 1971; 13: 221-38.

38. Bucci E. Contributo clinico e particolari di tecnica per la realizzazione di reimpianti e trapianti dentari. Arch Stomatol (Napoli) 1978; 19: 137-51.

39. Götsch F. Der interessante Fall - Ergebnis einer Replantation. Stomatol DDR 1978; 28: 678-79.

40. di Lauro F. Le indicazioni cliniche ai reimpianti e trapianti dentari. Arch Stomatol (Napoli) 1978; 19: 121-36.

41. Donnelly JC. Intentional replantation case update. J Endod 1982; 8: 471.

42. Donnelly JC. Intentional replantation: A case report of a mandibular first molar with a three-year follow-up. J Endod 1980; 6: 886-87.

43. Rosenberg ES, Rossman LE, Sandler AB. Intentional replantation: a case report. J Endod 1980; 6: 610-13

44. Weine FS. The case against intentional replantation. J Am Dent Assoc 1980; 100: 664-68.

45. Solomon CS. Intentional replantation: Report of case. J Endod 1981; 5: 317-20.

46. Stroner WF, Laskin DM. Replantation of a mandibular molar: Report of case. J Am Dent Assoc 1981; 103: 730-31.

47. Grossman LI. Intentional replantation of teeth: A clinical evaluation. J Am Dent Assoc 1982; 104: 633-39.

48. Kaufman AY. Intentional replantation of a maxillary molar. Oral Surg Oral Med Oral Pathol 1982; 54: 686-88.

49. di Lauro F, Bucci E, Matarasso S. Personal experience of dentai reimplantation. Clinical evaluations after 8 years. Minerva Stomatol 1982; 31: 569-75.

50. Lubin H. Intentional reimplantation: Report of case. J Am Dent Assoc 1982; 104: 858-59.

51. Goel BR, Satish C, Suresh C, Goel S. Clinical evaluation of gold foil as an apical sealing material for replantation. Oral Surg 1983; 55: 514-18.

52. Gray PP. Case report. Intentional replantation. Bull Aust Soc Endodontol 1983; 9: 18-19.

53. Manhart MJ. Reimplantation: The calcium hydroxide method. Gen Dent 1983; 3: 46-47.

54. Czonstkowsky M, Wallace JA. Replantation. Oral Surg Oral Med Oral Pathol 1984; 57: 558-59.

55. Nosonowitz DM, Stanley HR. Intentional replantation to prevent predictable endodontic failures. Oral Surg Oral Med Oral Pathol 1984; 57: 423-32.

56. Pouzanov VI, Shawa AM. The postponementary replantation of teeth. Odontostomatol Trop 1984; 7: 45-48.

57. Heiss J. Klinische und histologische Untersuchungen am replantierten Zahn. Z Stomatol 1944; 42: 73-91, 97-113.

58. Perint J. Tapasztalataim a replantatios müteték eredmenyeriol. Fogovosi Szemle 1948; 41: 135-44.

59. Schmidt H. Zum Thema Reimplantation. Dtsch Stomatol 1952; 2: 361-66.

60. Bielas I, Fuchs M, Horbal B, Pankiewictz Z. Die Bewertung der Replantation der Zähne auf Grund von 1030 experimentellen Versuchseingriffen. Schweiz Monatsschr Zahnheilk 1959; 69: 497-510.

61. Deeb E, Prietto DP, McKenna RC. Reimplantation of luxated teeth in humans. J S Calif Dent Assoc 1965; 28: 194-206.

62. Emmertsen E, Andreasen JO. Replantation of extracted molars. A radiographic and histological study. Acta Odontol Scand 1966; 24: 327-46.

63. Grossman LI. Intentional replantation of teeth. J Am Dent Assoc 1966; 72: 1111-18.

64. Kingsbury BC, Wiesenbaugh JM. Intentional replantation of mandibular premolars and molars. J Am Dent Assoc 1971; 83: 1053-57.

65. Gutner YI, Kushnir II Margulis RY. The remote results of replantation of teeth. Stomatologiia (Mosk) 1972; 51: 27-29.

66. Kumanov S. Causes for resorptive processes in reimplanted teeth in periodontitis. Stomalogia (Sofia) 1976; 59: 43-47.

67. Kumanov S. Possibilities for postponed teeth replantation in acute and exacerbated chronic periodontitis. Stomatologiia (Sofia) 1977; 59: 165-68.

68. Grossman LI. Intentional replantation of teeth. In: Robinson PJ, Guernsey LH, eds. Clinical tranplantation in dental specialities. St Louis, Mosby, 1980: 65-76.

69. Raasch HG. Die Replantation von Prämolaren und Molaren. Eine klinische und röntgenologische Studie (Thesis). University of München 1984.

70. Andreasen JO. Rud J. Modes of healing histologically after endodontic surgery in 70 cases. Int J Oral Surg 1972; 1: 148-60.

71. Andreasen JO. Treatment of fractured and avulsed teeth. J Dent Child 1971; 38: 29-48.

72. Stein G. Replantation of deciduous teeth. J Dent Res 1937; 16: 340-41.

73. Sakellariou PL. Replantation of infected deciduous teeth: A contribution to the problem of their preservation until normal shedding. Oral Surg Oral Med Oral Pathol 1963; 16: 645-53.

74. Sakellariou PL. Replantation of infected deciduous teeth: A contribution to the problem of their preservation until normal shedding. Preliminary report. Oral Surg Oral Med Oral Pathol 1963; 16: 645-53.

75. Rönning O, Koskinen L, Isotupa K. Replantation of non-vital deciduous molars. Proc Finn Dent Soc 1976; 72: 48-52.

76. Lam RV. Effect of root implants on resorption of residual ridges. J Prosthet Dent 1972; 27: 311-23.

77. Simon JHS, Kimura JT. Maintenance of alveolar bone by the intentional replantation of roots. A pilot study. Oral Surg Oral Med Oral Pathol 1974; 37: 936-45.

78. Simon JHS, Jensen JL, Kimura JT. Histologic observations of endodontically treated replanted roots. J Endod 1975; 1: 178-80.

79. Gound T, O'Neal RB, del Rio CF, Levin MP. Submergence of roots for alveolar bone preservation. II. Reimplanted endodontically treated roots. Oral Surg Oral Med Oral Pathol 1978; 46: 114-22.

80. Von Wowern N, Winther S. Submergence of roots for alveolar ridge preservation. A failure (4-year follow-up study). Int J Oral Surg 1981; 10: 247-50.

81. Mattison GD, von Fraunhofer JA, Delivanis PD, Anderson AN. Microleakage of retrograde amalgams. J Endod 1985; 11: 340-45.

82. Andreasen JO. Effect of various retrograde root filling techniques upon periapical healing. An experimental study in monkeys. 1990: In preparation.

83. Kos WL, Aulozzi DP, Gerstein H. A comparative bacterial micro leakage study of retrofilling materials. J Endod 1982; 8: 355-58.

84. Luomanen M, Tuompo H. Study of titanium screws as retrograde fillings, using bacteria and dye. Scand J Dent Res 1985; 93: 555-59.

85. Dryden JA. Ten-year follow-up of intentionally replanted mandibular second molar. J Endod 1986; 12: 265-67

86. Lu DP. Intentional replantation of periodontally involved and endodontically mistreated tooth. Oral Surg Oral Med Oral Pathol 1986; 61: 508-13.

87. Dehis M, Sabry M, Badawy MS. Implantation of autogenous roots for preservation of healed residual alveolar bone. Egypt Dent J 1985; 31: 235-45.

88. Loeck M, Becke J, Reichart P. Zur Problematik des apicalen Verschlusses bei therapeutischen Replantationen. Dtsch Zahnärztl Z 1987, 42:208-210.

89. Will R. Replantation. Das Wiedereinsetzen von Zähnen. Quintessenz Verlags-GmbH. Berlin, 1983.

Chapter 4
Autotransplantation of molars

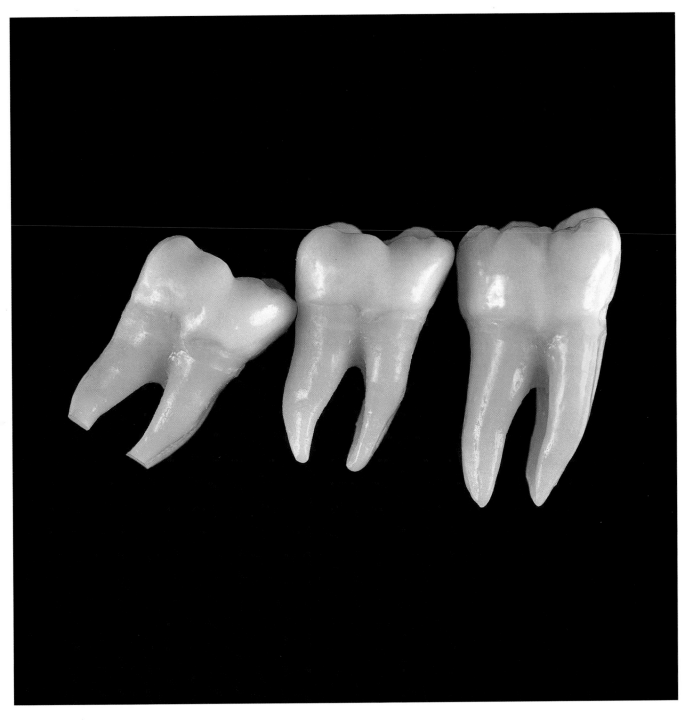

Indications

Third molar transplantations were pioneered in the USA in the beginning of the 1950s by Apfel[36] (1950) and Miller[31] (1951). Larger series of molar transplants were subsequently reported by Nordenram[11] (1963) and Walker & Shaeffer[74] (1964). All permanent molars can be transplanted, at least at certain stages of root development. But for obvious reasons it is the third molar which is normally used as a graft. The most common reason for third molar transplantation is the replacement of first molars where gross caries, marginal or periapical complications, or fractures have made conventional treatment impossible (Figs. 4.1 and 4.2).[1-3] A less frequent reason for transplantation is the replacement of impacted first or second molars.

Fig. 4.1. Various indications for third molar transplantation
A. Gross dental caries. B and C. External root resorption or periapical inflammation. D. Aplasia of premolars. E. Crown-root fracture. F. Non-eruption of first or second molars.

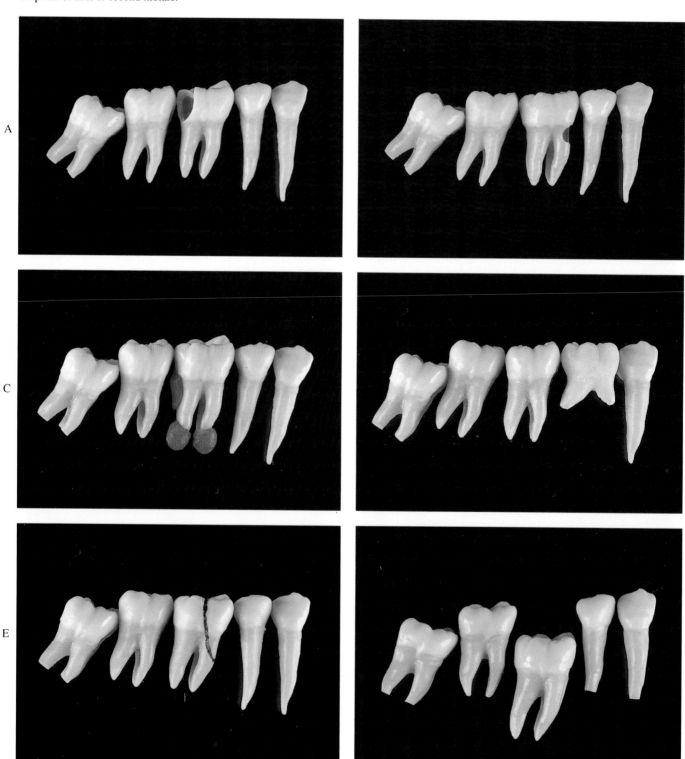

A

C

E

F

112

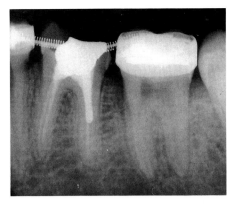 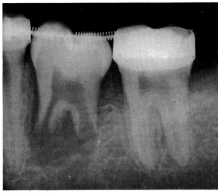 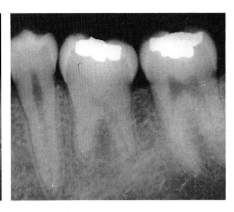

| 0 days | 0 days | 2 years |

Fig. 4.2. Mandibular third molar transplant used to treat a nonrestorable first molar (lingual crown-root fracture).

Finally, in some cases transplantation of third molars can also be indicated in the treatment of premolar aplasia, especially in the second premolar region (Fig. 4.3).

In some cases transplantation of third molars with small root dimensions can be used in the treatment of accidental loss of maxillary incisors.[4-7, 98]

Treatment planning

A radiographic and clinical examination should reveal the dimensions of the transplant and the space available in the recipient region.

Fig. 4.3. Premolar replacement (0 days)
Maxillary third molar transplants used in the treatment of mandibular premolar aplasia.

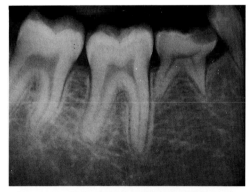 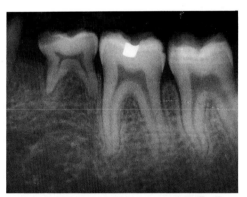

Postoperative condition (0 days)
The grafts have been rotated 90⁰.

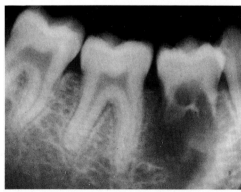 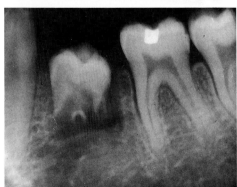

Condition after 1 year
Root formation completed.

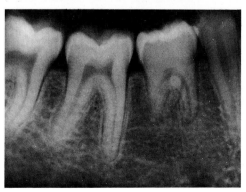 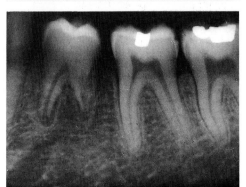

Recipient site analysis

With a sliding caliper the mesiodistal dimension at crown level can be determined directly in the mouth. The cervical buccolingual dimension of the alveolar process can also be calculated. The available socket dimension is calculated by subtracting the thickness of the mucosa, which normally amounts to 2 mm. For example a 14 mm alveolar ridge leaves a 12 mm width of alveolar bone. Surgical preparation should preferably leave the outer cortical bone plates intact and not thinner than 0.5 mm. The potential width of the socket can therefore be estimated to be 11 mm. In this regard it should be remembered that there should be some room around the transplant in order to prevent ankylosis. The potential graft should therefore have root dimensions slightly less than the maximal socket size.

The available apicocoronal dimension is evaluated from an intraoral orthoradial radiograph. In the evaluation of the available space for the socket, the position of critical structures such as the mandibular canal, the mental foramen, and the maxillary sinus should be considered.

Donor tooth analysis

Donor tooth analysis relies almost entirely upon radiographs, as the third molars are usually in a stage of semi- or noneruption. The panoramic radiographic technique, which is commonly used in third molar diagnosis, magnifies vertical dimensions from 9% to 23 %, and horizontal dimensions from 52% to 64 %.[8] This degree of distortion makes the panoramic radiographic technique unreliable for dimensional analysis.[8] A reliable radiographic evaluation is, therefore, dependent upon intraoral orthoradial and/or axial exposures. In the mandible, it is usually possible to obtain reliable orthoradial and axial exposures, whereas these projections are more difficult to achieve in the maxilla. In the analysis of intraoral radiographs, two factors should be considered: First, whether the exposure is actually orthoradial. If this is not the case the mesiodistal dimensions will be inflated. Secondly, the effect exposure geometry has on the enlargement factor. In this regard the film-tooth-focus distance determines the degree of magnification. The film-tooth distance is usually identical during these procedures; it is normally the tooth-focus distance which varies. If this distance is known, the exact magnification can be determined (see Appendices 5 and 6, p. 294 and 295).

The mesiodistal and apicocoronal dimensions of the graft are both determined from orthoradial exposures, whereas the buccolingual dimension is determined from axial exposures. The exposure technique for axial radiographs is illustrated in Fig 4.5 Apart from the above-mentioned tooth dimensions, root anatomy and graft position should also be evaluated, as these factors generally determine the extent of trauma caused by graft removal.

Donor tooth selection

When dimensions of the graft and the recipient site have been found to match, either by placing the potential graft in a normal or 90° rotated position (which is usually necessary for maxillary third molars because of their frequently large buccolingual dimension) the stage of root development has to be evaluated. In general, 2/3 to 3/4 root length is to be preferred. Furthermore, in the case of maxillary third molars the occlusal surface of the crown should lie at the level of the neck of the second molar in order to ensure an uncomplicated and therefore atraumatic graft removal. If the third molar is impacted with completed root formation, it is not a candidate for transplantation because of the high risk of ankylosis (see p.130).

Usually several third molars are available as potential donor teeth. Apart from the stage of root development the decisive factor in graft selection is the adaptation of crown and root anatomy to the existing conditions at the recipient site. To evaluate this the following guidelines are suggested. If a mandibular molar is to be replaced, the usual third molar graft preference is: an ipsilateral mandibular third molar, a contralateral mandibular third molar rotated 180°, a contralateral maxillary third molar in anatomic position, or an ipsilateral maxillary third molar rotated 180°.

If a maxillary molar is to be replaced, the preferred third molar replacements are: an ipsilateral maxillary third molar (Fig 4.4) or a contralateral maxillary third molar rotated 180° (Fig 4.6).

Fig. 4.4. Transplantation of a third molar from the same quadrant as replacement for a first maxillary molar.

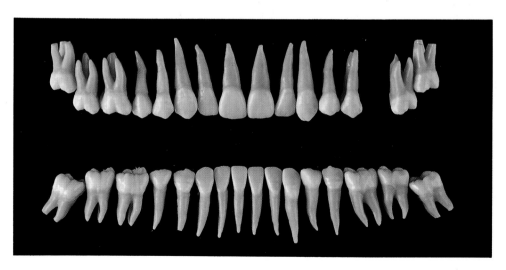

Surgical procedure

The recipient area is first prepared for the potential transplant. If a tooth is present it is extracted. In this context, it is important to split divergent roots and remove them individually in order not to injure the bone septa separating adjacent teeth.

The application of elevators should be restricted to the interradicular area in order not to traumatize the periphery of the socket. Apical granulation tissue, if present, is removed with a curette.

Fig. 4.5. **Axial exposure of the maxillary third molar.** An occlusal film is placed as far distally as possible. The central beam is directed from the midpoint at the base of the nose to the opposite maxillary third molar region (arrows).

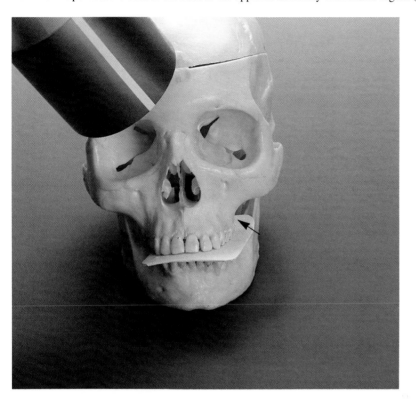

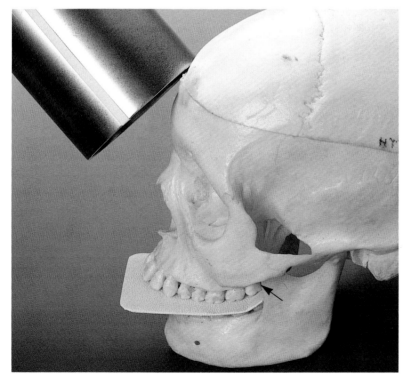

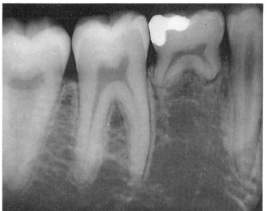

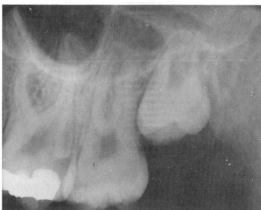

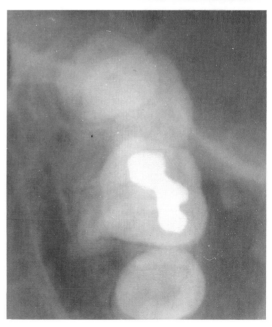

The septum in the socket is removed with a surgical bur down to the base of the socket. If necessary, the periphery of the socket is expanded. During this procedure it is important not to penetrate the septum separating adjacent teeth or the buccal or lingual cortical bone plates. Finally, the socket area is rinsed with a copious flow of saline in order to remove all debris, whereafter the socket is immediately covered with a gauze sponge to prevent saliva contamination while the coagulum is formed.

The next phase is the removal of the third molar. The goal here is to remove the graft atraumatically with an intact follicle or periodontal ligament (PDL). This requires specific techniques for the mandible and the maxilla (Figs. 4.7 and 4.8).

Fig. 4.6. A maxillary third molar transplanted to the opposite first molar site has been rotated 180⁰ in order to improve occlusal and proximal contacts.

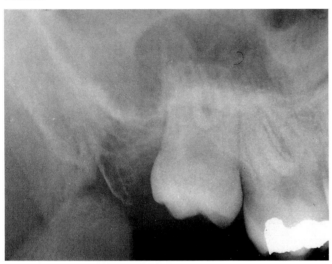

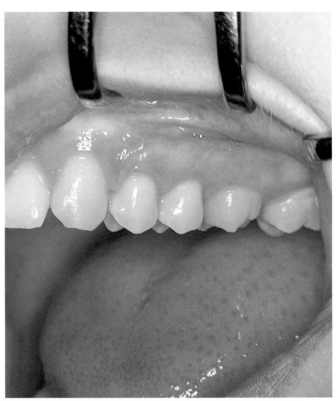

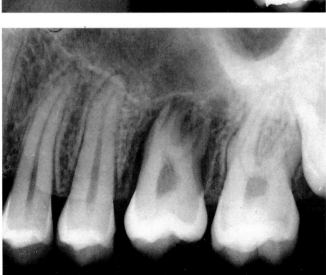

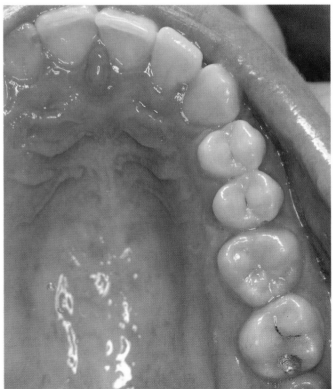

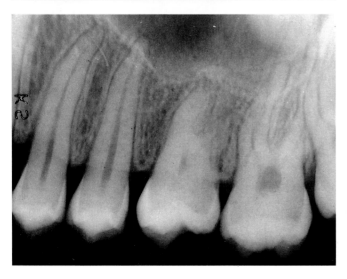

Fig. 4.7. Mandibular third molar transplantation

The indication for transplantation in this case was a complicated lingual crown-root fracture and periapical inflammation.

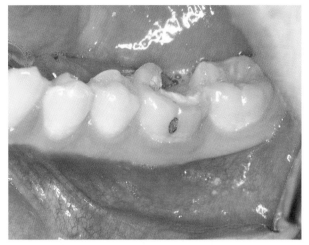
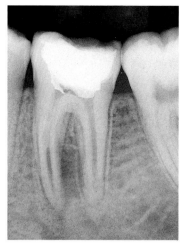

Extraction and preparation of the socket

The interradicular septum is removed and the socket enlarged using a contra-angle piece and a bur with internal cooling (see Appendix 7, p. 296). Thereafter the socket is rinsed with saline and covered with a gauze sponge.

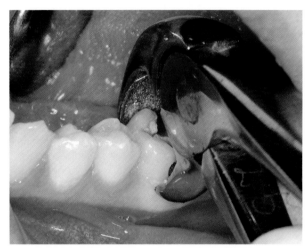
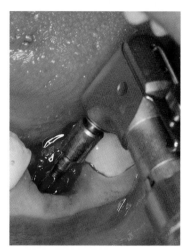

Incision and elevation of a flap

An incision is made at the height of the alveolar process from the ramus to the distal surface of the second molar. From there the incision follows the distal and buccal surfaces of the second molar. A buccal flap is then raised starting mesially. In the third molar region it is important that the mucosa is dissected free of the third molar follicle.

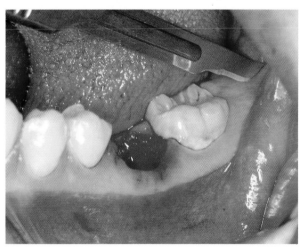
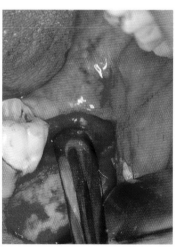

Exposure of the graft

Thereafter bone covering the periphery of the graft is removed with burs or chisels so that an axial and thereby atraumatic removal of the third molar is possible. If burs are used, the follicle should be shielded by insertion of an amalgam carver between the follicle and the bony socket. It is normally necessary to remove a considerable amount of bone buccally, distally, and sometimes also lingually.

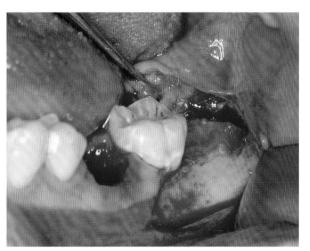
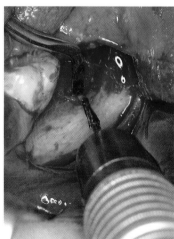

Fig. 4.7. Continued.

Separation of the follicle
Before any attempts are made at luxating the graft, it should be certain that the follicle is completely separated from adjacent connective tissue. This is best accomplished by inserting an amalgam carver in the space between the follicle and the bony socket and by separating the inserting fibers which are concentrated in the cervical region. If this step is omitted, the entire follicle could be torn away during tooth removal.

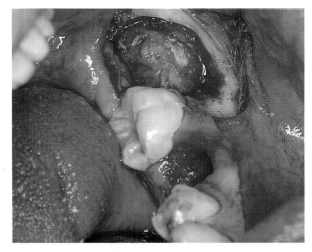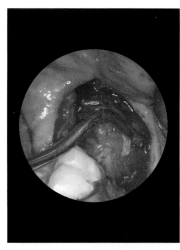

Removal of the graft
The tooth is luxated with an elevator placed interproximally between the second and third molars. It is important that the elevator does not contact the root surface but only the crown of the graft. When the molar is loose it is removed with forceps and inspected for defects in the follicle and the apical part of the pulp.

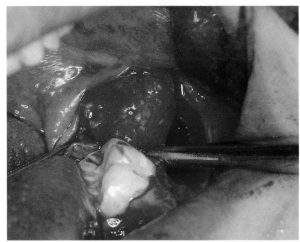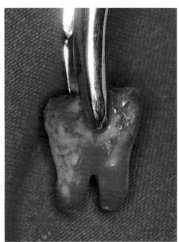

Testing the transplant
The transplant is then tried in its new socket. It should be possible to rotate the tooth slightly in the socket as an indication of a loose fit. The graft should be transplanted to the same level of eruption as it occupied at the donor site or slightly more erupted, as in this case. However, if there are defects in the follicle, its crown should not be placed below bone level, as this may lead to ankylosis and non-eruption.

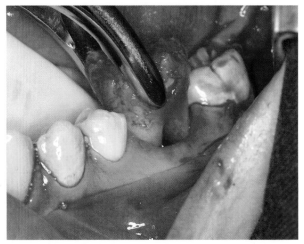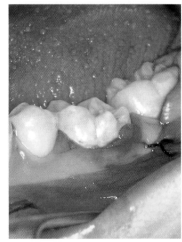

Splinting
Once occlusion has been checked, a suture is placed from the buccal to the oral gingival margin across the occlusal surface. If there is any tendency to displacement, it is important to consider that a suture splint is not sufficient. Instead an acid-etch/resin or wire splint should be used.

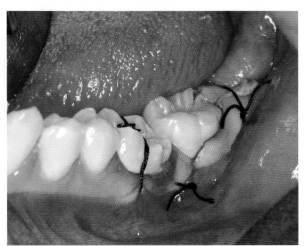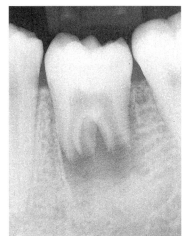

Fig. 4.8. Maxillary third molar transplantation

The indication for transplantation was in this case unsuccessful endodontic therapy combined with extensive breakdown of the crown.

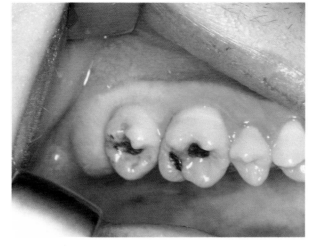
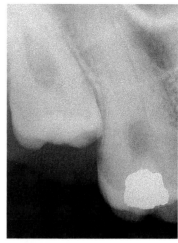

Incision and elevation of flap

The incision is started distally and continued palatally along the gingival sulcus of the second molar. A similar incision is made buccally to the region of the first molar, where an incision is made up to the vestibular sulcus. Flap elevation is initiated mesially and is then carried distally, where a careful dissection is made separating the follicle from adjacent connective tissue.

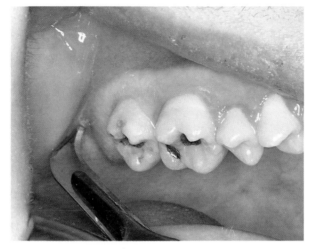
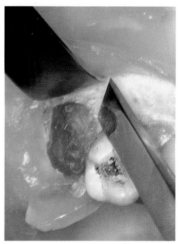

Surgical exposure

(Shown on a model)
The removal of bone in the maxilla is best performed with hand instruments. An osteotomy is made first using a chisel immediately distal and buccal to the second molar. A thin periosteal elevator can then be used to fracture the very thin bone covering the crown buccally, distally, and palatally.

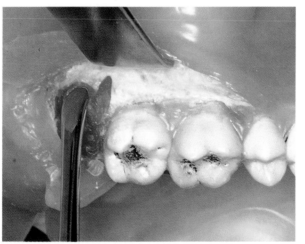
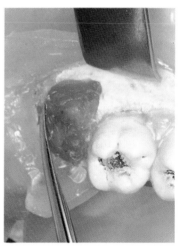

Separation of the follicle

Complete separation of the follicle from adjacent connective tissue is checked with an amalgam carver.

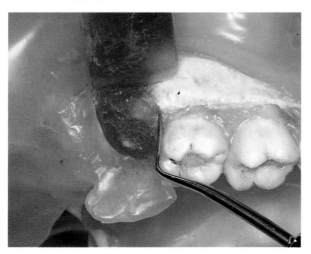
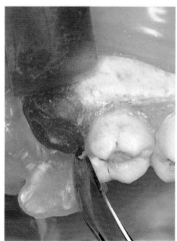

Fig. 4.8. Continued.

Loosening the graft
The third molar can then be luxated with an elevator placed between the second and the third molars. The graft is removed with forceps (shown on a model) and inspected for damage to the apical pulp and the PDL.

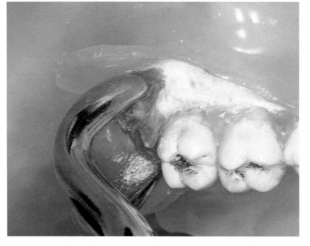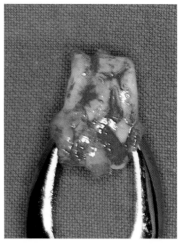

Preparing the graft site
In this case the graft region is an edentolous site. The mucosa is incised according to the size of the graft.

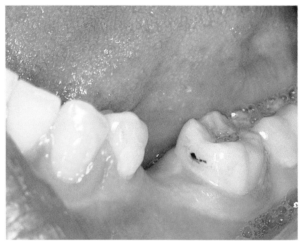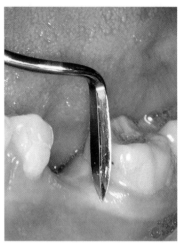

Transplantation
After creating a new socket with a bur, the graft is positioned in its new socket free of occlusal contact.

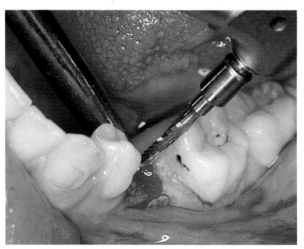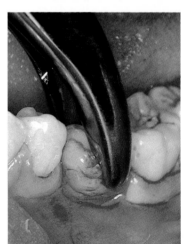

Splinting
One suture placed over the occlusal surface serves as a splint. Alternatively, a 0.2 mm wire spanning the occlusal surface from the second premolar to the second molar can provide a more stable form of fixation.

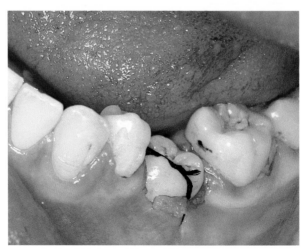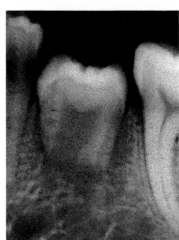

Special cases

Lack of space at the recipient site

If the pretransplant analysis reveals lack of space the optimal solution appears to be initial orthodontic treatment to create sufficient space (Fig. 4.9). If this is not possible, reduction of the proximal surface of the graft by grinding can be considered. The proximal surfaces can be reduced 0.5 mm by grinding without exposing dentin. This procedure should be done with a rotating diamond while the tooth is submerged in saline, or the tip of the bur is cooled under a constant flow of saline. It is very important that no heat is transmitted to the pulp during crown reduction.

Treatment of premolar aplasia

Transplantation of third molars to the premolar region is sometimes indicated. This can arise in cases with aplasia or loss of one or two permanent premolars. Because of the rather small buccolingual dimension of the alveolar process in the premolar region it is normally only maxillary molars which can be used and only those whose mesiodistal dimension is small enough. In these instances the graft should be rotated 90° mesially to accommodate for the palate root (Fig. 4.10).

The surgical procedures in the recipient site follow the guidelines outlined previously for the molar region. Due to uncertainty about graft size it is usually worthwhile postponing recipient site preparation until the third molar has been removed and direct measurements can be made. Transplantation can then be completed if these measurements are compatible with the recipient site.

Replacement of maxillary incisors

In rare cases a developing maxillary third molar has such a root anatomy that it can replace a lost maxillary central incisor (see Chapter 11, p. 283).[4-6, 98] In these instances it is necessary to expand the maxillary alveolar process during transplantation, a procedure described in Chapter 5, p. 157.

Replacement of molars due to juvenile periodontitis

This type of periodontal disease affects young individuals and results in a rapid loss of alveolar bone out of proportion to the amount of local irritants present, and especially involving permanent first molars and incisors.[14-16]

Fig. 4.9. Mandibular third molar transplantation used in the treatment of gross caries extending below the gingival margin. Due to the mesiodistal dimension of the third molar, additional space was created orthodontically prior to transplantation (0 days).

0 days   0 days

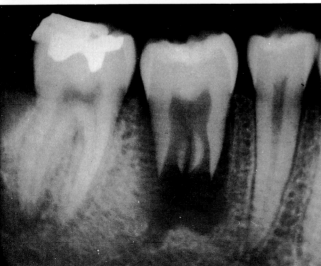
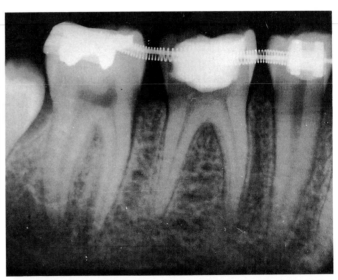

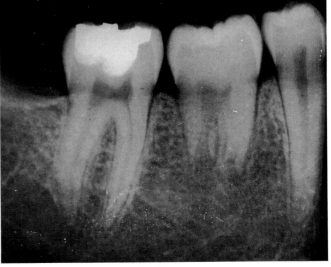

2 months   1 year

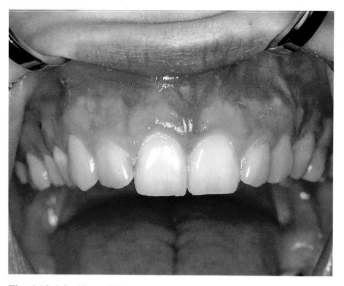
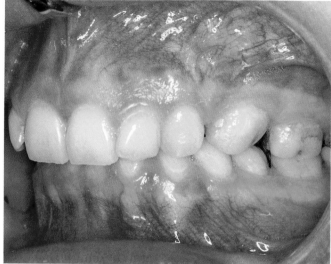

Fig. 4.10. Maxillary third molar transplantation used to treat aplasia of two maxillary premolars.

In several studies, autotransplantation of third molars has been used as a replacement for the affected first molars.[2,3,16-19] It has been shown that transplantation stimulates new formation of alveolar bone in the recipient site (Fig. 4.11). This is possibly related to the osteogenic effect of the vital PDL and the follicle (see Chapter 1, p. 45).

The surgical procedure follows the guidelines already outlined for molar transplantations. Concerning postoperative healing, it has been found in a follow-up study of 15 autotransplanted third molars that root formation continued in all cases and no root resorption or pulp necrosis occurred. Most important, none of the transplants showed pocket depths exceeding 3 mm.

Redressement forcé

In cases where an erupting second or third molar is locked under the cervical area of an adjacent tooth, surgical tilting can be performed (Fig. 4.12).[9-10] Long-term prognosis based on larger patient material is not available at the present time.

Transplantation to edentulous sites

The prognosis for transplantation of molars to edentulous sites apparently does not differ from that for transplantation to dentulous sites.[11-12] The preparation of the recipient site is begun with the removal of the mucosa covering the height of the alveolar process. The area of mucosa should be slightly less than the neck of the graft.

Two-stage transplantation procedure

Recently a new technique has been devised whereby a socket is prepared and left to heal for 14 days, whereafter transplantation is carried out. The motivation for this approach is that the transplant should be placed in a well-vascularized tissue bed.[89] Although the initial results are promising, this approach lacks a control group of conventionally transplanted teeth.

Apicoectomy in teeth with closed apices

In a recent study apicoectomy was attempted in order to favor revascularization of the pulp. This was, however, not found to occur.[91]

Fig. 4.11. Transplantation of a mandibular third molar in the treatment of juvenile periodontitis. From Borring-Møller & Frandsen, 1978.[2]

| 0 days | 0 days | 2 months | 1 year |

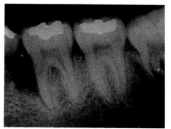
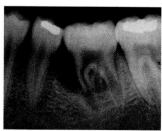
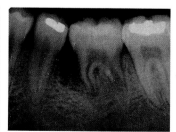
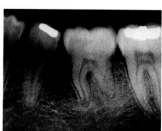

Fig. 4.12. Surgical tilting of a second mandibular molar

An incision is made corresponding to the mesial surface of the crown of the second molar.

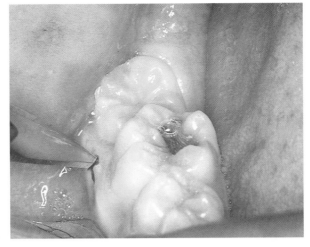 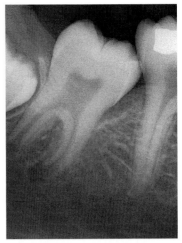

Placing the elevator

A straight elevator is inserted through the incision.

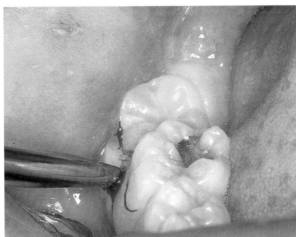 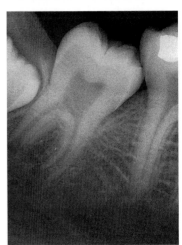

Uprighting the molar

The second molar is uprighted with a slow rotation of the elevator. An acid-etch splint should be applied for 4 weeks to prevent relapse.

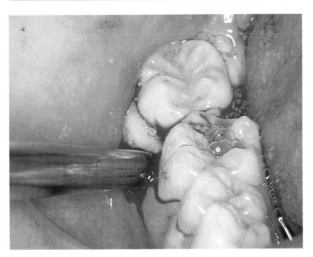 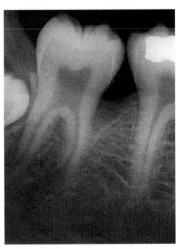

Postoperative healing

Normal sulcus depth is found after 4 weeks. The radiograph taken 1 year later shows no root resorption and initial pulp canal obliteration.

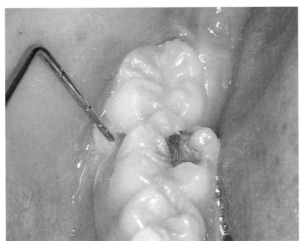 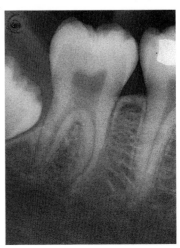

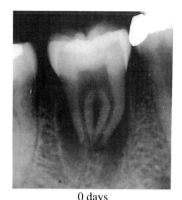
0 days

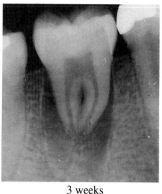
3 weeks

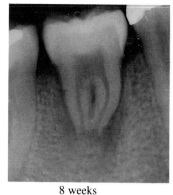
8 weeks

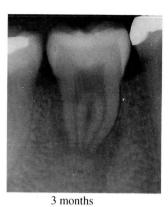
3 months

Fig. 4.13. Partial formation of the lamina dura 8 weeks after transplantation.

Postoperative follow-up

The patient is seen after 1 week, at which time the suture splint is removed. If firm splinting (e.g., acid-etch or wire splint) was indicated due to lack of supporting bone, 4 weeks is necessary to stabilize the transplanted tooth. Radiographic controls should be performed after 3 and 8 weeks. In cases with completed root formation, extirpation of the pulp is performed after 4 weeks; calcium hydroxide is then placed in the root canal (see Chapter 2, p. 62).

PDL healing

PDL healing as evidenced by lamina dura formation can be seen as early as 1 month and is usually present 2 to 4 months after transplantation (Fig. 4.13).

Pulpal healing

With regard to pulpal healing, the transplanted teeth begin to react to sensibility tests after 3-4 months;[20-21] the majority of cases will react positively after 6-8 months.[20-22]

Pulp canal obliteration

Signs of initial pulp canal obliteration can be seen as early as 1 month after transplantation and are usually present after 4 months (Fig. 4.14).[8,17,21] Another form of pulpal reaction to transplantation is sometimes seen, where bone extends through the apical foramen into the pulp chamber, creating an internal PDL (Fig. 4.15).[11,22] This finding indicates severe trauma to the Hertwig's epithelial root sheath (see Chapter 1, p. 43).

Fig. 4.14. Pulp canal obliteration is evident 2 months after transplantation.

0 days   2 months   6 months   1 year

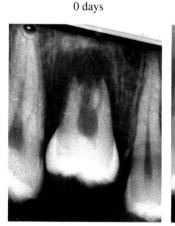
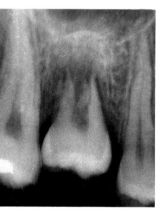
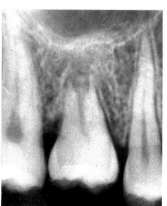
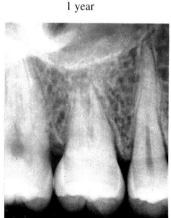

Fig. 4.15. Invasion of bone and and PDL into the pulp chamber in a transplanted maxillary third molar.

0 days   1 month   1 year   2 years

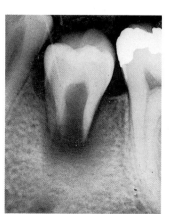
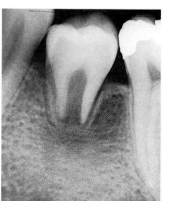
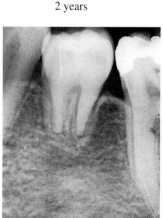

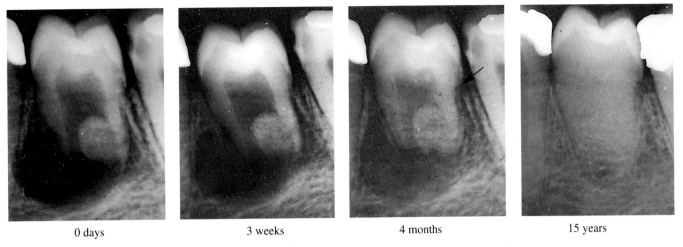

0 days	3 weeks	4 months	15 years

Fig. 4.16. Development of surface resorption (arrow) subsequent to transplantation of a maxillary third molar.

Root resorption

Root resorption is usually diagnosed 1 to 6 months after transplantation. In this regard it is essential to differentiate between surface (Fig. 4.16), inflammatory (Fig. 4.17), and replacement resorption (Figs. 4.18 and 4.19) as each of these resorption types requires either no or specific treatments (see p. 129).

Fig. 4.17. Development of inflammatory resorption (arrows) after transplantation of a mandibular third molar.

0 days	1 month	6 months	9 months

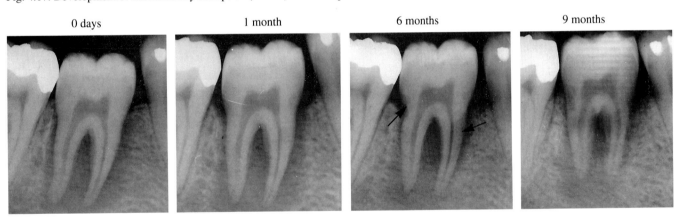

Fig. 4.18. Development of replacement resorption subsequent to transplantation of a maxillary third molar. Note the disappearance of the PDL space.

0 days	1 year	3 years	4 years

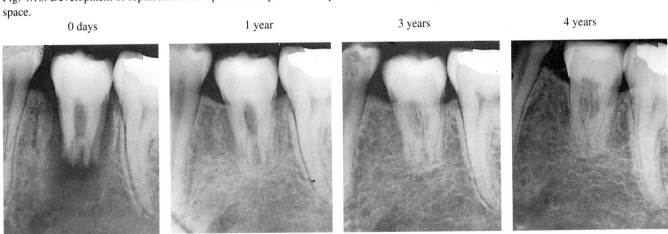

125

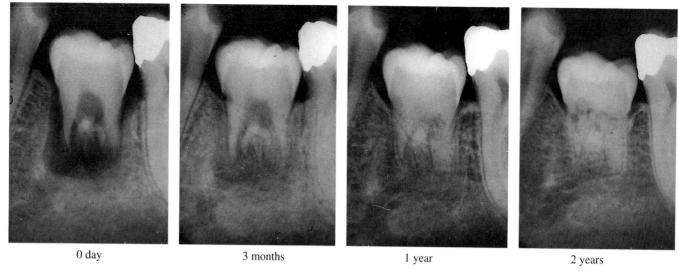

| 0 day | 3 months | 1 year | 2 years |

Fig. 4.19. Development of replacement resorption subsequent to transplantation of a maxillary third molar. Note the progressive infra-occlusion.

Root growth

Radiographic evidence of root growth is usually seen after 4 months; its extent at this time ranges from 1 to 2.5 mm (Fig. 4.20).[21] Continued root growth can be expected over a period of approximately 3 years.

Eruption

Eruption of the transplant is especially noticeable in the first postoperative month and is possibly aided by healing processes in the socket area which tend to push the transplanted tooth into the oral cavity.[21,24]

Prognosis

The results of third molar transplantation have been described in several review articles,[25-30,113-121] case reports,[31-72,98-112] and a number of clinical studies based on larger materials.[11,20-24,73-97,126] In Table 4.1 the results are listed for clinical studies where one or more complications have been adequately documented. As expected, the success rate varies considerably, first of all because of great variations in case selection (incomplete versus complete root formation), but presumably also because of differences in techniques and observation periods. However, several long-term studies have shown that stable healing results can be obtained (Figs. 4.21 and 4.22).

Fig. 4.20. Sequence of root development subsequent to transplantation of a maxillary third molar.

| 0 days | 6 months | 1 year | 2 years |

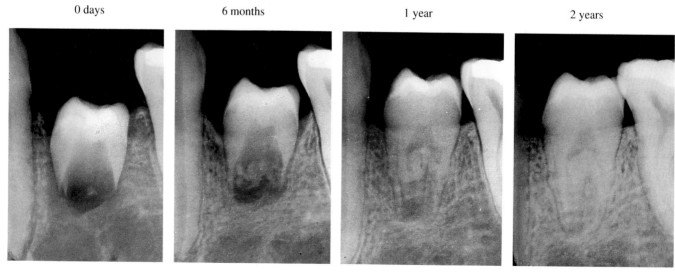

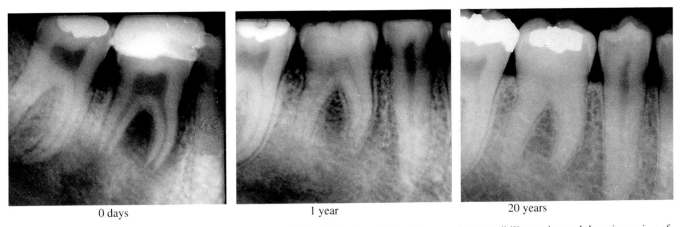

0 days	1 year	20 years

Fig. 4.21. The long-term result of transplantation of a mandibular third molar. The tooth responds to sensibility testing and there is no sign of root resorption.

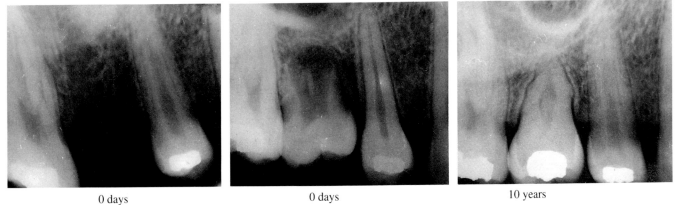

0 days	0 days	10 years

Fig. 4.22. The long-term result of transplantation of a mandibular third molar. The tooth reacts to sensibility testing at the last control. There is

Table 4.1. Long-term results of autotransplantation of third molars

	Observation period		Age of patients		Number of teeth	Stage of root formation*	Tooth survival	PDL healing**	Pulp healing		Gingival healing
									Sensibility	Canal obliteration	
	yr.	(mean)	yr.	(mean)			%	%	%	%	%
Nordenram, 1963[11]	0.5-7		13-22	(17.2)	61	I	79	85	56	52	77
Galanter & Minami, 1968[23]	1-10		15-23		31	I	74	94	84		100
Andreasen & al., 1970[22]	0.7-6		13-23		18	I	95	94	50	56	84
			19-46		56***	C	96	21			50
Sing & Dudani, 1970[21]	(0.4)		13-17		25	I			76	84	84
Hovinga, 1986[85]	2-10	(6.0)	14-21	(17.5)	16	I	100	100			
Nethander & al., 1988[89]	1-5		13-65	(30.7)	57****	I	89	79			
Andreasen 1990[86]	0.5-20	(4.7)	15-21	(17.9)	151	I,C	96	81			93

*   Third molars with incomplete root formation = I
*   Third molars with complete root formation = C
**   PDL healing without any sign of root resorption
***   Impacted third molars endodontically treated at time of surgery
****   All teeth transplanted with a two-stage technique

Fig. 4.23. Tooth survival of 219 autotransplanted third molars with different stages of root formation at the time of surgery. From Andreasen, 1990.[86] Note that there is only 5 years observation period for teeth with closed apices.

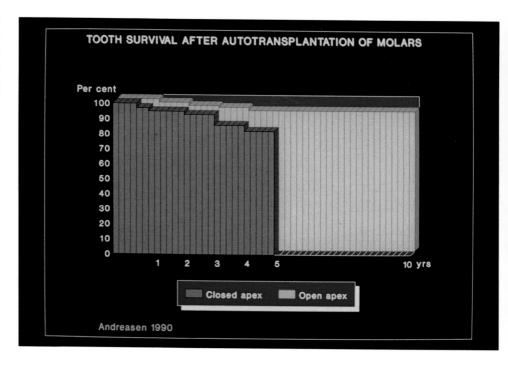

Tooth survival

One reliable indicator of the success appears to be transplant survival. In the studies shown in Table 4.1 the frequency of graft survival was 74% to 100%, with any graft loss usually occuring within 5 years. Only a single factor has been related to graft loss so far; namely root formation at the time of transplantation (Fig. 4.23). It appears from several studies that transplantation at very early and very late root development stages results in increased graft loss.[83,86] Thus, complete root formation at the time of transplantation appears to lead to an increase in graft loss compared to transplantation at earlier stages. In the following, postoperative complications will be described.

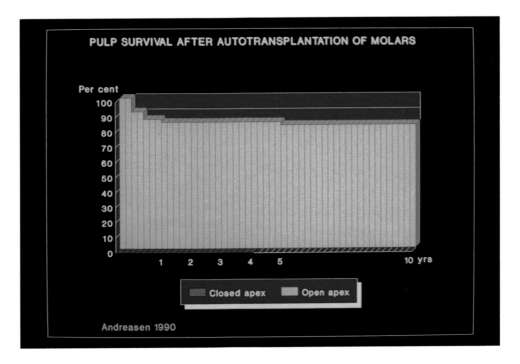

Fig. 4.24. Pulpal healing of 209 autotransplanted third molars with different stages of root formation at the time of surgery. From Andreasen, 1990.[86]

Pulpal healing and pulp necrosis

Reports on pulpal revascularization in transplanted third molars are usually based on sensibility testing. The figures range from 50% to 84% in the studies cited in Table 4.1. If pulp canal obliteration is used as proof of pulpal revascularization, similar figures are obtained. A strong relationship is found between root development and pulp revascularization. Thus, among molars transplanted with incomplete root formation (stages 1 to 4) revascularization takes place in 80% to 90% of the cases, whereas pulp necrosis is quite common in teeth transplanted with more mature root formation (Fig. 4.24).

Pulp necrosis usually becomes evident after 1 to 6 months and is seen as a periapical radiolucency, lack of pulp canal obliteration, and lack of sensibility response. A pathognomonic sign of pulp necrosis is external inflammatory root resorption. Early endodontic treatment (i.e. after 3-4 weeks) has been shown to increase the longevity of the transplant in cases with complete root formation.[92,126]

Finally internal resorption (i.e., resorption processes originating from the pulp canal) is sometimes found and is usually related to the development of partial pulp necrosis after transplantation (Fig. 4.25). In this regard it should be considered that inflammatory resorption affecting the labial and lingual parts of the root may simulate internal resorption.

PDL healing and root resorption

The rate of PDL healing without root resorption has been examined in only a few studies and frequencies range from 79% to 100% among teeth transplanted without immediate endodontic treatment (Table 4.1).

Relatively sparse information exists about clinical factors related to development of root resorption. In one study it appeared that an age factor was in operation. Thus among third molars transplanted before 18 years of age, less root resorption was seen than in transplantations performed at later ages.[11]

Fig. 4.25. Partial pulp necrosis and internal root resorption (arrow) following transplantation of a mandibular third molar.

| 0 days | 2 months | 6 months | 5 years |

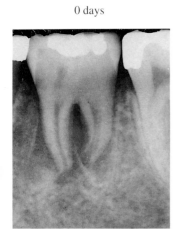
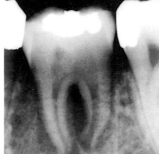
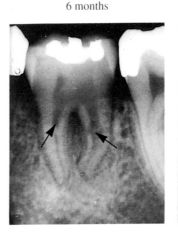
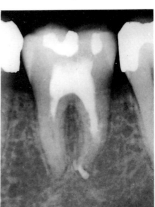

Fig. 4.26. PDL healing of 209 autotransplanted molars with different stages of root formation at the time of surgery. From Andreasen, 1990.[86] Note that there is only 5 years observation period for teeth with closed apices.

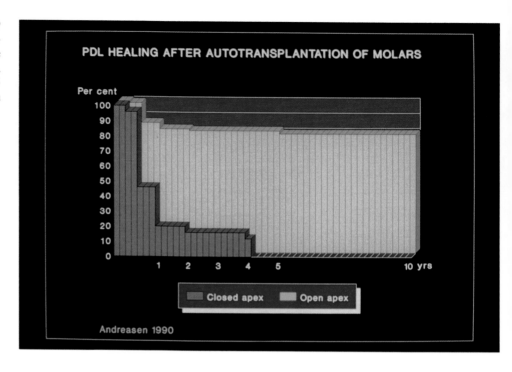

The relationship of PDL healing to various stages of root development is shown in Fig. 4.26. According to the results of this clinical study, stages 2 and 3 appear to be optimal with regard to PDL healing. Transplantation at stages 5 and 6 bears with it a considerable risk of root resorption.[86, 125] In other clinical studies where impacted third molars with completed root formation were transplanted after extra-alveolar root filling, root resorption was found to affect almost all transplants (Fig. 4.27).[22,58]

Fig. 4.27. Replacement resorption following the transplantation of an impacted third molar with completed root formation. From Andreasen & al., 1970.[22]

| 0 days | 1 year | 3 years | 5 years |

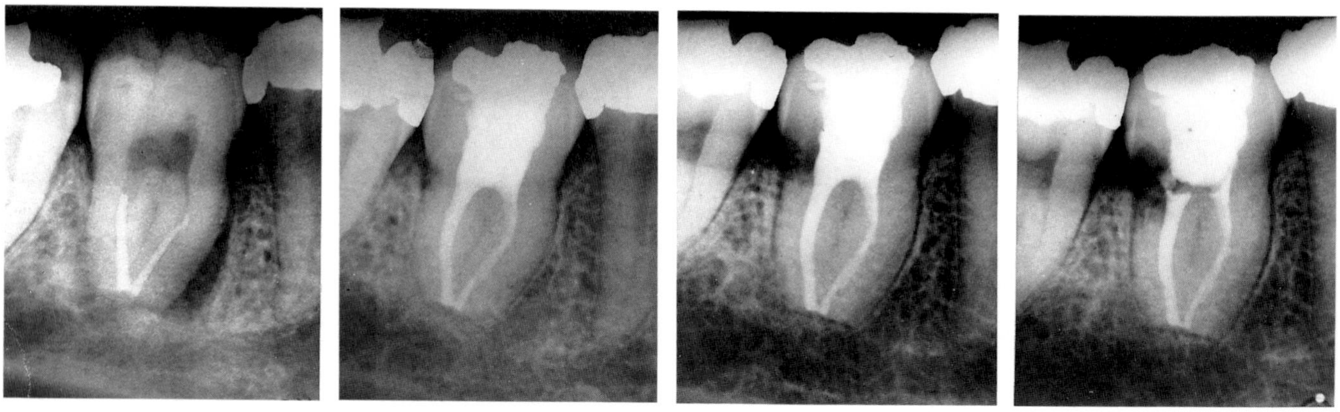

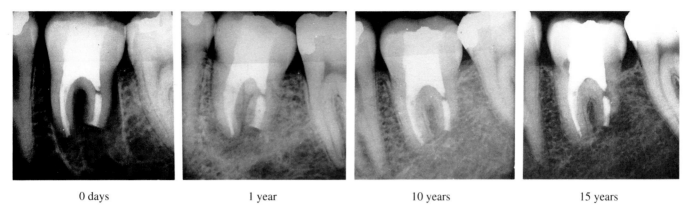

0 days	1 year	10 years	15 years

Fig. 4.28. Replacement resorption following the transplantation of a mandibular third molar in a 20-year-old man. Over a 15-year observation period, there is only slight progression of the resorption process.

This phenomenon is possibly an expression of atrophy of the PDL which is typical of impacted teeth and which makes them vulnerable to traumatic injuries during graft removal. In older individuals the replacement resorption can take a very protracted course (Fig. 4.28).

When ankylosis affects the labial or the lingual part of the root it may simulate internal root resorption (Fig. 4.29).

Fig. 4.29. Ankylosis affecting the labial or lingual part of the root imitating internal root resorption following transplantation of a maxillary third molar.

0 days	1 year	2 years	3 years

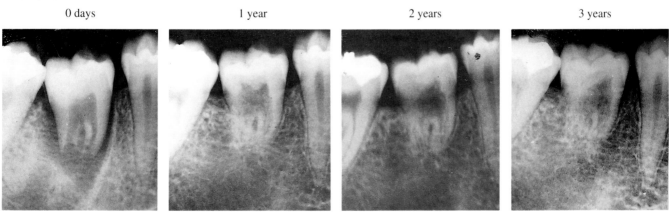

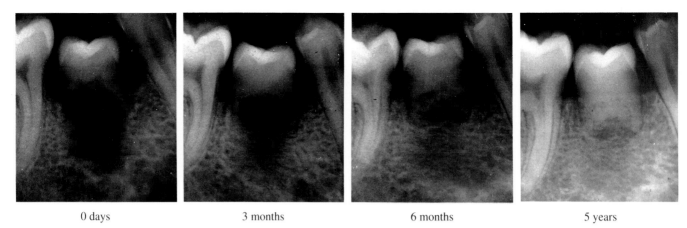

| 0 days | 3 months | 6 months | 5 years |

Fig. 4.30. Arrested root formation of a maxillary third molar which was transplanted at a very early stage and placed too superficially in the prepared socket.

Root development and developmental disturbances

Disturbances in root development have been examined in a number of studies and found to be significantly related to the stage of root development at the time of transplantation (Fig. 4.32).[21,36,76-79,86] Thus transplantation of third molars at a stage of initial root formation, as was commonly practiced in the early 1950s, often resulted in no root growth after transplantation.[22,24,36,42,50,56,65,76-79,85,86] Furthermore a superficial orientation of the transplant at this stage of root development in all cases led to a complete arrest of root formation while a deeper position resulted in restricted root formation (Fig. 4.30).[36]

Studies on the extent of root formation subsequent to third molar transplantation have generally shown that in most cases an increase in root length of approximately 1-2 mm can be expected. However, great variations have been found, ranging from arrested root formation up to an increase of 6 mm.[20-23,76] Only sparse information exists on factors determining root formation apart from the stage of root formation at time of transplantation[21,36,76-79,86] and an expected relationship between the length of the observation period and increase in root length.[23,76]

An analysis of the figures published by Alvarez & al.[76] (1968) seems to indicate that in order to achieve a satisfactory root length after transplantation of for example, 10 mm (which will ensure reasonable firmness of the transplant), the stage of root development should be approximately 8-9 mm, which amounts to two-thirds of the expected root length for third molars. If earlier stages of root development are chosen, such as half root formation, slightly more root growth can be expected in some cases; however, a risk of arrest of root formation is present.

Lack of root growth leads to excessive mobility of the transplant due to the unfavorable crown-root ratio. Thus, figures published by Galanter & Minami[23] (1968) demonstrate that a final root length of 7 mm or less led to a considerable increase in mobility. In conclusion, the transplantation of third molars with approximately 2/3 to 3/4 root formation (stage 3) appears to best if optimal root length is to be achieved.

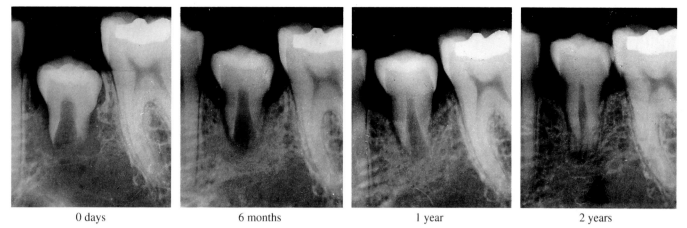

| 0 days | 6 months | 1 year | 2 years |

Fig. 4.31. Loss of marginal attachment subsequent to the transplantation of a maxillary third molar.

Gingival healing and loss of marginal attachment

This factor has been examined in studies of third molar transplants with immature root formation. A general finding has been that loss of marginal attachment is rare after transplantation of teeth with incomplete root formation (Fig. 4.31).[21-23] However, when endodontically treated teeth with completed roots were transplanted, this loss became a prominent feature, affecting up to half of the transplanted teeth (Table 4.1).

Caries susceptibility

In a study reported by Nordenram[11] (1963) it was examined whether caries disposition of a third molar is altered when it is transplanted to a new site, compared to its nontransplanted antemire. In this study it was found that 16 out of 18 examined pairs of third molars showed less caries in the transplanted position. Thus, there appears to be a strong relationship between the position of the transplant and caries susceptibility.

Healing related to graft selection

In Fig. 4.33 a synopsis is shown on the relation between stage of root development at time of transplantation and the various healing parameters. It appears that 3/4 to 4/4 root formation with an open apex is to be preferred.

Fig. 4.32. Synopsis of the relation between stage of root development and various healing parameters. It appears that three-quarter to full root development with wide open apices offers maximum security for an acceptable healing result regarding all healing parameters. From Andreasen, 1990.[86]

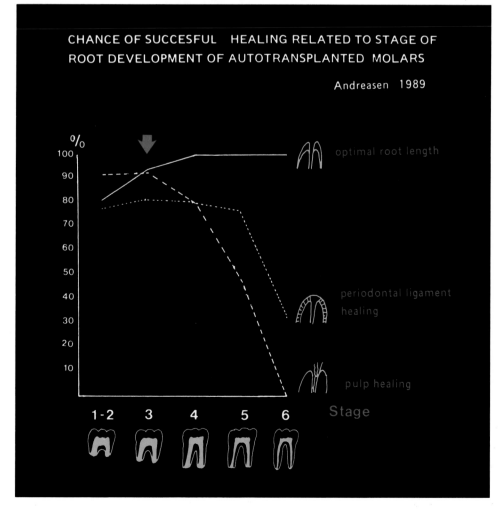

Essentials

Indications

Extraction of molars
Aplasia of premolars
Loss or aplasia of incisors

Treatment planning

Preoperative radiographs
Space evaluation

Surgical procedure (Figs. 4.6 and 4.7)

1. Administer antibiotic therapy and local anesthesia.
2. Extract the tooth to be replaced.
3. Prepare the socket.
4. Remove transplant.
5. Place the transplant within the socket at a level identical to that which it previously occupied.
6. Use preferentially a suture splint.
7. Take a postoperative radiograph.

Follow-up

(See Appendix 2, p. 290)

Prognosis

Tooth survival (5 years)

Incomplete root formation	90%
Complete root formation	82%

Pulpal healing

Incomplete root formation	82%
Complete root formation	0%

PDL healing

Incomplete root formation	79%
Complete root formation	12%

References

1. Marzola C, Filho HN. Transplant of dental germs and frequency of exodontia. Estomatol E Cultura 1968; 2: 57-70.

2. Borring-Møller G, Frandsen A. Autologous tooth transplantation to replace molars lost in patients with juvenile periodontitis. J Clin Periodontol 1978; 5: 152-58.

3. Borring-Møller G, Frandsen A. Autolog tandtransplantation som en metode til erstatning af parodontalt destruerede molarer på patienter med juvenil parodontitis.Tandlægebladet 1979; 83: 111-14.

4. Kristerson L. Unusual case of tooth transplantation: Report of case. J Oral Surg 1970; 28: 841-44.

5. Kristerson L, Nederfors T. Autotransplantation vid omfattande traumatiska tandförluster. Tandläkartidningen 1980; 72: 18-22.

6. Kristerson L, Kvint S. Autotransplantation av tänder - en klinisk behandlingsmetod. Tidsskr Tandlæger 1982; 2: 7-14.

7. Kragh Madsen I. Autotransplantation i privat praksis. Tandlægebladet 1984; 88: 373-74.

8. Lund TM, Manson-Hing LR. A study of the focal troughs of three panoramic dental x-ray machines. Part II. Image dimensions. Oral Surg Oral Med Oral Pathol 1975; 39: 647-53.

9. Laskin DM, Peskin S. Surgical aids in orthodontics. Dent Clin North Am 1968; July: 509-24.

10. Peskin S, Graber TM. Surgical repositioning of teeth. J Am Dent Assoc 1970; 80: 1320-26.

11. Nordenram Å. Autotransplantation of teeth. Acta Odontol Scand 1963; 21: Suppl 33.

12. Conklin WW. Transplantation of third molar into edentulous site. Oral Surg Oral Med Oral Pathol 1974; 38: 193-97.

13. Brauer MK. Autogenous tooth root transplant: A case report. Periodont Case Rep 1980; 2: 9-12.

14. Levine RA. Twenty-five month follow-up of an autogenous third molar transplantation in a localized juvenile periodontitis patient: A case report. Compend Contin Educ Dent 1987;8:560-77.

15. Saxen L. Juvenile periodontitis. J Clin Periodontol 1980; 7: 1-19.

16. Hörmand J. Juvenil parodontitis In: Hjørting-Hansen E.(ed). Odontologi 1979. Copenhagen : Munksgaard, 1979; 113-24 .

17. Baer PN, Gamble JW. Autogenous dental transplants as a method of treating the osseous defect in periodontosis. Oral Surg Oral Med Oral Pathol 1966; 22: 405-10.

18. Hoffman ID. Familial occurrence of juvenile periodontitis with varied treatment of one of the siblings with five year follow-up. Case reports. J Periodontol 1983; 5 : 44-48.

19. Rubin MM, Berg M, Borden B. Autogenous transplants in the treatment of juvenile periodontitis (periodontosis). J Am Dent Assoc 1982; 105: 649-51.

20. Clark HB, Tam JC, Mitchell DF. Transplantation of developing teeth. J Dent Res 1955; 34: 322-28.

21. Singh KK, Dudani IC. Autogenous transplantation of developing mandibular third molars. J Indian Med Assoc 1970; 42: 199-212.

22. Andreasen JO, Hjørting-Hansen E, Jølst O. A clinical and radiographic study of 76 autotransplanted third molars. Scand J Dent Res 1970; 78: 512-23.

23. Galanter DR, Minami RT. The periodontal status of autografted teeth. A pilot study of thirty-one cases. Oral Surg Oral Med Oral Pathol 1968; 26: 145-59.

24. Miller HM. Transplantation and reimplantation of teeth. Oral Surg Oral Med Oral Pathol 1956; 9: 84-95.

25. Hale ML. Autogenous transplants. J Am Dent Assoc 1954; 49: 193-98 .

26. Nordenram Å. Tandtransplantationer. Svensk Tandläkar Tidskr 1964; 57: 55-72.

27. Nordenram Å. Tandtransplantationen, dess värde ur klinisk och vetenskaplig synvinkel. Göteborgs Tandläkar-Sällskaps Årsbok 1965; No 329: 1-20.

28. Nordenram Å. "Reservdelsmänniskan" från oralkirurgisk synpunkt. Tandläkartidningen 1982; 74: 560-67

29. Sveen K, Vindenes H. Autotransplantasjon av tenner, indikation, teknikk og prognose. Nor Tandlægefor Tid 1979; 89: 481-87

30. Slagsvold 0. Transplantasjon av tenner ved ortodontisk behandling. In: Holst JJ,Nygaard Østby B, Oswald 0, eds. Nordisk Klinisk Odontologi (15-x-1) Copenhagen: A/S Forlaget for Faglitteratur 1979: 1-18.

31. Miller HM. Transplantation. A case report. J Am Dent Assoc 1950; 40: 237-38.

32. Miller HM. Transplantation of teeth. NY State Dent J 1951; 17: 382-86.

33. Miller HM. Tooth transplantation. Report of case. J Oral Surg 1951; 9: 68-69.

34. Miller HH. Third molar transplantation. Int Dent J 1952; 3: 42-44.

35. Miller HM. Reimplanting human teeth. Dent Survey 1953; 29: 1439-43.

36. Apfel H. Autoplasty of enucleated prefunctional third molars. J Oral Surg 1950; 8: 289-96.

37. Apfel H. Preliminary work in transplanting the third molar to the first position. J Am Dent Assoc 1954; 48: 143-50.

38. Apfel H. Transplantation of the unerupted third molar tooth. Oral Surg Oral Med Oral Pathol 1956; 9: 96-98.

39. Collings GJ. Dual transplantation of third molar teeth. Oral Surg Oral Med Oral Pathol 1951; 4: 1214-19.

40. Siegel MT. Third molar transplantation. J Am Dent Assoc 1952; 45: 698

41. McMahon HT. Transplantation of a viable and incompletely formed third molar: report of case. J Oral Surg 1952; 10: 345-46.

42. Noble FP. Autotransplantation: report of three cases. J Oral Surg 1954; 12: 54-59.

43. Erwig R, Hahn W. Autotransplantation von 3. Molaren. Dtsch Zahnärtzeblatt 1955; 9: 767-68.

44. Tam JC. Autogenous transplantation of a partially formed tooth. Report of a case. Oral Surg Oral Med Oral Pathol 1956; 9: 71-75 .

45. Hale ML. Autogenous transplants. Oral Surg Oral Med Oral Pathol 1956; 9: 76-83.

46. Weiner E. Transplantation of teeth. Transplant Bull 1956; 3: 97-99.

47. Fong CC, Agnew RG. Transplantation of teeth: clinical and experimental studies. J Am Dent Assoc 1958; 56: 77-86.

48. Meyer W. Die Begriffsbestimmungen bei der Pflanzung von Zähnen. ZWR 1957; 60: 152- 55.

49. Goldberg H. Transplantation: report of a case. J Am Dent Assoc 1961; 63: 833.

50. Hühne S. Zahnkeimtransplantationen bei Kindern. Dtsch Stomatol 1961; 11: 302-09.

51. Nordenram Å. Autoplastic tooth transplantation: its clinical applicability. Oral Surg Oral Med Oral Pathol 1962; 15: 1489-94.

52. Nordenram Å. The unerupted, partially erupted or erupted tooth. A potential autograft. Swed Dent J 1971; 64: 293-309.

53. Hayton-Williams DS. Transplantation of lower third molar to first molar site. Dent Pract 1963; 13: 317-18.

54. Müller EE. Transplantation of impacted teeth. J Am Dent Assoc 1964; 69: 449-59.

55. Metro PS. Bilateral simultaneous transplantation with a modified surgical technique. Oral Surg Oral Med Oral Pathol 1965; 20: 159-65.

56. Caprioglio D, de Risky S, Nidoli G. Autotrapianti di germi di III molare inferiore. Riv Ital Stomatol 1967; 22: 641-62.

57. Marano PD. Dental transplantation simplified. Oral Surg Oral Med Oral Pathol 1967; 24: 567-72.

58. Lindholm K, Westerholm N. Transplantation of endodontically treated third molars. Proc Finn Dent Soc 1973; 69: 17-20.

59. Bolton R. Autogenous transplantation and replantation of teeth: Report on 66 treated patients. Br J Oral Surg 1974; 12: 147-65.

60. Conklin WW. Autogenous dental transplants. Oral Surg Oral Med Oral Pathol 1969; 28: 17-25.

61. Conklin WW. Long-term follow-up and evaluation of transplantation of fully developed teeth. Oral Surg Oral Med Oral Pathol 1978; 46: 477-85.

62. Marzola C. Dental germs transplantation - a modification in the surgical technique. Estomatologia E Cultura 1972; 6: 86-97.

63. Marzola C. Transplantes seu estudo em odontologia. Sao Paulo: Universidade de Sao Paulo, Brazil 1975.

64. Brown KH. Vital tooth transplants: report of cases. J Am Dent Assoc 1973; 87: 655-60.

65. Pantera TG, Pantera RL. Intraoral third molar transplants: report of three cases and long-term follow-up. J Am Dent Assoc 1978; 97: 486-90.

66. Martina R, di Lauro F, Bucci E. Valutazione ortodontica di alcuni trapianti dentari. Arch Stomatol 1978; 19: 287-302.

67. Danziger F. An autogenous tooth transplant: report of case. J Am Dent Assoc 1978; 96: 105-06

68. Northway WM, Konigsberg S. Autogenic tooth transplantation: "The state of the art". Am J Orthod 1980; 77: 146-62.

69. Müller W, Zinner R. Zahnkeimtransplantation in ein vorbereitetes Gewebelager. Stomatol DDR 1981; 31: 305-09.

70. Eskici A. Zahn- und Zahnkeimtransplantation im Rahmen der kieferorthopädischen Behandlung. Öster Z Stomatol 1980; 77: 458-60.

71. Eskici A. Replantation und Transplantation von Zähnen und Zahnkeimen. Dtsch Zahnärztl Z 1980; 35: 343-45.

72. Eskici A. Tierexperimentelle Untersuchungen und klinische Ergebnisse der Zahnkeimtransplantation. Fortschr Kiefer Gesichtschir. 1983; 28: 100-02

73. Fong CC. Transplantation of the third molar. Oral Surg Oral Med Oral Pathol 1953; 6: 917-26.

74. Walker RV, Schaffer R. Transplantation of teeth. (Series of 50 tooth transplantations) Baylor. Dent J 1964; 14: 4-9.

75. Logan TH. A simplified surgical techique for autogenous lower third molar transplants. NZ Dent J 1966; 62: 189-97.

76. Alvarez N, Biolcati EL, Bracco OC. Trasplantes autogenos de germenes de terceros molares. Rev Assoc Odont Argent 1968; 56: 189-200.

77. Marzola C. Autoplasty of the preformed lower third molars. Surgical methodology. Rev Arqo Cent Est Rac Odont 1969; 6: 105-16.

78. Marzola C. Autotransplantation of tooth germs - clinical and roentgenologic study of 69 cases. Rev Brasil Odontol 1969; 26: 47-60.

79. Marzola C. Dental transplantation - criteria and standards for analysing results. Rev Arq Cent Est Fac Odont 1969; 6: 173-85.

80. Marzola C. Ortotopic homovital autogenous transplantation of human lower third molars germs; clinical and radiographic study. Rev Fauchard (Argentina) 1970; 1: 324-33.

81. Nordenram Å. Autotransplantation of teeth. A clinical investigation. Br J Oral Surg 1970; 7: 188-195.

82. Mugnier A, Bordais P, Gineste P, Marchand J, Serafinowska A. Contribution a la transplantation des dents de sagesse inferieures. Experience de 6 ans. Rev Stomatol (Paris) 1976; 77: 541-56.

83. Kristerson L, Kvint S. Autotransplantation av tänder - 10 års erfarenheter. Tandläkartidningen 1981; 73: 598-606.

84. Andreasen JO. Long term prognosis of autotransplanted third molars. An analysis of 209 transplants 1990; In preparation.

85. Hovinga J. Autotransplantatie van kiemen van derde molaren. Resultaten van voortgezette observatie. Ned Tijdschr Tandheelkd 1986; 93: 235-37.

86. Andreasen JO. Third molar autotransplantation, relation between successful healing and stage of root development at time of grafting. Presented at the annual meeting in Scandinavian Association of Oral and Maxillofacial Surgeons, August 15-19, 1990, Nyborg, Denmark.

87. Schwartz O, Bergmann P, Klausen B. Autotransplantation of human teeth. A life-table analysis of prognostic factors. Int J Oral Surg 1985; 14: 245-58.

88. Kahnberg KE. Autotransplantation of teeth. I. Indications for transplantation with a follow-up of 51 cases. Int J Oral Maxillofac Surg 1978; 16: 577-85.

89. Nethander G, Andersson JE, Hirsch JM. Autogenous free tooth transplantation in man by a 2-stage operation technique. A longitudinal intra-individual radiographic assessment. Int J Oral Maxillofac Surg 1988; 17: 330-36.

90. Khoury F. Erfahrung mit einer modifizierten Methode zur Weisheitzahntransposition (autologe Weisheitzahntransplantation). Dtsch Zahn-Mund-Kiefer Gesichtschir 1985; 9: 265-68.

91. Khoury F. Grundlagen und klinische Aspekte der autologen Zahntransplantation (Zahntransposition). ZWR 1986; 95: 1036-46.

92. Eliasson S, Laftman AC, Strindberg L. Autotransplanted teeth with early-stage endodontic treatment: A radiographic evaluation. Oral Surg Oral Med Oral Pathol 1988; 65: 598-603.

93. Menezes AC, Marcal P, Chaves Filho ES, Menezes MHM. Transplantes autogenos de terceiros molares com rizogenese completa em humanos. R Cent Ci Biomed Univ Fed Uberlandia 1986; 2: 49-63.

94. Jacobs HG, Rost-Dickmann I. Die autologe Zahntransplantation - Prinzipien und Nachuntersuchungsergebnisse. Quintessenz Int 1988; 39: 817- 26.

95. Jewan J, Pennig J. Autotransplantation von Zahnen zum Ersatz der Sechsjahr-molaren. Zahnärztl Prax 1985; 9: 338- 42.

96. Henrichvark C, Neukam FW. Indikation und Ergebnisse der autogenen Zahntransplantation. Dtsch Zahnärztl Z 1987; 42: 194-97.

97. Fasen D. Die Erfolgsaussichten der autologen Zahnkeimtransplantation. Eine klinische, röntgenologische und histologische Nachuntersuchung. Dtsch Zahnärztl Z 1983; 38: 139-41.

98. Dermaut L, De-Pauw G. L'autogreffe de dents: une dimension supplémentaire dans la practique dentaire. Rev Belge Med Dent 1989; 44: 85-98.

99. Murganic Z. Zahntransplantation nach Molarenverlust (I). Quintessenz Int 1986; 37: 1319-27.

100. Murganic Z. Zahntransplantation nach Molarenverlust (II). Quintessenz Int 1986; 37: 1481-89.

101. Conklin WW. Transplantation of mandibular third molar in seventh decade: Long-term follow-up and evaluation. Oral Surg Oral Med Oral Pathol 1987; 64: 407-10.

102. Stoll P, Härle F, Schilli W. Transplantation eines Weisheitzahnes in ein autologes Beckenkammtransplantat am Unterkiefer. Fallbericht. Dtsch Zahn-Mund-Kiefer Gesichtschir 1978; 11: 5-7.

103. Artis JP, Brissard P. La transplantation des germes de troisieme molaire: notre point de vue. Inf Dent 1987; 69: 2403-07.

104. Smith JJ, Wayman BE. Successful autotransplantation. J Endod 1987; 13: 77-80.

105. Rakusin H, Jurosky KA, Gutmann JL. A five-year follow-up of autogenous tooth transplantation: a case report. Int Endod J 1988; 21: 327-32.

106. McDonald F. Transplantation after failure of eruption. J Clin Orthod 1988; 22: 176-79.

107. Hernandez SL, Cuestas-Carnero R. Autogenic tooth transplantation: A report of ten cases. J Oral Maxillofac Surg 1988; 46: 1051-55.

108. Pital ML. Use of a cantilevered acrylic splint in the autogenous transplantation of a third molar: report of case. J Am Dent Assoc 1988; 117: 329-31.

109. Rahn R. Transplantation impaktierter Weisheitzahne. Quintessenz Int 1987; 38: 7-19.

110. Saravia ME, Mercuri LG, Mourino AP. Autogenous third molar transplantation: report of a case. J Dent Child 1985; 52: 455-8.

111. Hofmann B, Didier D. Utilisation d'un greffon dentaire dans une mentoplastie. A propose d'une observation. Rev Stomatol Chir Maxillofac 1988; 89: 132-4.

112. Zinner R. Transplantation von Zähnen. Stomatol DDR 1986; 36: 300-05.

113. Feldmann G. Voraussetzungen, Vorgehen, Erfolge bei der Zahntransplantation. Zahnärztl Mitt 1985; 75: 2532-42.

114. Hartmann HJ. The transplant of vital 3. molars. J Oral Implant 1987; 13: 54-69.

115. Eskici A. Autogene Zahnkeimtransplantationen. Klinische und tierexperimentelle Untersuchungen. Z Stomatol 1987; 84: 357-66.

116. Eskici A. Klinische und tierexperimentelle Untersuchungen zur Autotransplantation von Zahnkeimen (I). Quintessenz Int 1987; 38: 565-70.

117. Eskici A. Klinische und tierexperimentelle Untersuchungen zur Autotransplantation von Zahnkeimen (II). Quintessenz 1987; 38: 737-51.

118. Eskici A. Klinische und tierexperimentelle Untersuchungen zur Autotransplantationen von Zahnkeimen (III). Quintessenz Int 1987; 38: 913-24.

119. Eskici A, Droschl H, Bantleon H, Permann I. Die Entwicklung des Parodontiums nach Zahnkeimtransplantationen im Rahmen der kieferorthopädischen Behandlung. Fortschr Kieferorthop 1989; 50: 285-93.

120. Khoury F. Chirurgische Möglichkeiten zur Erhaltung der Kauebene im Molaren-bereich. ZWR 1985; 94: 726-33.

121. Khoury F. Die Spättransposition von Weisheitzahnen. Dtsch Zahnärztl Z 1986; 41: 1061-64.

122. Khoury F. Die Transposition von vollentwickelten Weisheitzähnen nach Resektion ihrer Wurzelspitzen. Dtsch Zahn-Mund-Kiefer Gesichtschir 1986; 10: 184-90.

123. Al-Himdani K. L'auto-transplantation: Indications - Technique operatoire. Bilan clinique. Rev Odonto-stomatol 1986; 15: 95-107.

124. Zinner R. Transplantation von Zähnen. Stomatol DDR 1986; 36: 300-05.

125. Heinrichvark C, Neukam FW. Indication und Ergebnisse der autogenen Zahntransplantation. Dtsch Zahnärztl Z 1987; 42: 194-197.

126. Kahnberg K-E. Autotransplantation of teeth. (I). Indications for transplantation with a follow-up of 51 cases. Int J Oral Maxillofacial Surg 1987; 16: 577-585.

Chapter 5
Autotransplantation of premolars

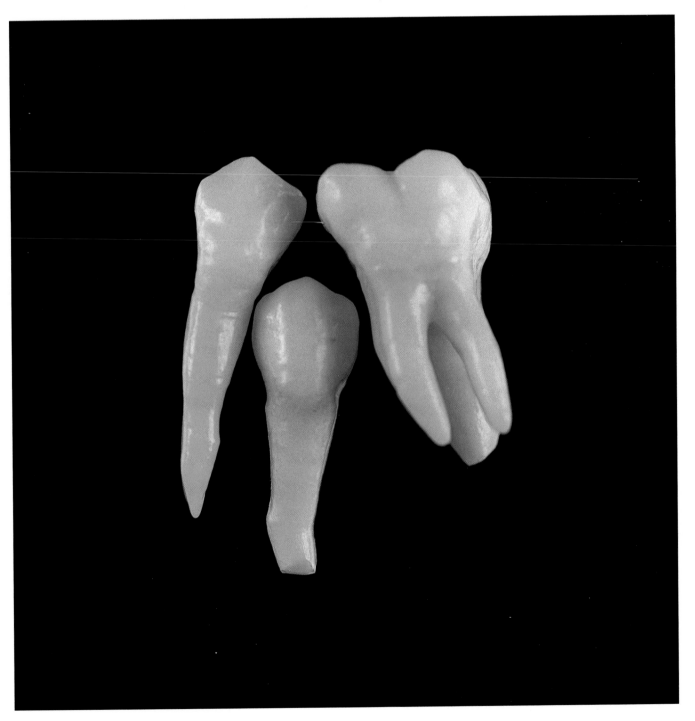

Indications

Within the past 20 years it has been found that premolar transplantation is a very reliable procedure which can be used in various situations (Fig. 5.1). The most frequent indication for premolar transplantation appears to be agenesis of permanent premolars, a condition which is seen in 6%-10% of the population (see also Chapter 10, p. 258).[1]

Fig. 5.1. Various indications for premolar transplantation.
A. Ectopic position of the premolar. B. Aplasia of permanent premolars. C. Loss of second molars. D to F. Congenital or accidental loss of anterior or posterior teeth.

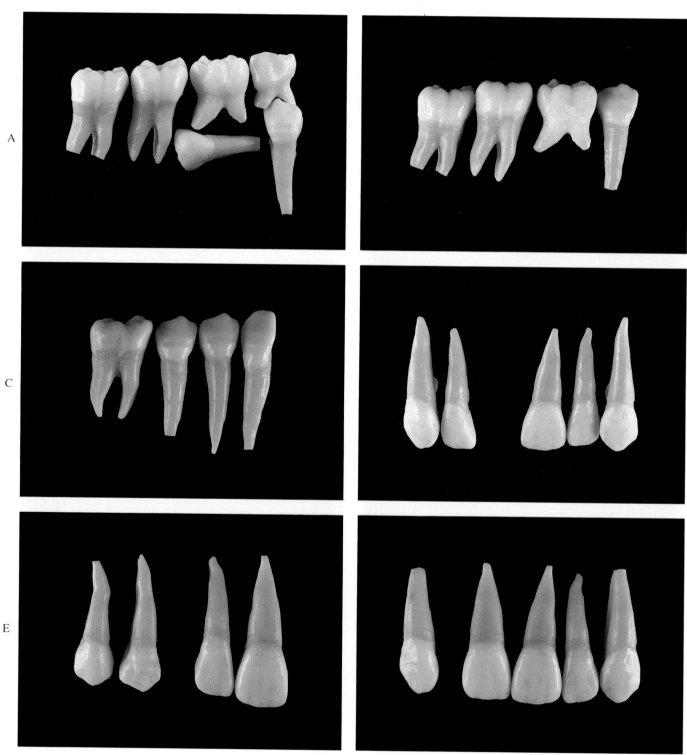

A

C

E

140

Fig. 5.2. Aplasia treated by transplantation

Transplantation of a maxillary second premolar in a case of aplasia of a second mandibular premolar. At the last control, the tooth reacts normally to sensibility testing; there is no sign of root resorption and there is normal completion of root development.

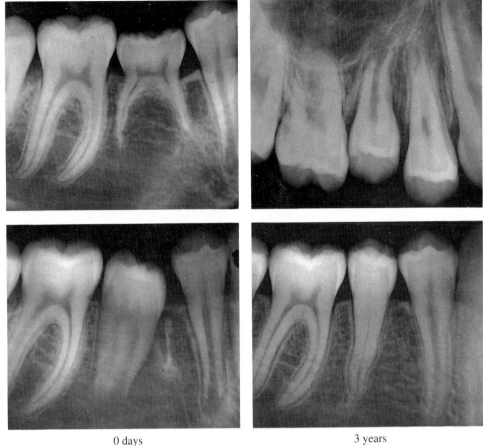

0 days   3 years

In these cases, transplantation of premolars from the opposite jaw to the aplasia site is often indicated (Figs. 5.2).

Other indications for premolar transplantation appear in connection with premolar ectopia or impaction, conditions which particularly affect second premolars (Figs. 5.3 and 5.4). The overall frequency of premolar impaction has been reported to be 0.5%.[2] The frequency of *maxillary* second premolar impaction has been found to range from 0.1% to 0.3% and for *mandibular* premolar impaction from 0.2% to 0.3%.[3,4]

Fig. 5.3. Transplantation of an ectopic mandibular second premolar.

0 days   0 days   10 years

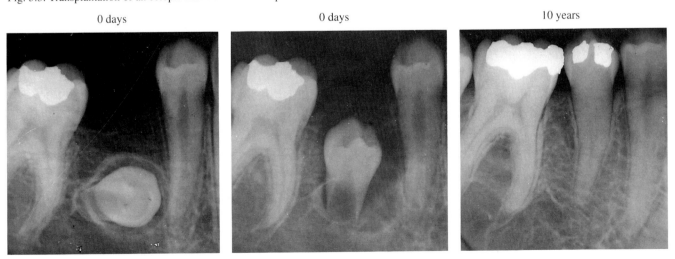

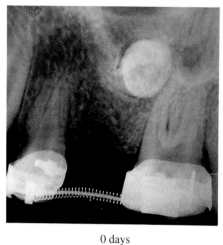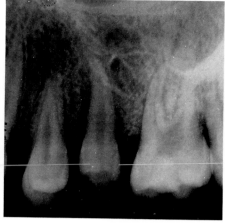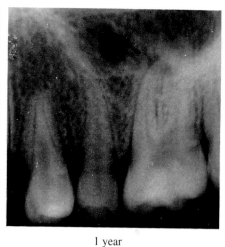

0 days   0 days   1 year

Fig. 5.4. Transplantation of an ectopic maxillary second premolar.

Another indication for premolar transplantation is congenital or accidental loss of anterior teeth, where transplanted premolars which are subsequently restored can replace missing anterior teeth (Fig. 5.5).[5,27,28,33,35,48-51] Avulsion of anterior permanent teeth due to trauma has been found to affect 0.2% of school-age children;[5,46] and congenital lack of lateral incisors is found with a frequency of 2% in the general population.[6]

Before transplantation is carried out in any of the above-mentioned situations, it is essential that a careful orthodontic analysis is made, confirming the indication for this procedure (see also Chapter 10, p. 258). Included in this analysis is a clinical and radiographic evaluation of the potential graft(s) and the recipient site in order to determine whether they are compatible.

Fig. 5.5. External root resorption of an incisor treated by transplantation

A replanted incisor shows extensive resorption (ankylosis). A second mandibular premolar was used as replacement and subsequently restored with composite resin.

0 days

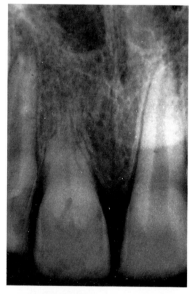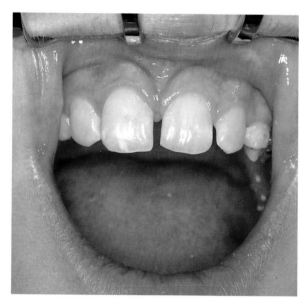

5 years

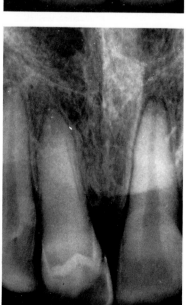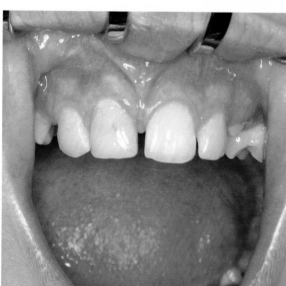

Fig. 5.6. Space evaluation
The mesiodistal dimension is evaluated in the premolar region with a sliding caliper.

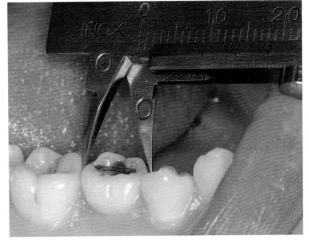

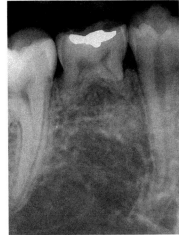

Labiolingual analysis
The width of the alveolar process is evaluated cervically.

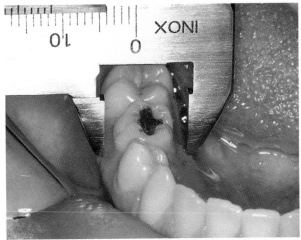

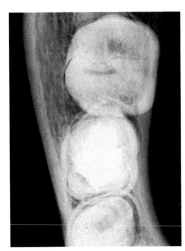

Treatment planning

Aplasia

In these cases, the premolar to be transplanted is usually found in its normal position in the jaw; a single orthoradial radiograph of the potential graft is therefore usually sufficient for estimation of the mesiodistal dimension of the crown as well as the root length. However, the radiographic estimation of the crown width should be carried out with caution, as it has been shown that this measure is often 1-2 mm greater than the true crown width, presumably due to slight rotation of the developing premolars.[7] Information from tables of average tooth dimensions is therefore more reliable concerning this measure (see Appendix 4, p. 292). Concerning the labiolingual dimension of the graft, this can be estimated in the mandible by taking an axial radiograph. In the maxilla a similar radiograph can be taken; however, because of the difficulty of this technique in this region, it is seldom indicated. Instead a table of average tooth measurements should be used (see Appendix 4, p. 292).

A radiograph of the recipient site is also necessary in order to evaluate the mesiodistal dimension of bone available. In the mandible, it is also important to evaluate the position of the mandibular canal and in the maxilla, the location of the sinus. The labiolingual dimension of the recipient site can be evaluated directly in the oral cavity (Fig. 5.6). The width of the alveolar process is measured cervically with a sliding caliper and the following calculation is made: Assuming that the

actual width is 15 mm, the thickness of the alveolar mucosa is deducted, which amounts to 2 mm, leaving a 13 mm width of the alveolar process. Due to the fact that the labial and lingual cortical bone plates should be left intact, another 1 mm should be subtracted, leaving 12 mm buccolingually for the new alveolus. Finally it should be considered that there should be some space around the transplant. Thus the potential graft should have a root dimension slightly less than this measure.

Concerning graft choice, all premolars can be used. However, the first maxillary premolar is the least suitable because of its divergent roots, which can complicate an atraumatic graft removal. As a general rule, premolars from the maxilla should be transplanted to the opposite side of the mandible (and vice versa) in order to create optimal occlusal and proximal relations.

The optimal stage of root development for transplantation is 3/4 root formation (see p. 172). However, clinical conditions might require transplantation in earlier stages. Thus, close proximity of the sinus to the recipient site could necessitate transplantation in stages with initial root formation. Furthermore an atrophic alveolar process might indicate transplantation at an early stage of tooth development, at which time the transplanted tooth could induce growth of the alveolar process.[8]

Fig. 5.7. Location of ectopic pre-molars

Axial exposure reveals the lingual position of the ectopic second premolar.

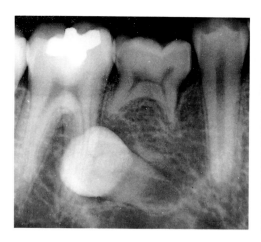

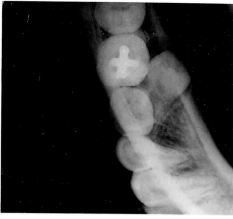

Ectopia

In these cases, it is important to evaluate whether denudation or autotransplantation is the optimal treatment, as denudation of the tooth eventually supplemented with orthodontic traction is a safer treatment (see Chapter 10, p. 258). The position of the ectopic mandibular premolar should be determined radiographically by both orthoradial and axial exposures.

In most cases the tooth germ is placed with its crown tilted lingually[9] (Fig. 5.7). In the maxilla, the position of the premolar is usually determined by orthoradial and eccentric exposures, which will reveal the position of the tooth in relation to other teeth (Fig. 5.8). If necessary, an axial view will accurately depict the anatomic relationship between the ectopic premolar and adjacent teeth. Finally the space conditions at the recipient site should be evaluated as described above. In general, the stage of root development which is ideal for repositioning ectopic premolars is 3/4 root formation; however, very close proximity to adjacent teeth could indicate earlier graft removal (see p. 172).

Trauma

After trauma, where a premolar transplant has been decided upon to replace a lost incisor, radiographic and clinical examination should determine the actual space available at the recipient site. All premolars can be used to replace incisors, although the first maxillary premolar is not ideal. The transplants can be placed in normal position or rotated 45^0-90^0 according to the width of the tooth to be replaced (see also Chapter 10, p. 280) Concerning the replacement of maxillary lateral incisors, the first mandibular premolar has the optimal root and crown anatomy for this location. It is very important that the crown can fit into the space available and that the width of the transplanted tooth in the cervical area leaves a minimum of 1 mm interdental bone between the transplant and adjacent teeth. The labiolingual dimension is also important. In these cases, it should be decided whether there is room enough within the alveolus or whether the alveolus should be expanded in relation to the surgical procedure (see later).

Surgical procedure

In the following figures, the surgical procedures of various types of premolar transplantations will be illustrated:

Maxillary premolar graft removal and mandibular recipient site preparation (Fig. 5.9)

Mandibular premolar graft removal (Figs. 5.10 and 5.11)

Fig. 5.8. Eccentric exposures used to determine the position of a maxillary premolar. A-C. Distoeccentric, orthoradial, and mesioeccentric exposures respectively. Note the shift in the position of the crown in relation to the first premolar, indicating the palatal position of the tooth (i.e., the tooth follows the direction of the tube).

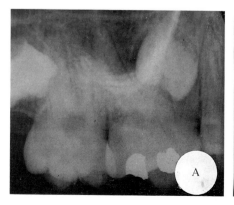

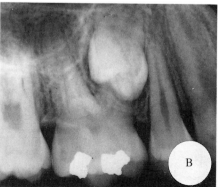

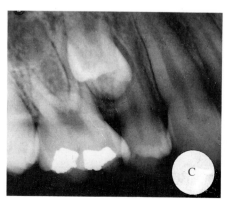

Fig. 5.9. Maxillary premolar transplantation to the mandible

In this case a maxillary second premolar was transplanted due to aplasia of the mandibular second premolar.

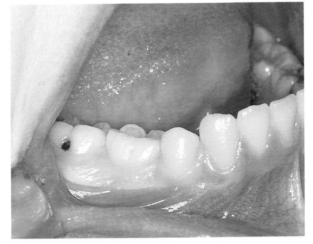
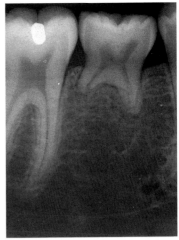

Extraction of primary molar

During the last phase of the luxation procedure, the tooth should be rotated 45° so that the divergent apices do not damage interdental bone and the interdental papillae. In the case of ankylosed molars it is only necessary to remove those fragments which interfere with the creation of the new socket. The remaining ankylosed fragments will be resorbed.

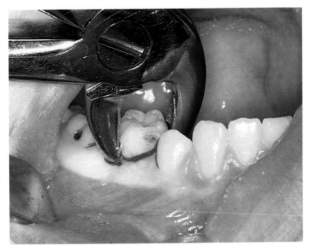
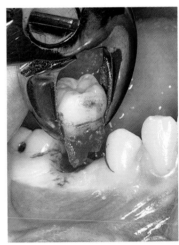

Preparation of the socket

A surgical bur, preferably with internal cooling (see Appendix 7, p. 296), is directed axially at the interdental septum until the desired socket depth is achieved. This should not exceed the radiographic graft length by more than 1-2 mm. The socket is then enlarged laterally. It is usually an advantage to rotate the graft distally to confine the transplant to the limits of the alveolar bone.

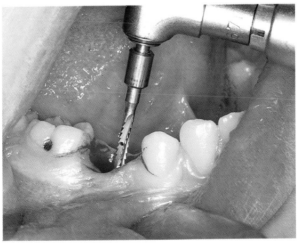
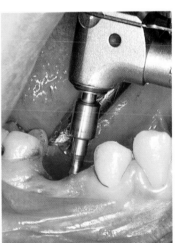

Rinsing the socket

Distorotation, in contrast to mesiorotation, lessens the risk of damage to the mental artery and nerve. Furthermore, when the socket has been enlarged sufficiently, it is rinsed thoroughly with saline and covered with a gauze sponge to prevent saliva contamination. This position ensures a minimal distance from the surrounding gingiva and thus optimizes gingival healing.

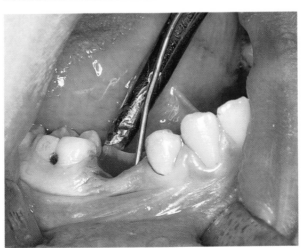
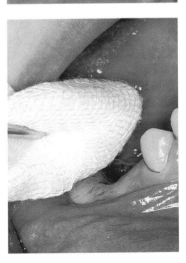

Fig. 5.9. Continued.
Removing the maxillary graft

If the premolar has not yet erupted, the primary molar is extracted first and a marginal incision from the first molar region to the canine region is made severing the interdental papillae in the graft region. If the graft has erupted, the PDL is incised with a special surgical blade (see p. 296) as deeply as possible and the tooth is then extracted with a forceps. During this procedure, it is essential to use only slight luxating movements.

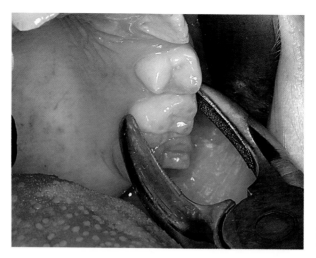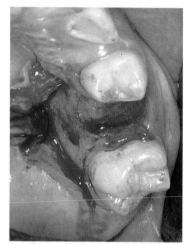

Raising a flap

A flap is first raised distally. Because almost all maxillary premolars are located with their crown tilted palatally, it is necessary to remove palatal bone in order to permit atraumatic graft removal.

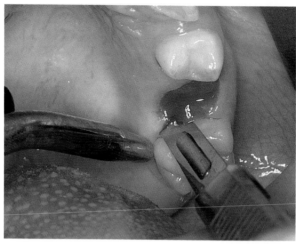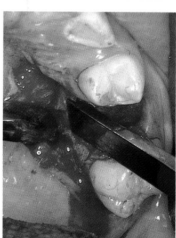

Bone removal

The bone covering the palatal root of the primary molar is removed with a bone cutter or a chisel.

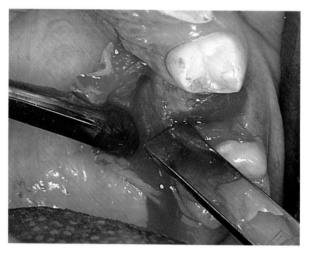

Uncovering the graft

All bone covering the occlusal surface of the graft must be removed. This is done preferably with chisels which can work close to adjacent teeth.

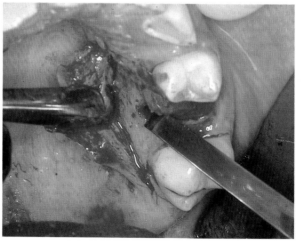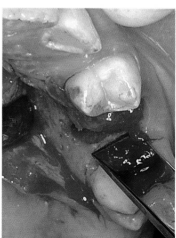

Fig. 5.9. Continued.

Enlarging the follicle

A thin periosteal elevator is then inserted at the labial aspect of the follicle. Space is created by displacing the bone plate labially. In order not to separate the follicle from the graft, it is important that all collagenous attachments are severed. This can be accomplished with an amalgam carver.

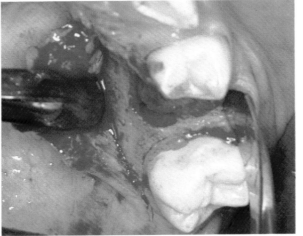 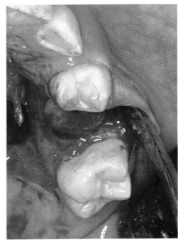

Separating the follicle and removing the graft

The graft is loosened by using a thin periosteal elevator placed labially. The tooth is then grasped with a forceps and removed. If not freed entirely from its socket, the entire follicle could inadvertently be stripped from the tooth. If separation of the follicle is noted, the final phase of tooth removal should be made by grasping the follicle with a hemostat and completing the extraction procedure by drawing out both the tooth and the follicle.

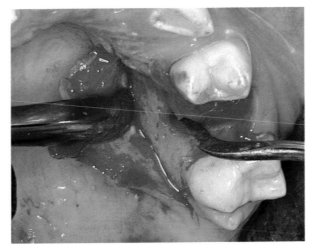 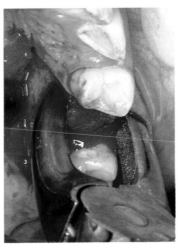

Inspecting the graft

Once the graft has been removed, it should be inspected for the presence of defects in the follicle. It should also be noted whether the apical pulp is intact. If that structure is missing, arrested root formation can be expected (see text).

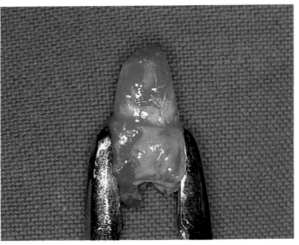 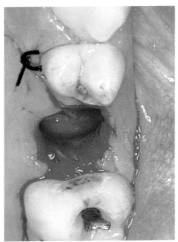

Transplanting the graft

The graft is then cleansed with saline and positioned in its new socket. It is grasped with two fingers and rotated slightly to ensure adequate space for the transplant. If there is not, the socket should be enlarged. As a rule, the tooth germ should be transplanted to an apicocoronal level in the recipient site identical with the site from which it was taken. After placing the transplant, the tooth is stabilized by a suture splint. In the case of 45⁰ rotation, a suture across the occlusal surface will maintain the tooth in its new position.

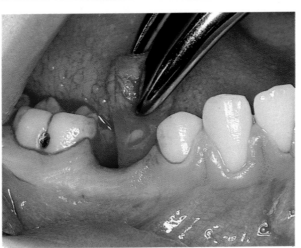 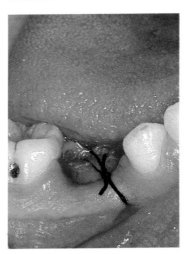

Fig. 5.10. Mandibular premolar transplantation to the maxilla

In this case a mandibular second premolar was transplanted to the maxilla due to aplasia of the maxillary second premolar.

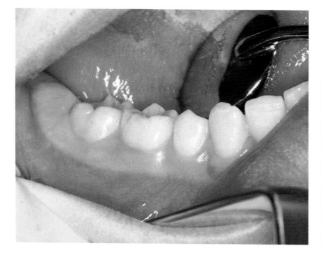 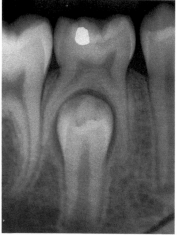

Extraction of the primary molar

The primary molar is extracted with an attempt not to injure the interdental papillae.

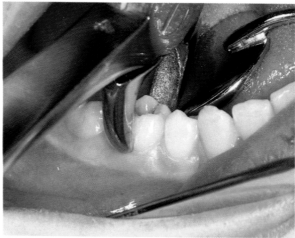 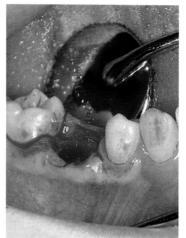

Raising the flap

A flap is raised from the first premolar to the molar region.

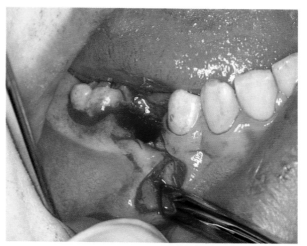 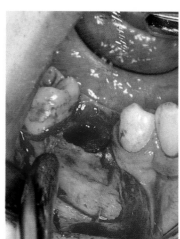

Osteotomy of the buccal bone plate

An osteotomy that corresponds to the bone covering the coronal half of the graft is made.

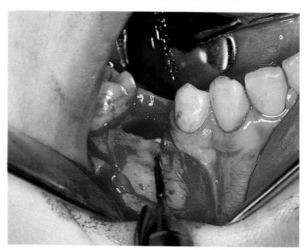

Fig. 5.10. Continued.

Removing the buccal bone plate

The buccal bone plate is removed with a chisel.

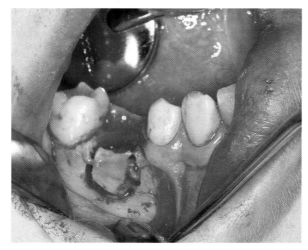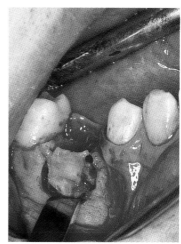

Loosening the follicle

The follicle attachment to the bone is loosened with an amalgam carver.

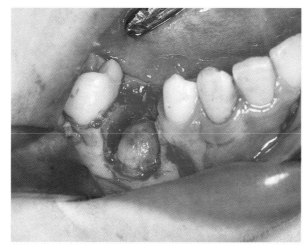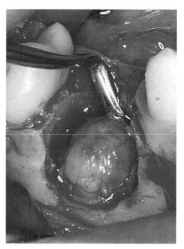

Removing the graft

The tooth germ is raised with two excavators placed below the proximal cervical areas. If resistance is met lingually, a periosteal elevator may guide the tooth in the labial direction.

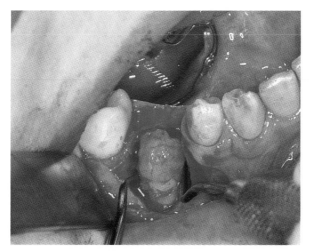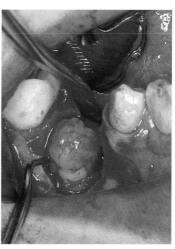

Removed graft

The graft shows an intact follicle. The flap is then repositioned and sutured.

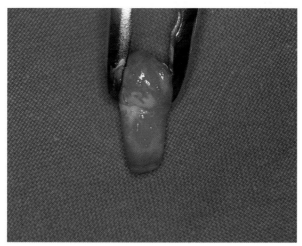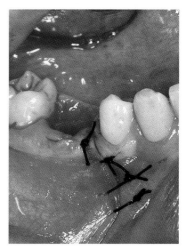

Fig. 5.11. Mandibular premolar graft removal

In this case an erupted mandibular premolar is removed for grafting.

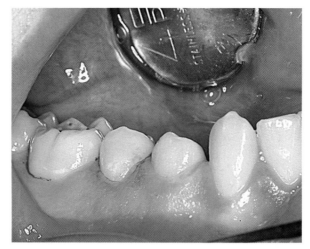
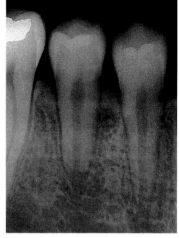

Incision of the PDL

A surgical blade no. 15 has been ground down to a narrow stylet which can sever the PDL to a depth of 4-8 mm (see Appendix 7, p. 296).

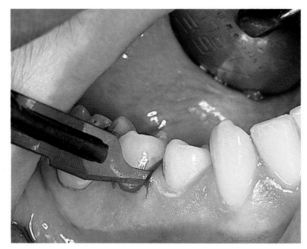
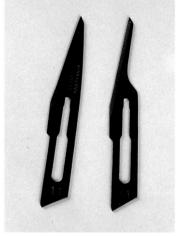

Extracting the graft

The tooth is extracted using slight rotating movements.

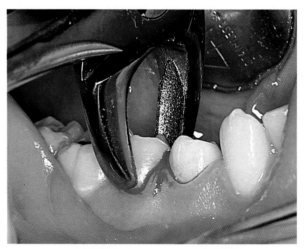
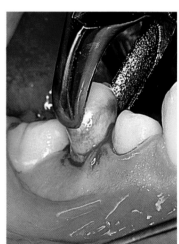

Inspecting the graft

The graft is inspected for defects in the PDL cover as well as the apical pulp.

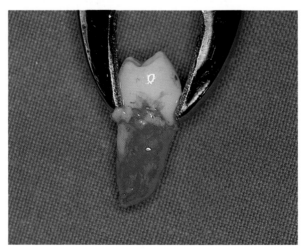

Fig. 5.12. Transplanting to the maxillary incisor region

The left central incisor has developed extensive root resorption after trauma. Transplantation of a maxillary second premolar was therefore indicated.

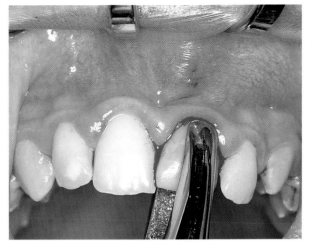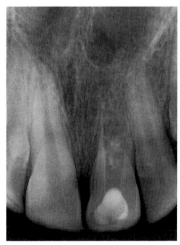

Raising a flap and osteotomy

In this case where space conditions do not allow rotation of the graft, it is necessary to expand the labiolingual dimension of the socket by removing and replanting the labial socket wall. A rhomboid flap is raised which should not interfere with the proximal gingiva. Thereafter two cuts are made with a thin surgical bur through the labial bone plate mesial and distal to the potential socket. A stop cut is then placed apically, corresponding to the position of the root apex of the transplant.

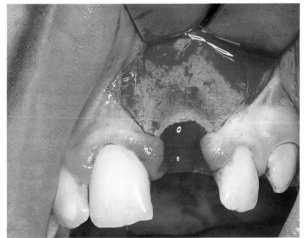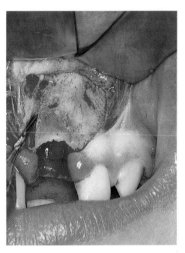

Removing the bone plate

The entire labial bone plate can be removed with a chisel (see Appendix 7, p. 296). The bone plate is then placed in physiologic saline.

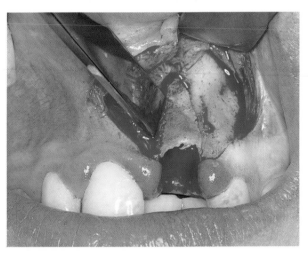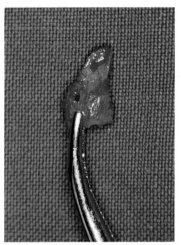

Preparing the socket

The socket is enlarged using a bur with internal cooling (see Appendix 7, p. 296). It is essential that the bone septum against the adjacent teeth has a minimum thickness of 1 mm in order not to jeopardize the vitality of this structure.

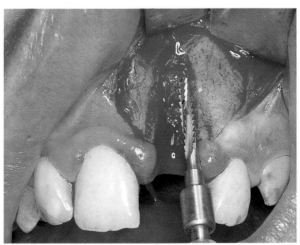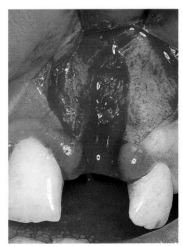

Fig. 5.12. Continued.

Removing the graft

The graft is half erupted. The PDL is therefore incised as high up as possible with a stylet in order to sever the new fiber insertions (see Appendix 7, p. 296). The tooth is then extracted with forceps.

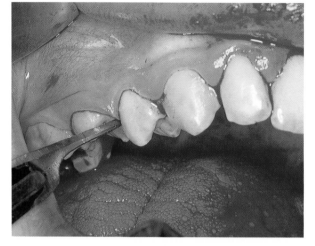 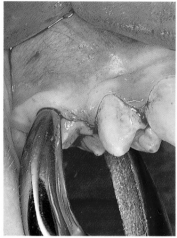

Positioning the graft

The graft is tested in its new position and fastened to the palatal gingiva by a cervical suture.

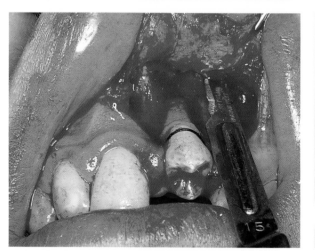 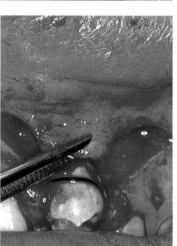

Testing the labial flap

The labial flap is repositioned. If correct positioning causes any tension, it is necessary to elongate the flap. Because of its rhomboid shape, there is no problem in moving the flap coronally. The periosteal fibers are transected with a surgical blade no 11. (see Appendix 7, p. 296) at the base of the flap, allowing elongation of the flap.

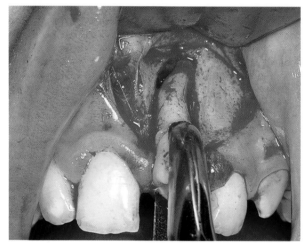 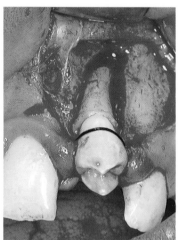

Replanting the bone plate

The labial bone plate, which has been stored in physiologic saline, is cut lengthwise with heavy scissors and placed with its cortical surface against the root, covering the labial surface. Cortical and not cancellous bone is placed against the root surface so that minimal osteogenic bone contacts the root surface in order to prevent ankylosis. Sectioning the bone plate facilitates revascularization of the PDL labially.

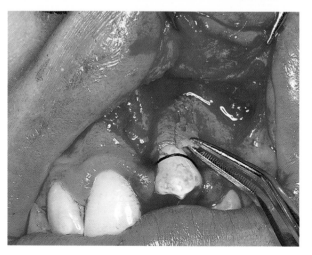 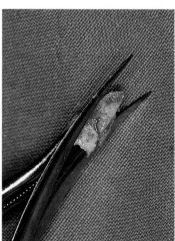

Fig. 5.12. Continued.

Repositioning the flap
The flap is repositioned and two sutures are placed at the gingival margin mesially and distally. The remaining incision is then closed with sutures.

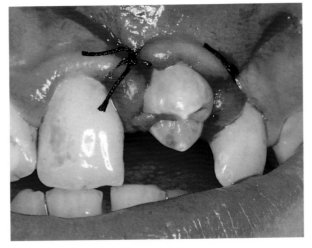 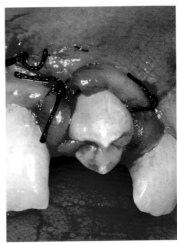

Splinting
A thin 0.2 mm wire is twisted around the central incisor, traversing the occlusal surface of the graft and anchored around the lateral incisor. To prevent apical movement, the wire is fastened to the labial surface of the two incisors with composite resin using an acid-etch technique.

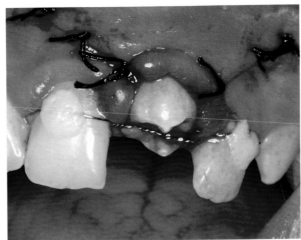 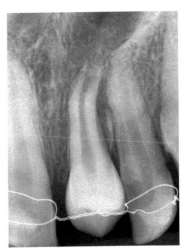

Follow-up
The transplanted tooth responds to sensibillity testing at the 6 months, control.

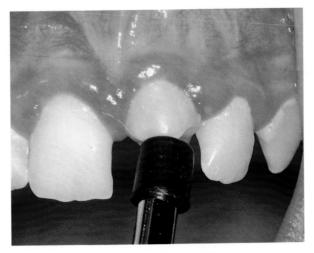 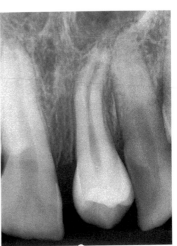

Orthodontic movement
The tooth is rotated 45⁰ in order to increase the mesiodistal dimension at the graft.

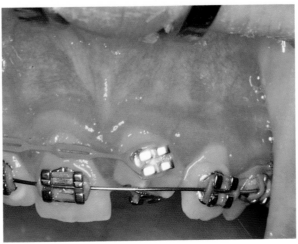 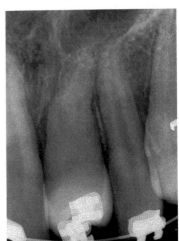

Fig. 5.13. Multiple incisor loss and alveolar atrophy treated by premolar transplantation

This 11-year-old boy had had four incisors avulsed 1 year previously. The patient had a class I malocclusion whereby two first mandibular premolars could be used as lateral incisor replacements. Two maxillary second premolars were then used as central incisors.

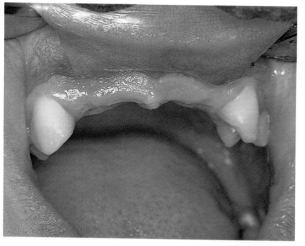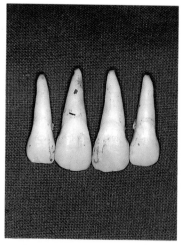

Preparing the socket in the lateral incisor region

The outline of the socket is demarcated with a 6-mm punch biopsy instrument. Thereafter an alveolus is created with a bur with internal cooling (see Appendix 7, p. 296).

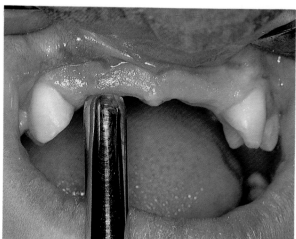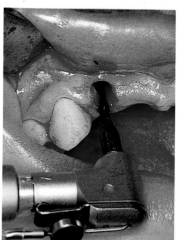

Transplanting to the lateral incisor region

The two mandibular premolars are transplanted to the lateral incisor region and splinted with sutures.

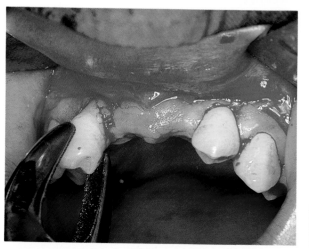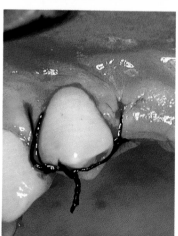

Transplanting to the central incisor region

Four months later, two maxillary second premolars are transplanted. Due to marked atrophy of the labial bone, an open procedure is used with removal and replantation of the labial bone plate.

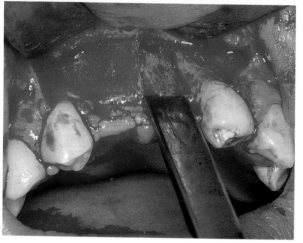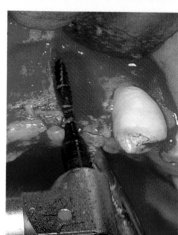

Fig. 5.13. Continued.

Positioning and splinting

The second premolars are fastened with a cervical suture. The previously removed cortical bone is used to cover the labial aspects of the roots.

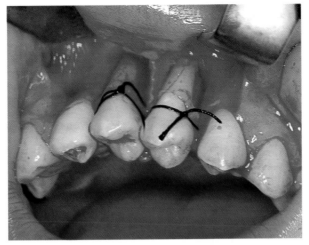
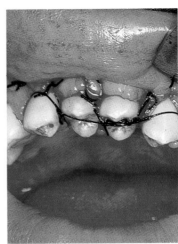

Analyzing the graft before restoration

A labial and axial evaluation of the graft reveals that the labial cusps of the "lateral incisors" must be reduced, as well as the lingual cusps of the "central incisors."

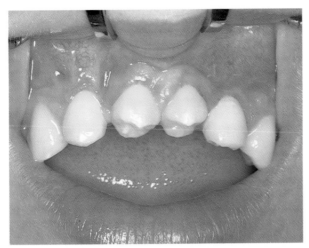
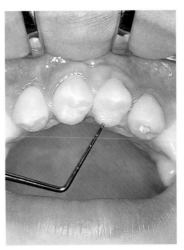

Restoring the transplanted teeth

The transplanted premolars are restored. In this case it was not necessary to expose dentin.

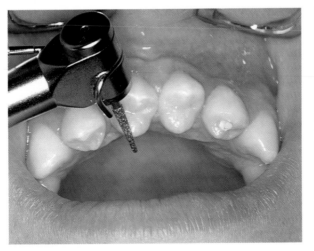
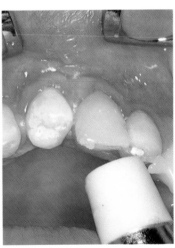

Condition after restoration

Six months after transplantation, the "incisors" were restored with composite resin. Details of the restorative technique are described in Chapter 11, p. 280. From Andreasen & al., 1989.[48]

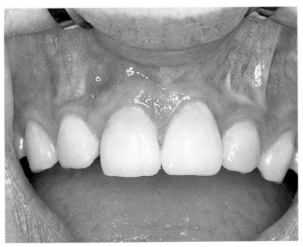
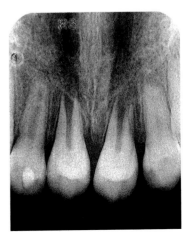

Fig. 5.14 Palatal tilting of a maxillary graft

Due to the extension of the sinus, normal positioning of a premolar graft is not possible.

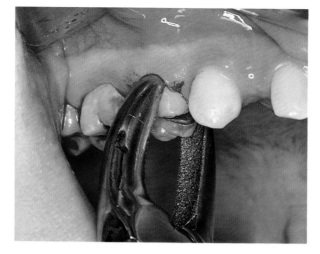 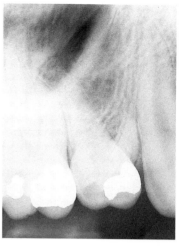

Preparation of the socket

The preparation of the new socket follows the outline of that part of the existing socket which was occupied by the palatal root of the primary molar.

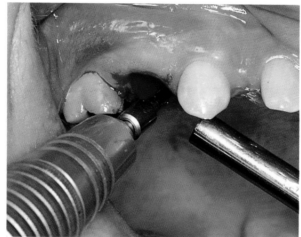 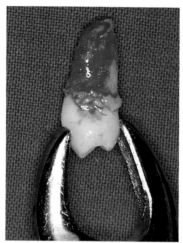

Positioning of the graft

The graft is positioned in the enlarged palatal socket.

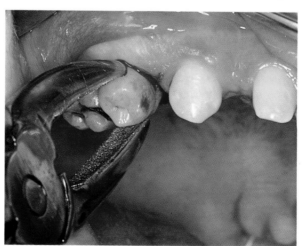 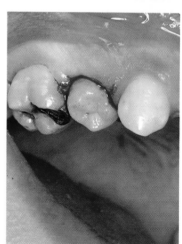

Splinting

A suture is placed across the occlusal surface to prevent extrusion (See also Fig. 5.16).

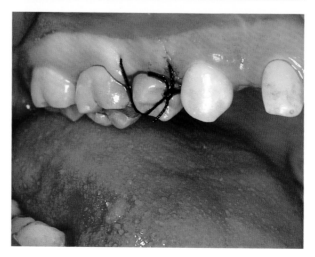 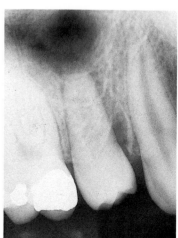

Special cases

Transplantation to a site with labio-lingual bone atrophy

In cases where there is atrophy of the alveolar process, it is usually necessary either to rotate the premolar 90° or to expand the socket area. The alveolar process can be expanded either by fracturing the labial bone lamella or by temporarily removing the bone and later replacing it (Figs. 5.12 and 5.13). In the first instance, two vertical cuts are made with a thin surgical bur placed within the socket and drilling through the bone mesially and distally according to the size of the root of the potential transplant. A suitable instrument (e.g., needle holder) is then placed in the socket and the labial bone wall fractured thereby gaining approximately 2-3 mm (see Chapter 6, p. 193). If more space is needed, it is necessary to remove the entire labial wall by raising a mucoperiosteal flap and then temporarily removing the labial bone plate while the new socket is prepared. The bone plate is then replanted once the graft has been positioned. This technique is shown in Figs. 5.12 and 5.13.

Transplantation to the maxillary anterior region (Figs. 5.12 and 5.13)

If a maxillary central incisor is to be replaced, it is important to first consider the indication for transplantation (see Chapter 10, p. 267) and if decided upon, to evaluate the size of the potential transplant.[48-51] The mandibular premolars will usually fit into the maxillary anterior region after only minor adjustments, whereas maxillary premolars will usually require surgical alterations in the socket area, including expansion of the socket. Irrespective of the potential transplant, occlusion should be considered. In the case of mandibular premolars, occlusal interference is generally not a problem, regardless of the position of the future transplant, whether placed normally or rotated. In the case of maxillary premolar transplants, occlusal considerations are decisive. If a maxillary second premolar is to be used and one wishes to increase the mesiodistal aspect of the transplant, rotation of 45° or 90° can be desirable. The socket should then be enlarged to accommodate the root. If this is not possible, a labial flap can be raised and the bone plate removed as described earlier. Thereafter the new socket is prepared and the labial socket wall repositioned after splitting it lengthwise with heavy scissors or rongeurs.

In the case of maxillary lateral incisor replacements, the mandibular first premolars are ideal, and it is usually possible to place the transplant within the alveolar process without removing the labial bone plate (Fig. 5.13).

Transplantation to the maxillary premolar region

A frequent obstacle to transplantation in the maxilla is a large sinus extension. In these cases, it is important to measure the length of the potential transplant with respect to the distance available in the maxilla from the bottom of the sinus to the level of marginal bone. In some cases, it is possible to choose the stage of transplantation which allows the tooth to be placed in the maxilla without interference with the sinus. However, in most cases, the length of the potential transplant will exceed the space available. Two possibilities exist to circumvent this problem (Fig. 5.15). The tooth can be tilted either palatally or buccally. Selection of the tilting direction depends upon regional anatomy; thus if the sinus bulges buccally, the tooth is tilted palatally and vice versa. The tooth´s position can be corrected later orthodontically if necessary.

Palatal or buccal tilting of the graft (Fig. 5.15)

With palatal tilting preparation of the socket should follow the direction of the palatal root of the primary molar. In this direction there is enough room for the new socket (Fig. 5.14). In the case of buccal tilting preparation of the socket implies perforation of the cortical bone plate. However, this approach should only be used if there is a minor discrepancy between the length of the root and the distance available to the sinus. In most instances, it is advantageous to raise a mucoperiosteal flap buccally and remove the labial bone plate and then prepare the new socket. When the graft has been positioned the bone plate is replaced.

Surgical repositioning of ectopic premolars (Fig. 5.16)

In these cases, which are most often seen in the mandible, radiographic verification of the graft position is essential. The usual position of both mandibular and maxillary premolars is lingual, which again dictates the direction of the surgical approach level. After surgical exposure the tooth is repositioned to a position which is equivalent to its stage of development.

Fig. 5.15. Palatal or buccal tilting of a graft in order to avoid the sinus.

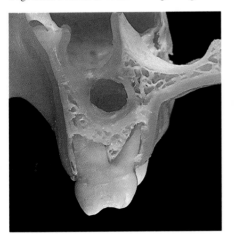
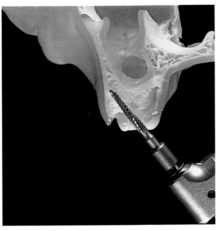
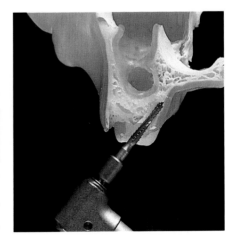

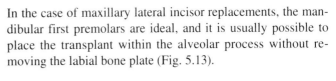

Fig. 5.16. Repositioning of an ectopic mandibular premolar

In this case, an ectopically placed second premolar is surgically repositioned. The radiographic examination reveals the lingual position of the graft.

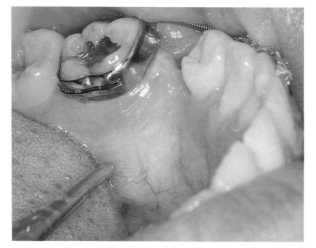

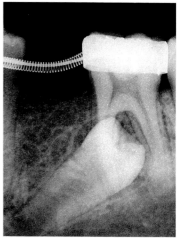

Raising a flap

A lingual flap extends from the lateral incisor to the second molar region. The second primary molar is extracted. A broad wound retractor (see Appendix 7, p. 296) is inserted as far apically as possible. A bulge in the bony contour is usually seen corresponding to the crown of the tooth.

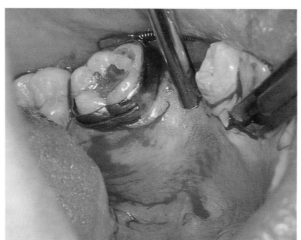

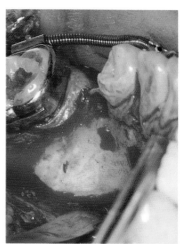

Uncovering the graft

The occlusal surface of the impacted tooth is now exposed with chisels or burs. If the tooth is not placed very superficially, it is usually necessary, as in this case, to remove the lingual bone plate from the cervical margin to the occlusal surface of the ectopic premolar in order to visualize the graft.

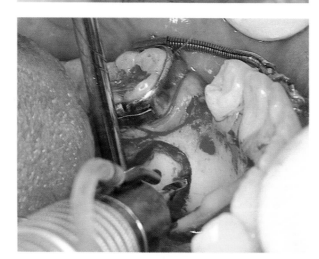

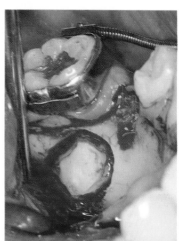

Loosening the follicle

If the crown is tilted towards the base of the mandible, it is necessary to remove considerably more bone lingually and apically in order to allow the tooth to be removed. The follicle is loosened with an amalgam carver and the graft loosened with an excavator.

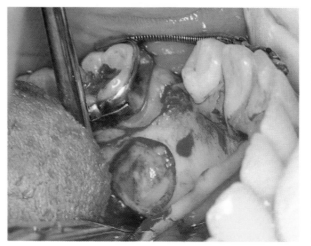

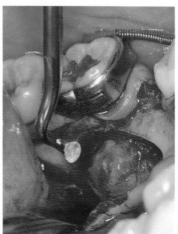

Fig. 5.16. Continued.

Removal of the graft
The graft is loosened with a thin, slightly angled periosteal elevator placed below the exposed crown. The graft can then be lifted out of the socket with forceps.

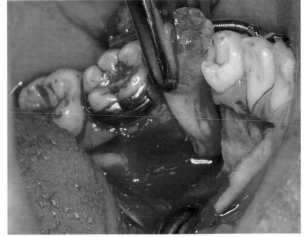 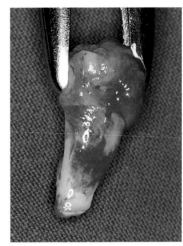

Preparing the new socket
The new socket is prepared preferably with a bur with internal cooling. The socket will usually lack the lingual bone plate due to graft removal.

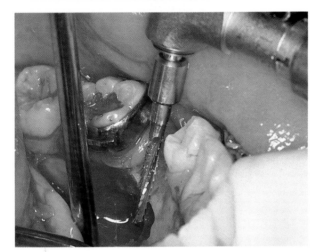 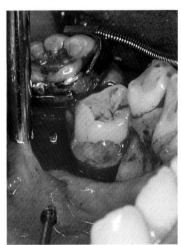

Positioning of the graft
After removal, the tooth is transplanted to a position which is equivalent to its stage of root development. If there are parts of the follicle covering the crown which are missing it is important that this portion is not placed below bone level because of the risk of ankylosis. The flap is then repositioned and sutured.

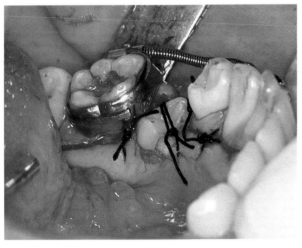 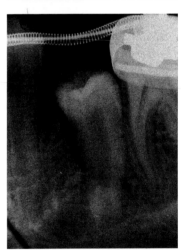

Follow-up
The tooth has begun to erupt 1 month after surgery.

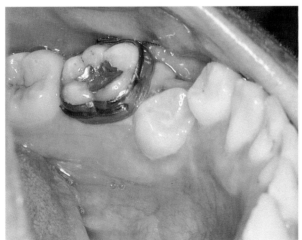 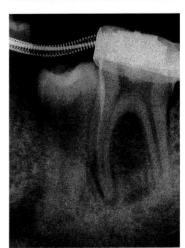

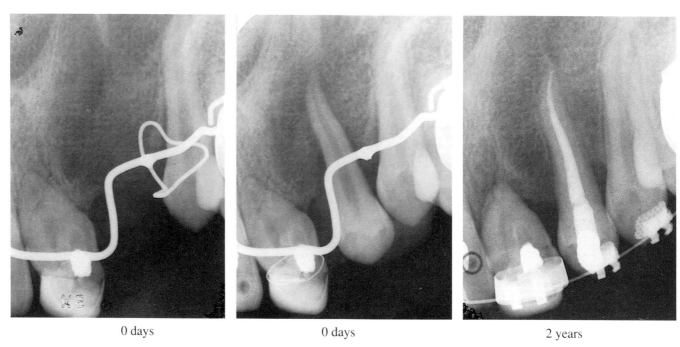

| 0 days | 0 days | 2 years |

Fig. 5.17. A cleft palate patient treated by transplantation of a mandibular second premolar to the bone graft site. From Hillerup & al., 1987.[54]

Cleft palate cases

Recently secondary grafting of iliac bone has become a common procedure.[54] If the canine is present at the cleft site it will normally erupt through the grafted bone. If teeth are missing in the cleft area premolars can be succesfully transplanted to the region. Apparently the grafted bone responds to the tooth graft as normal alveolar bone (Fig. 5.17).[54] However, a recent experimental study indicates that an interim period of at least 4 months should elapse before tooth transplantation in order to limit the risk of root resorption.[55,56]

Splinting types

There is experimental evidence that firm splinting does not promote either pulpal or periodontal healing. In most premolar transplantations, a suture splint provides sufficient stabilization in the initial healing period. When a premolar is rotated 45[0], a suture from the buccal to the lingual gingiva and retained in the central fissure is sufficient for splinting. If the premolar is not rotated, a figure-of-eight suture should be used. If there is a tendency to displacement, more stable splinting can be achieved with an occlusal 0.2 mm wire in a figure-of-eight application (Fig. 5.18), or an acid-etch splint can be used.

Fig. 5.18. When there is a tendency for displacement e.g. when the labial bone plate has been removed and replaced, an occlusal 0.2 mm wire fastened to the adjacent teeth and transversing the occlusal surface can stabilize the transplant and still allow a minimum of mobility. To prevent the wire from moving coronally the position can be ensured by application of composite resin after etching. If there is need for greater stability, a conventional acid-etch/composite splint can be used.

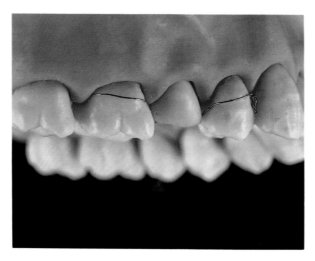

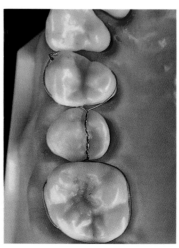

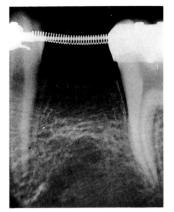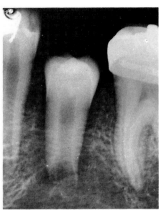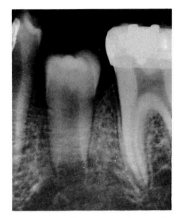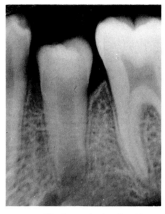

Fig. 5.19. Radiographic progression of PDL healing after transplantation of a maxillary second premolar to a mandibular aplasia site. From Andreasen & al., 1990.[46]

Postoperative follow-up

Sutures should be removed 1 week after transplantation. In the case of transplantation of premolars with completed root formation, endodontic therapy is initiated 3 weeks after transplantation, at which time the transplant is reasonably consolidated in its socket.

PDL healing

PDL healing evidenced by reformation of lamina dura is seen in isolated areas around the root after 1 month and is usually complete after 2 months (Fig. 5.19).[11,46] If the transplant is placed next to the median suture, a delay in the reformation of the lamina dura can be expected (Fig. 5.20).[46]

Pulpal sensibility

Pulpal sensibility can in rare cases be demonstrated after 1 month, but is usually found after 4 to 6 months.[44,45] However, later return of sensibility may occur (Figs. 5.21 and 5.22). It should be borne in mind that in some cases there is radiographic evidence of pulpal revascularization (pulp canal obliteration) whereas no sensibility reaction can be elicited. When the first response appears it is usually a lower response level than the nontransplanted contralateral antimere.[45]

Pulp necrosis

Pulp necrosis is usually diagnosed 4-8 weeks after transplantation based on the presence of a periapical rarefication and/or inflammatory root resorption.[46] The tooth usually shows tenderness to percussion and negative sensibility. The diagnostic value of the latter sign is limited, however, as it usually takes 4-6 months before sensibility returns in cases with pulpal healing (Fig. 5.22).[46] In cases of partial pulp necrosis the typical features are unchanged pulp canal dimensions, premature closure of the apical foramen, and periapical radiolucency (Fig. 5.23).

Pulp canal obliteration

Pulp canal obliteration can be seen after 2 months and is normally very prominent 6 months after transplantation, especially in the crown.[45] The process usually progresses to total pulp canal obliteration in the part of the pulp canal formed prior to transplantation (Fig. 5.23).[45]

Fig. 5.20. Delay in formation of a lamina dura due to interference with the median suture. From Andreasen & al., 1990.[46]

0 days	1 month	2 months	5 months

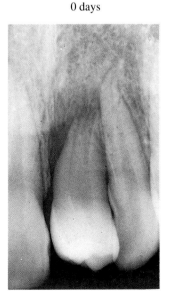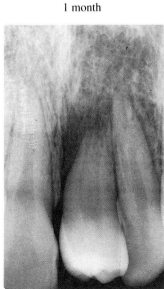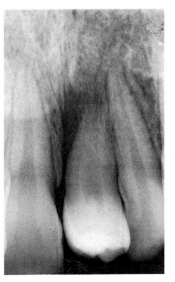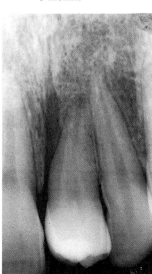

Fig. 5.21. Percentage of transplanted premolars reacting to sensibility
testing at varying observation periods after transplantation. From
Andreasen & al., 1991.[45]

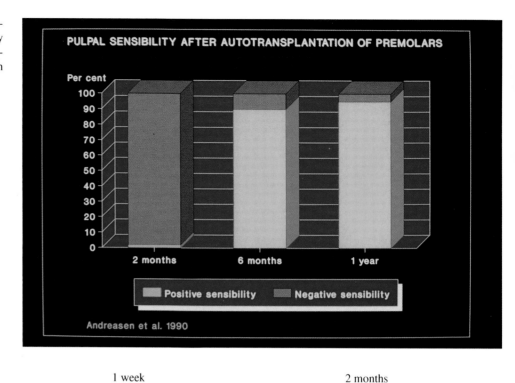

PULPAL SENSIBILITY AFTER AUTOTRANSPLANTATION OF PREMOLARS

Positive sensibility Negative sensibility

Andreasen et al. 1990

1 week   2 months

Fig. 5.22. Vital sensibility response
elicited 2 months after transplantation of a maxillary second premolar. From Andreasen & al., 1990.[45]

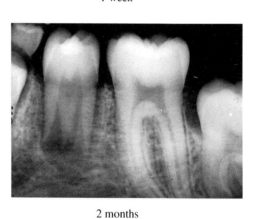

2 months   2 years

Fig. 5.23. Partial pulp necrosis after
transplantation of a maxillary
second premolar. Typical features
are unchanged pulp canal dimensions, premature closure of the
apical foramen, absent or limited
root growth, and periapical radiolucency. From Andreasen & al.,
1990.[45]

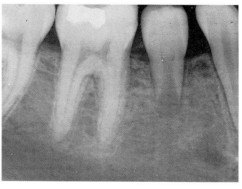

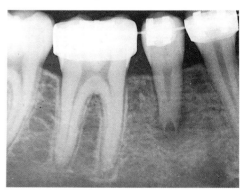

5 years   5 years

Fig. 5.24. Partial and total pulp
canal obliteration developed after
transplantation of two mandibular
second premolars (same patient).

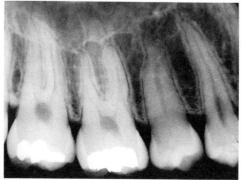

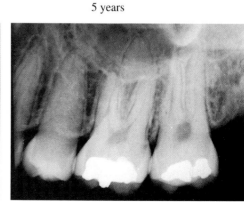

Fig. 5.25. Normal sensibility response and no sign of pulp canal obliteration in a maxillary second premolar transplanted to the mandibular region. Such a condition is rare. The homologous second premolar is shown on the right. From Andreasen & al., 1990.[45]

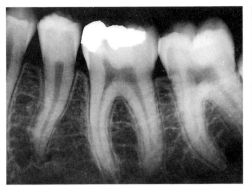

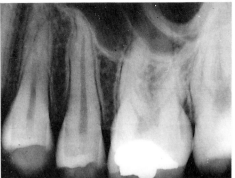

| 2 years | 3 years |

Pulp canal obliteration develops in almost all teeth with pulpal revascularization after transplantation (Fig. 5.25).[45] In rare cases secondary pulp necrosis may develop, which in most instances is related to untreated caries, extensive crown preparation (see Chapter 11, p. 279) or traumatic luxation injury (Fig. 5.26).[39,45]

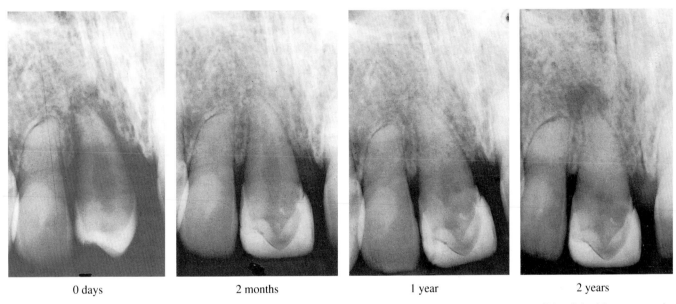

| 0 days | 2 months | 1 year | 2 years |

Fig. 5.26. Pulp canal obliteration with secondary pulp necrosis of a transplanted mandibular first premolar, possibly elicited by a traumatic injury sustained 2 years after transplantation. From Andreasen & al., 1990.[45]

Fig. 5.27. Surface resorption (arrow) subsequent to transplantation of a maxillary second premolar. The cause of resorption could be collision between the graft and the mesial socket wall cervically. From Andreasen & al., 1990.[46]

| 0 days | 6 months | 5 years |

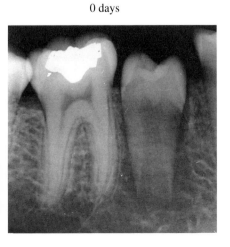

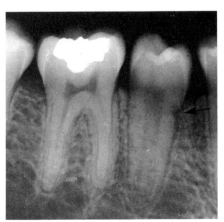

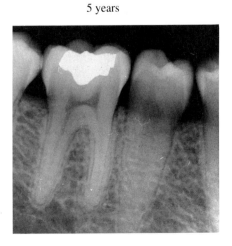

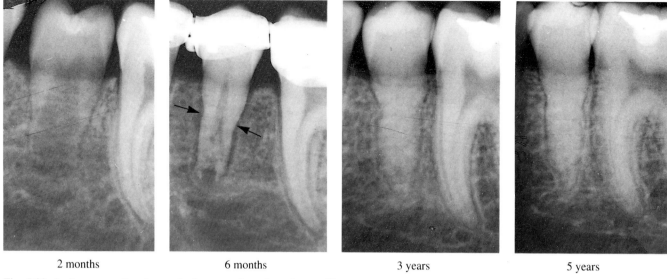

| 2 months | 6 months | 3 years | 5 years |

Fig. 5.28. Surface resorption (arrows) after transplantation of a maxillary second premolar. The cause of resorption is possibly orthodontic treatment of the transplanted tooth. From Andreasen & al., 1990.[46]

Root resorption

Root resorption can usually be diagnosed 1 to 6 months after transplantation[46] and may appear as surface resorption (Figs. 5.27 and 5.28), inflammatory resorption (Figs. 5.29 and 5.30), or replacement resorption (Fig. 5.31). The diagnostic features of these three resorption types are illustrated in Chapter 2.

If inflammatory resorption develops, it is very important to initiate endodontic therapy immediately in order to prevent progression of the resorption process[46] (Fig. 5.30).

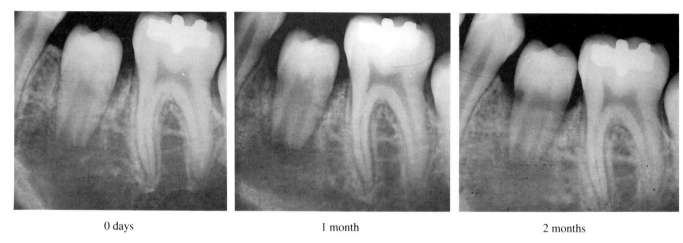

| 0 days | 1 month | 2 months |

Fig. 5.29. Inflammatory resorption after transplantation of a maxillary second premolar. Note the undermining nature of the resorption cavity and the associated breakdown of the lamina dura. From Andreasen & al., 1990.[46]

Fig. 5.30. Inflammatory resorption affecting the cervical area of a transplanted maxillary second premolar. Note that the buccally or lingually positioned resorption cavities show up as punched out radiolucencies (arrows). After extirpation of necrotic and infected pulp tissue and the use of a calcium hydroxide dressing, the resorptive process is arrested. From Andreasen & al., 1990.[46]

| 0 days | 3 months | 4 months |

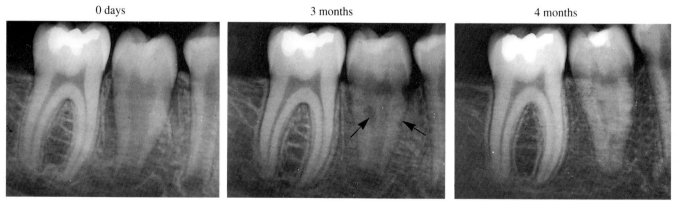

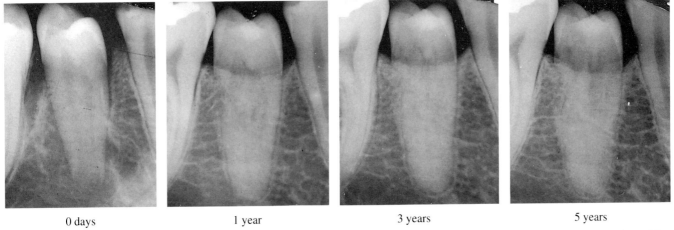

| 0 days | 1 year | 3 years | 5 years |

Fig. 5.31. Replacement resorption affecting the cervical area of a transplanted second maxillary premolar. Note the rapid progression of the resorption process and the infraposition of the transplant. From Andreasen & al., 1990.[46]

If replacement resorption develops, diagnosed clinically (hard metallic percussion tone) and/or radiographically, it is worthwhile to luxate and extrude the transplant (Fig. 5.32).[46] This procedure is described in Chapter 2, p. 87.

Root growth

Root growth can be demonstrated after 2 months and in some cases has been found to continue unimpeded after transplantation.[47] At the site where root formation begins after transplantation, a thickening of the root is often seen due to hyperactivity of the root sheath immediately after transplantation (Fig. 5.33).

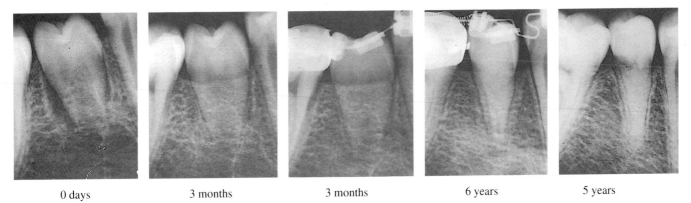

| 0 days | 3 months | 3 months | 6 years | 5 years |

Fig. 5.32. Replacement resorption of a transplanted second maxillary premolar successfully treated by luxation and immediate orthodontic extrusion of the infrapositioned tooth. From Andreasen & al., 1990.[46]

Fig. 5.33. Normal root length subsequent to transplantation of a second mandibular premolar. Note the slight cementum hyperplasia (arrows) developed after transplantation. From Andreasen & al., 1990.[47]

| 0 days | 2 months | 1 year | 2 years |

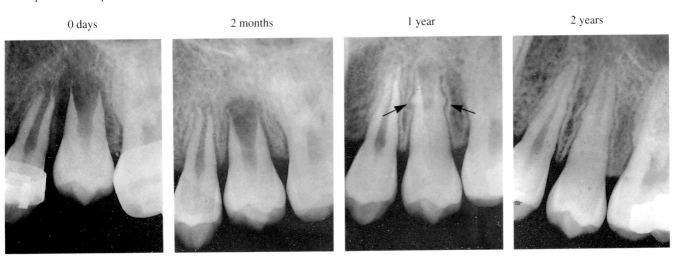

Fig. 5.34. Comparison of root growth between transplant and control
Preoperative radiographs. The ectopically positioned left second premolar was transplanted to an upright position.

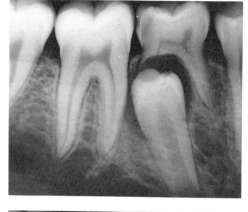 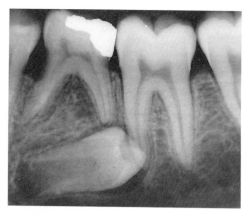

Condition after 1 year
The right second premolar has not yet achieved completed root development.

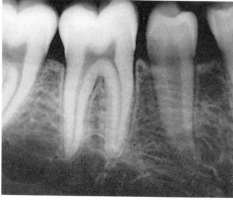 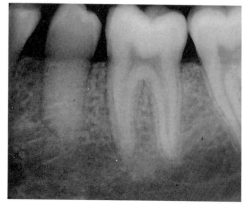

Condition after 2 years
There is a slightly reduced root length of the transplanted premolar compared to its homologous control. From Andreasen & al., 1990.[47]

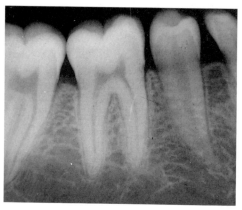 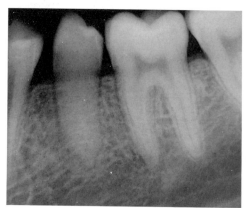

Root growth of a transplanted molar is in some cases very similar to that of a nontransplanted molar (Fig. 5.34). However, there is usually a certain reduction in the antici- pated root growth and sometimes complete arrest.[34,39,47] (Fig. 5.35)

Fig. 5.35. Complete arrest of root formation after transplantation of a second maxillary premolar. Despite the very short root, the tooth shows only slight loosening and the situation has been stable over a 10-year period. From Andreasen & al., 1990.[47]

| 2 months | 2 years | 5 years | 10 years |

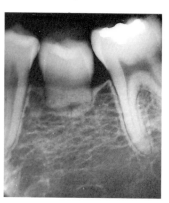 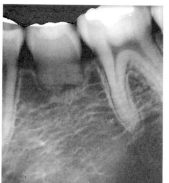 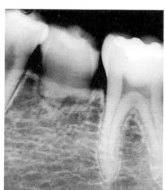

Fig. 5.36. Effect of loss of Hertwig´s epithelial root sheath

Condition immediately after transplantation of a second maxillary premolar to an aplasia site in the mandible.

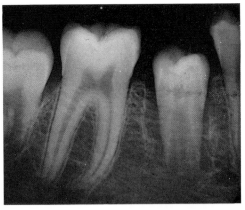
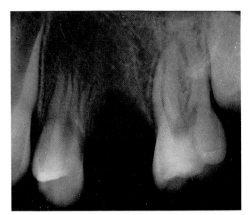

Condition after 1 year

Complete arrest of root formation after transplantation of a maxillary second premolar. A radiograph of the donor site reveals the formation of a root tip, presumably a result of the remnant of Hertwig's epithelial root sheath. From Andreasen & al., 1990.[47]

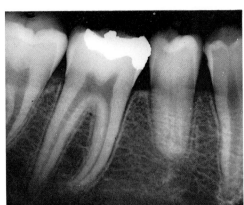
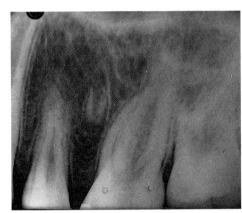

In the latter cases the explanation is usually that the Hertwig´s epithelial root sheath has been torn and left at the graft site (Fig. 5.36).[47] At later follow-up the formation of a new root apex can be demonstrated at the donor site. In cases where a complete arrest of root formation occurs the usual response of the periodontium is ingrowth of bone and PDL into the pulp chamber, forming an internal PDL.

Orthodontic movement is sometimes necessary to adjust the transplants orthodontically, especially in the case of rotated premolars. In these cases, it is possible to use light forces 3 months after transplantation, at which time revascularization of the pulp is optimal. If possible, orthodontic treatment of the transplant should be completed within 6 months after transplantation, when pulp canal obliteration becomes very prominent.

Restoration of transplanted teeth can be performed 3-6 months after surgery. Concerning the restorative technique, see Chapter 11, p. 278.

Prognosis

The results of premolar transplantation have been demonstrated in a number of case reports[12-29,48-53] as well as several clinical studies on the long-term prognosis 10 to 20 years after premolar transplantation (Table 5.1).[32-47] It appears from these studies that premolar transplantations have a very good long-term prognosis, especially if performed at the proper stage of root development.

In the following, the frequency of various complications will be described as well as their relation to various clinical factors.

Table 5.1. Long-term results of autotransplantation of premolars

	Observation period yr (mean)	Age of patients yr (mean)	Number of teeth	Tooth survival %	PDL healing %	Pulp healing Sensibility %	Canal obliteration %	Gingival healing %
Slagsvold & Bjercke, 1974[34],1978[35]	3-13 (6.2)	8-19 (11.8)	34	100	94		100	
Kristerson, 1985[39]	1-18 (6.3)	10-58 (6.3)	82*	96	89	70	87	
			18*	78	50	6	6	
Andreasen & al., 1990[44-47]	5	9-31	317*	95	90	96		99
			53**	98	60	15		99

* Incomplete root formation
** Complete root formation

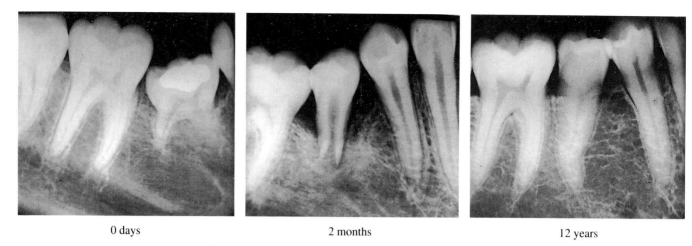

| 0 days | 2 months | 12 years |

Fig. 5.37. Long-term survival of a transplanted second maxillary premolar.

Fig. 5.38. Survival of 370 auto-transplanted premolars with different stages of root development at the time of surgery. From Andreasen & al., 1990.[44]

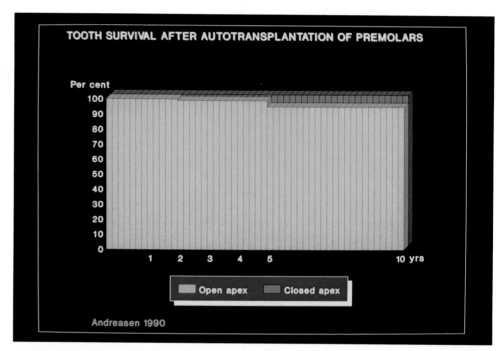

Fig. 5.39. Pulpal healing of 370 autotransplanted premolars with different stages of root development at the time of surgery. From Andreasen & al., 1991.[45]

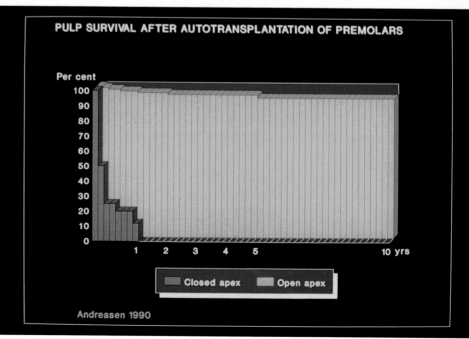

Fig. 5.40. PDL healing of 370 autotransplanted premolars with different stages of root development at the time of surgery. From Andreasen & al., 1990.[46]

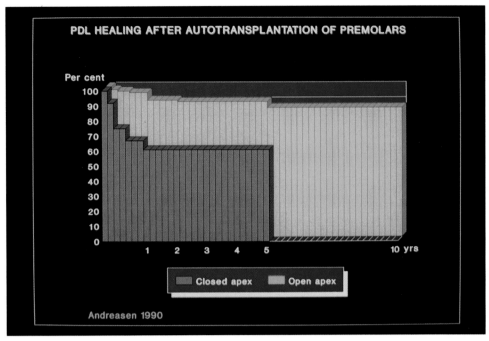

Tooth survival

The results from various clinical studies appear in Table 5.1. In the author's material, a 5-year survival rate of 95%-100 % was found according to stage of root formation at the time of transplantation (Fig. 5.37).[44] When transplants are lost it usually occurs 3-5 years after transplantation and is normally caused by the progression of ankylosis.

Pulpal healing and pulp necrosis

The risk of pulp necrosis is very closely related to the stage of root development at the time of transplantation (Fig. 5.39).[45] Thus transplantation of teeth with almost mature or mature root development is followed by a considerable risk of pulp necrosis (Fig. 5.39).[45] In a multivariate statistical analysis, the only clinical factor that appeared to influence revascularization was the stage of root development. With regard to ensuring pulpal revascularization, transplantation should not be performed later than stage 4 (full root length and wide open apical foramen). If endodontics is performed immediately after transplantation, the tooth can be transplanted at stage 6. Due to the wide root canal, which may lead to endodontic problems if revascularization does not occur, teeth in stage 5 should not be transplanted (Fig. 5.46).

PDL healing and root resorption

Root resorption is a rare complication after premolar transplantation, especially when teeth are transplanted with incomplete root formation. In a statistical analysis of the influence of various clinical factors upon the development of root resorption, it was found that both stage of root development and position of the graft (unerupted, impacted, semierupted, or erupted) were closely related to the risk of root resorption.[46] Due to the close association between these two factors, both of them were generally good in predicting root resorption. It appears from Fig. 5.40 that the risk of complicating root resorption increases with completion of root development.

Root development and developmental disturbances

A close correlation between the length of the transplanted tooth and the contralateral nonoperated premolar has also been found, indicating that the growth potential of a tooth has a strong capacity to express itself and that genetics controls root growth to a great extent[47] (Fig. 5.41).

Fig. 5.41. Root growth is to a large extent genetically determined. The graph shows the difference in tooth length of 20 homologous premolars compared to 20 randomly chosen premolars. From Andreasen & al., 1990.[47]

Comparison of actual and radiographic tooth length of 21 paired (homologous) premolars.

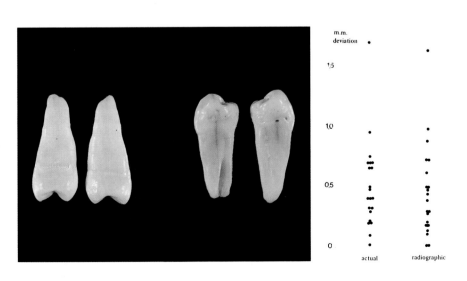

Fig. 5.42. Normal root growth
Identical root growth is found in a transplanted and a nontransplanted second premolar. From Andreasen & al., 1990.[47]

0 days

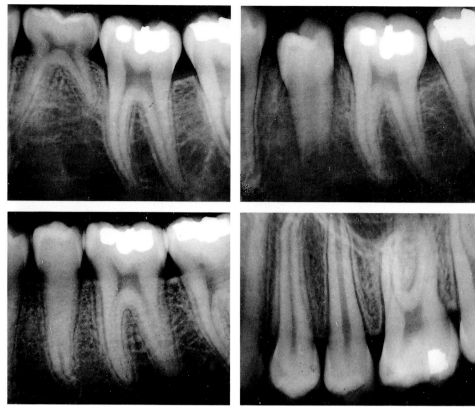

2 years

Root growth after autotransplantation has been studied in various longitudinal studies. It has been found that transplanted teeth usually show radiographic evidence of diminished root development. Thus, in comparison with contralateral nontransplanted teeth, the transplanted teeth have been found on average to be 1 to 3 mm shorter. An ectopic position of the graft before transplantation appears to be related to a significant risk of reduced root growth after transplantation (Fig. 5.43).

Finally, it has been found that there is a close correlation between final tooth length and tooth length at the time of transplantation (Fig. 5.44).

Fig. 5.43. Reduced root growth
Slightly reduced root formation of a transplanted ectopic second premolar compared to the non-transplanted contralateral premolar. From Andreasen & al., 1990.[47]

0 days

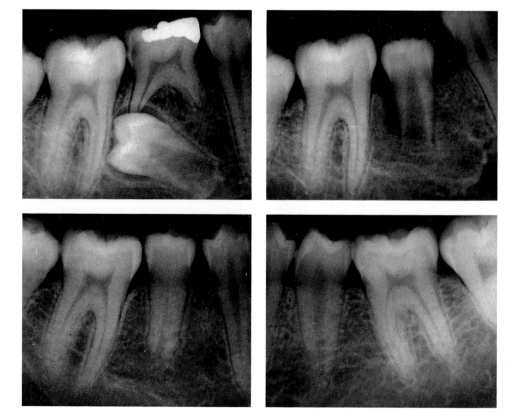

5 years

Fig. 5.44 Root growth after transplantation (black part of the bars) related to stage of root development at the time of surgery. From Andreasen & al., 1990.[47]

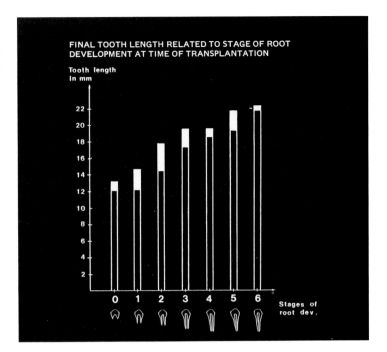

A reasonable goal for transplantation could be that the premolar transplant should attain at least two-thirds of the expected root length, amounting to about 10 mm root support. If this goal is pursued, it appears that the transplantation should generally be performed with approximately two-thirds root formation (Figs. 5.44 and 5.46).

Gingival healing and marginal attachment loss

As suggested by Table 5.1, loss of marginal attachment is a very rare complication. It is usually caused by a too superficial placement of the graft in the socket or food impaction in the proximal areas after surgery (Fig. 5.45).

Fig. 5.45. Loss of marginal attachment after transplantation of a maxillary second premolar. From Andreasen & al., 1990.[46]

| 0 days | 0 days | 2 years |

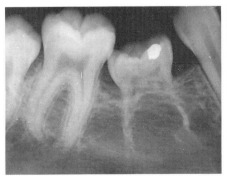
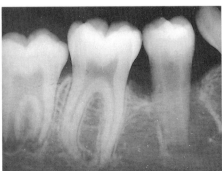
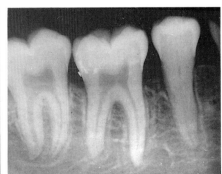

Healing related to graft selection

It appears from the above-mentioned survey of the various complications that they are very closely related to root development. With the goal of obtaining a graft with a maximum chance of periodontal and pulpal healing and reasonable root length (e.g., above 17 mm) it seems appropriate to choose teeth in stages 3 or 4 (i.e., 3/4 or 4/4 root formation with a wide open apex) (Fig. 5.46). If the graft has already passed that stage it is advisable to wait until stage 6 (root formation complete, apex closed) and then undertake endodontic therapy after transplantation. This will ensure a reasonably good prognosis. Due to the root canal anatomy, first maxillary premolars should generally not be used.

Fig. 5.46. Graft selection
Pulpal and periodontal healing and root growth after transplantation related to stage of root development at the time of grafting. It appears that 3/4 to full root length with open apices offers optimal healing results when all healing parameters have been considered. From Andreasen & al., 1990.[47]

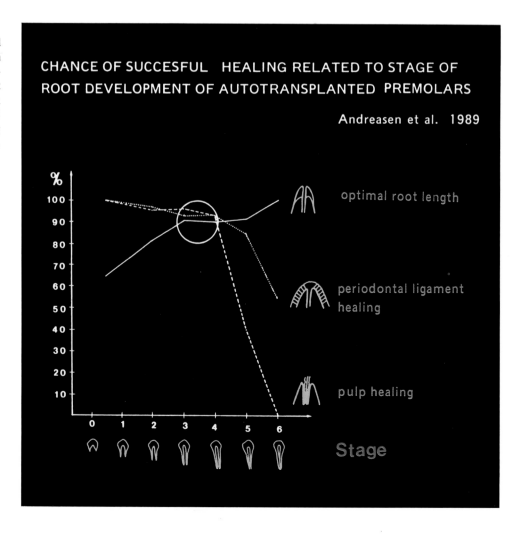

172

Essentials

Indications

Aplasia of premolars
Ectopia or impaction of premolars
Congenital or accidental loss of anterior teeth

Treatment planning

Preoperative radiographs
Space evaluation

Surgical procedure

1. Administer local anesthesia and antibiotics
2. Extraction of primary molars
3. Prepare the socket
4. Remove the transplant atraumatically
5. Place the transplant within the confines of the socket whenever possible. If there are space problems, rotate the transplant, fracture or transplant the labial bone lamella
6. If there are problems with the sinus extension, tilt the transplant buccally or palatally or displace the sinus mucosa
7. Place a suture splint
8. Take a postoperative radiograph

Follow-up

See Appendix 2, p. 290

Prognosis

Tooth survival (5 years)

Incomplete root formation	95%
Complete root formation	100%

Pulpal healing (5 years)

Incomplete root formation	94%
Complete root formation	12%

PDL healing (5 years)

Incomplete root formation	86%
Complete root formation	62%

References

1. Rølling S. Hypodontia of permanent teeth in Danish school-children. Scand J Dent Res 1980 ; 88 : 365-69.

2. Mead SV. Incidence of impacted teeth. Int J Orthod Oral Surg Radiogr 1930; 16: 885-93.

3. Sinkovits V, Polczer MG. Die Häufigkeit retinierter Zahne. Dtsch Zahnärztl Z 1964; 19: 389-96.

4. Tränkmann J. Häufigkeit retinierter Zähne der zweiten Dentition. Dtsch Zahnärztl Z 1973; 28: 415-20.

5. Andreasen JO, Ravn JJ. Epidemiology of traumatic dental injuries to primary and permanent teeth in a Danish population sample. Int J Oral Surg 1972; 1: 235-39.

6. Grahnén H. Hypodontia in the permanent dentition. A clinical and genetical investigation. Odont Rev 1956; Suppl. 3:1-100.

7. Lutz B. Untersuchungen über den Verzeichnisfaktor bei der enoralen röntgenologischen Darstellung Seitzahngebietes. Dtsch Stomatol 1969; 19: 767-75.

8. Hjortdal O, Bragelien J. Induksjon av kjevekamvekst ved hjelp av autotransplantat-sjon av tannanlegg. Nor Tannlægeforen Tid 1978; 88: 319-22.

9. Nordenram Å, Strömberg C. Positional relationships of the retained premolar. Acta Odontol Scand 1968; 26: 177-83.

l0. Bjerke B. Autotransplantasjon av tenner på barn. In: Hjørting-Hansen E, ed. Odontologi. Copenhagen: Munksgards Forlag, 1979: 7-25.

11. Andreasen JO, Paulsen HU. A comparison of damage to the Hertwig's epithelial root sheath using various extraction techniques 1990. In preparation.

12. Archer WH. Replantation of an accidentally extracted erupted partially formed mandibular second premolar. Report of a case. Oral Surg Oral Med Oral Pathol 1952; 5: 256-58.

13. Biederman W. Conserving impacted teeth. NY State Dent J 1965; 18: 57-66.

14. Collins GJ. Reimplantation of a tooth. Oral Surg Oral Med Oral Pathol 1955; 8: 44-46.

15. Henry CB. Examples of reimplantation of teeth in young subjects. Proc R Soc Med 1955; 48: 35-44.

16. Holland DJ. A technique of surgical orthodontics. Am J Orthod 1955; 41: 27-44.

17. Serling L. Surgical repositioning of an impacted mandibular bicuspid. J Am Dent Assoc 1959; 59: 553-54.

18. Hühne S. Zahnkeimtransplantationen bei Kindern. Dtsch Stomatol 1961; 11: 304-09.

19. Cook RM, Girt S. Transplant of left bicuspid to right side: Case report. J Am Dent Assoc 1962; 64: 723-24.

20. Reding JF, Ritchie DJ. Surgical removal of an unerupted second premolar and its transplantation into an artificially created socket in the dental arch. Aust Dent J 1962; 7: 457-59.

21. Mead KT, Monsen RM. Surgical repositioning of developing impacted teeth. J Am Dent Assoc 1965; 71: 621-25.

22. Tomlin AJ. Reimplantation of four impacted second premolars. Report of a case. Oral Surg Oral Med Oral Pathol 1966; 21: 286-93.

23. Anthony AJ. Vital tooth transplant into a surgically created socket. Oral Surg Oral Med Oral Pathol 1969; 27: 293-96.

24. Dixon DA. Autogenous transplantation of tooth germs into the upper incisor region. Br Dent J 1971; 131: 260-65.

25. Stewart RE, Merrill R, Porter DR. Unusual sequelae to surgical repositioning of an impacted premolar. Oral Surg Oral Med Oral Pathol 1974; 37: 688-91.

26. Dixon DA. The transplantation and surgical movement of developing teeth. Int Dent J 1975; 25: 46-52.

27. Brady J. Transplantation of a premolar to replace a central incisor with advanced resorption. J Dent 1978; 6: 259-60.

28. Shulman LB. Impacted and unerupted teeth: Donors for transplant tooth replacement. Dent Clin North Am 1979; 23: 369-83.

29. Northway WM, Konigsberg S. Autogenic tooth transplantation: "The state of the art". Am J Orthod 1980; 77: 146-62.

30. Smith GN, Adams RW, Smith SA. Premolar enucleation and autogenous transplantation. J Am Dent Assoc 1980; 101: 265-68

31. Azaz B, Steiman Z, Koyoumdjisky-Kaye E, Lewin-Epstein J. The sequelae of surgical exposure of unerupted teeth. J Oral Surg 1980; 38: 121-27.

32. Slagsvold O, Bjercke B. Autotransplantation av premolarer. Göteborgs Tandläkare-Sällskaps Årsbok 1967; No 351: 45-85.

33. Slagsvold O. Autotransplantation of premolars in cases of missing anterior teeth. Trans Eur Orthod Soc 1970; 66: 473-85.

34. Slagsvold O, Bjercke B. Autotransplantation of premolars with partly formed roots. A radiographic study of root growth. Am J Orthod 1974; 66: 355-66.

35. Slagsvold O, Bjercke B. Applicability of autotransplantation in cases of missing upper anterior teeth. Am J Orthod 1978; 74: 410-21.

36. Slagsvold O, Bjercke B. Indications for autotransplantation in cases of missing premolars. Am J Orthod 1978; 74: 241-57.

37. Kristerson L, Kvint S. Autotransplantation av tänder - 10 års erfarenheter. Tandläkartidningen 1981; 73: 598-606.

38. Rud J. Transplantation af præmolarer. Tandlægebladet 1981; 85: 612-25.

39. Kristerson L. Autotransplantation of human premolars. A clinical and radiographic study of 100 teeth. Int J Oral Surg 1985; 14: 200-213.

40. Schwartz O, Bergmann P, Klausen B. Resorption of autotransplanted human teeth: a retrospective study of 291 transplantations over a period of 25 years. Int Endod J 1985; 18: 119-31.

41. Deplagne H, Campagne J. Autotransplantation von Prämolarkeimen. Orthodontie und Kieferorthopädie 1985; 1: 71-81.

42. Kristiansen H, Kromann AM, Nyborg H, Wenzel A. En radiologisk vurdering af heling efter autotransplantation af tænder. Tandlægebladet 1986; 90: 664-68.

43. Pogrel MA. Evaluation of over 400 autogenous tooth transplants. J Oral Maxillofac Surg 1987; 45: 205-11.

44. Andreasen JO, Paulsen HU, Yu Z, Ahlquist R, Bayer T, Schwartz O. A long-term study of 370 autotransplanted premolars. Part I. Surgical procedures and standardized techniques for monitoring healing. Eur J Orthod 1990; 12: 3-13.

45. Andreasen JO, Paulsen HU, Yu Z, Bayer T, Schwartz O. A long-term study of 370 autotransplanted premolars. Part II. Tooth survival and pulp healing subsequent to transplantation. Eur J Orthod 1990; 12: 14-24.

46. Andreasen JO, Paulsen HU, Yu Z, Schwartz O. A long-term study of 370 autotransplanted premolars. Part III. Periodontal healing subsequent to transplantation. Eur J Orthod 1990; 12: 25-37.

47. Andreasen JO, Paulsen HU, Yu Z, Bayer T. A long-term study of 370 autotransplanted premolars. Part IV. Root development subsequent to transplantation. Eur J Orthod 1990; 12: 38-50.

48. Andreasen JO, Paulsen HU, Fjellvang H, Barfoed K. Autotransplantation af præmolarer til behandling af tandtab i overkæbefronten.Tandlægebladet 1989; 93: 435- 40.

49. Paulsen HU, Andreasen JO, Schwartz O. Behandling af tandtab i fronten med autotransplantation af tænder. Tandlæg Nye Tidsskr 1990; 5: 70-5.

50. Bowden DE, Patel HA. Autotransplantation of premolar teeth to replace missing maxillary central incisors. Br J Orthod 1990; 17: 21-28.

51. Oikarinen K. Replacing resorbed maxillary central incisors with mandibular premolars. Endod Dent Traumatol 1990; 6: 43-46.

52. Sussman HI. Creating a transplanted abutment. A case report. N Y State Dent J 1986; 52: 20-22.

53. Baudet-Pommel M, Collangettes-Peyrat D, Chouvet- Lejczyk V. Autotransplantation, résultats cliniques, radiographiques, orthodontiques, critéres de réussite. Actual Odontostomatol 1988; 163: 463-72.

54. Hillerup S, Dahl E, Schwartz O, Hjørting-Hansen E. Tooth transplantation to bone grafts in cleft alveolus. Cleft Palate J 1987; 24: 137-41.

55. Stenvik E, Semb G, Bergland O et al. Experimental transplantation of teeth to simulated maxillary alveolar clefts. Scand J Plast Reconstr Surg 1989; 23: 105-08.

56. Stoll P, Härle F, Schilli W. Transplantation eines Weisheitzahnes in ein autologes Beckenkammtransplantat am Unterkiefer. Dtsch Zahn-Mund-Kiefer Gesichtschir 1987; 11: 5-07.

Chapter 6
Autotransplantation of canines

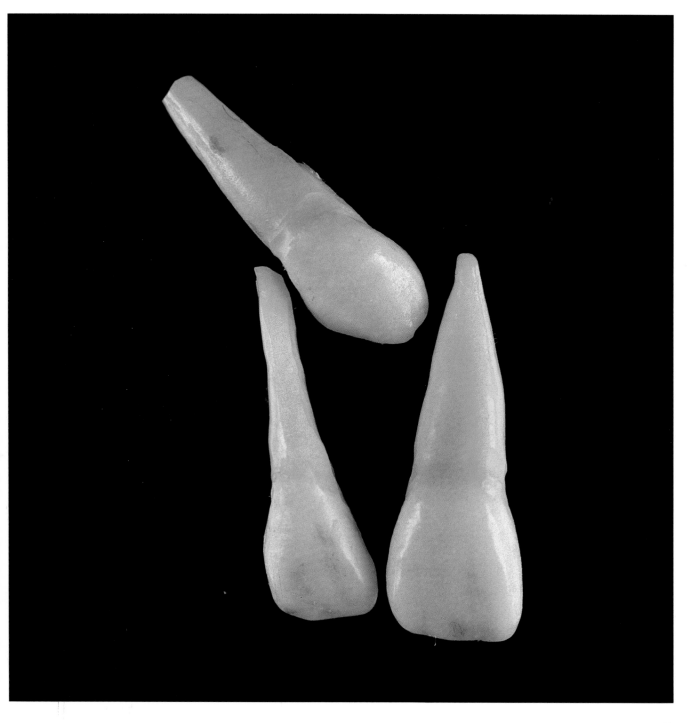

Indications

This technique, which is described for the treatment of ectopically placed canines, was pioneered at the beginning of this century by *Widman*[1,2] (1917, 1918). Indications for canine transplantation can be summarized as follows (Fig. 6.1):

Ectopic position where surgical exposure and/or subsequent orthodontic realignment are difficult or impossible to carry out (Fig. 6.2).

Cases where the eruption path of the canine has led to extensive root resorption of the lateral and/or the central incisor and where transplantation can save one or both of the resorbed teeth (Figs. 6.3 and 6.4).[117]

Fig. 6.1. Indications for canine transplantation
A-D. Ectopic position of the canine, where surgical exposure and subsequent orthodontic realignment would be difficult or impossible.

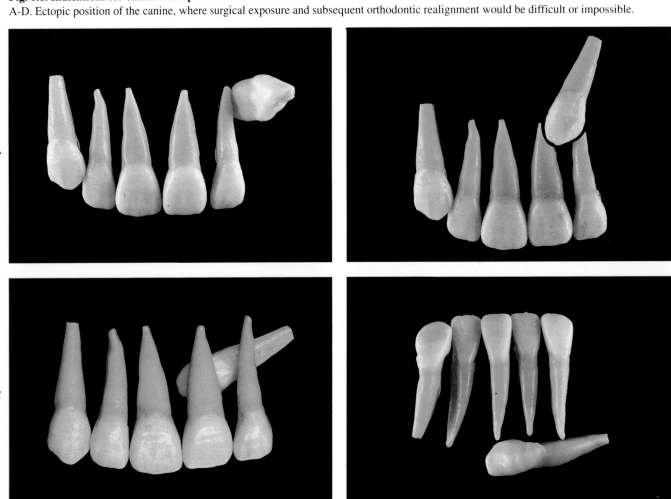

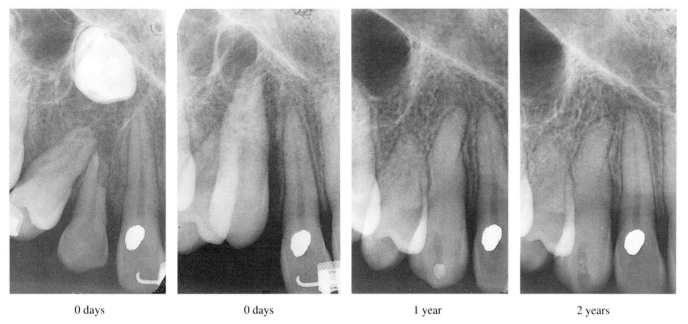

| 0 days | 0 days | 1 year | 2 years |

Fig. 6.2. Ectopic position of a maxillary canine treated by transplantation.

Etiology and frequency of impactions

Maxillary canines

The canine is the final tooth to erupt. This means that it has to force its way past incisors and premolars. The eruption path is very long and obstacles during this eruption sequence may lead to impaction.[3] Thus, lack of space in the anterior region has been found to be related to canine impaction labially or interproximally, whereas ectopic orientation of the canine tooth germs is perhaps the most important factor influencing palatal impactions.[4,5] Impaction of maxillary canines has been found to affect 0.8% to 2.4% of the population,[4,6-12] and appears to be slightly more common in girls,[3, 6-10,14-16] with the majority of the teeth being *unilaterally* impacted.[6,8,13,14] Palatal impactions appear to be two to three times more common than buccal impactions.[4,6,13-15] In the labially and palatally oriented teeth, the most frequent location of the canine crown is between the apex and the neck of the lateral incisor, with the long axis of the tooth placed at an angle to the sagittal plane. When the axis of the impacted tooth is vertical, the tooth can usually be found impacted in the middle of the alveolar process between the lateral incisor and premolar.[14]

Mandibular canines

Mandibular canines appear to be impacted less often than maxillary canines.[17] Reported frequencies of mandibular canine impactions range from 0.05% to 0.4%.[6,9-12] These teeth are usually impacted horizontally in labial position below the apices of incisors and with the crown positioned mesially, often crossing the midline.

Fig. 6.3. Transplantation of a canine where surgical exposure and orthodontic traction has been unsuccessful. Note extensive loss of supporting bone as well as cervical resorption of the canine elicited by the ligature. After transplantation, a certain amount of marginal bone has been reformed, possibly induced by the vital periodontal ligament (PDL) of the transplant. From Andreasen, 1987.[117]

| 0 days | 0 days | 1 year | 4 years |

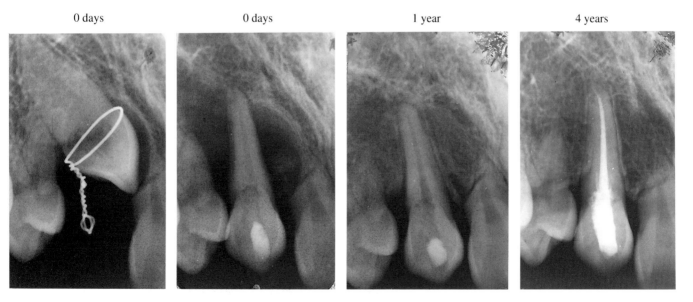

Treatment planning

The aim of the *clinical evaluation* is to reveal whether there is sufficient space mesiodistally and faciolingually to accommodate a canine transplant. The crown and root dimensions of the potential transplant cannot usually be evaluated from radiographs because of image distortion.[18] So unless a contralateral canine has erupted, dimensions have to be estimated using tables of average tooth dimensions (see Appendix 3, p. 292). An analysis of space conditions should include information about the following dimensions of the *transplant*: the maximum width of the crown, the mesiodistal and the labiolingual width of the root at the cervical margin, and the root length. The available mesiodistal width of the *recipient region* is then measured between the proximal surfaces of the lateral incisor and the first premolar. The labiolingual dimension of the alveolar process is also evaluated directly. In this context the width of the labial and lingual mucoperiosteum (usually amounting to 2 mm) should be subtracted from the total measure. The mesiodistal space cervically and the apicocoronal space conditions are evaluated from an orthoradial radiograph. In this context, surgical preparation of the socket must not come closer than 1 mm to the root surface of adjacent teeth. Finally, an analysis is made of the occlusal condi-

tions in the recipient region. In some cases overeruption of the antagonist has taken place, so that reduction or orthodontic correction of opposing teeth is necessary to accommodate the transplant. If the mesiodistal space conditions are not adequate, it is advisable to create more space orthodontically prior to transplantation. If this is not possible, minor adjustments can be made by grinding the mesial and distal surface of the crown (see p. 191) or by placing the transplant in labioversion and then later moving the canine into occlusion orthodontically when adequate space has been created. However, this procedure carries a risk of labial gingival retraction (see p. 201).

The *radiographic analysis* serves several purposes, each of which requires different projections. In the vertical plane, radiographs should reveal the depth of impaction and its relation to adjacent roots and anatomic structures, such as the nasal cavity. In the horizontal plane, the radiograph should localize the canine in relation to the labial and lingual bony plates and to other structures such as roots. Finally an orthoradial exposure should be made to determine the mesiodistal dimension of the potential transplant from the neck of the tooth to its apex. As each of the radiographic procedures varies from the maxilla to the mandible, each location will be described separately.

Fig. 6.4. Bilateral canine impactions treated with autotransplantation
Bilateral ectopic eruption of maxillary canines has resulted in loss of the lateral incisors and severe resorption of the two central incisors. The two canines were transplanted to the contralateral lateral incisor region so that the marked root curvature of the roots could fit the existing sockets. Endodontic treatment was subsequently performed. At the last control there is no sign of root resorption of the canines. The two centrals are only slightly loose and respond to sensibility testing. From Andreasen, 1987.[117]

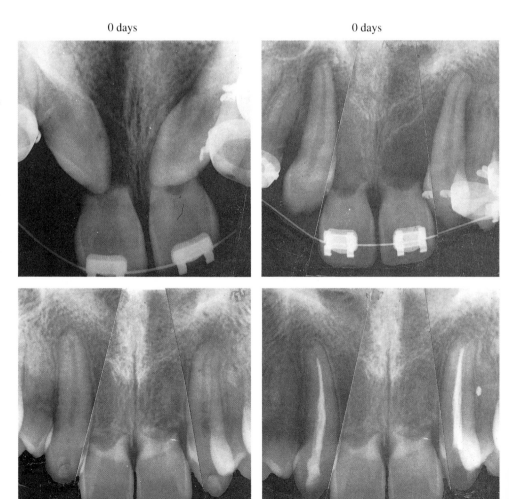

0 days   0 days

2 weeks   3 years

Maxillary impactions

Several radiographic techniques have been described for the impacted maxillary canine.[13,19-27] In the following, emphasis will be placed on exposures which fulfill the above-mentioned objectives for canine localization (Fig. 6.5).

A *panoramic exposure* gives valuable information about the depth of impaction and the relation between the crown and root apices and/or the nasal cavity.

An *orthoradial exposure* of the canine region will reveal finer details in the relation between the crown of the canine and adjacent apices. Furthermore, important information is obtained with respect to the mesiodistal space and the apico-coronal dimensions of the future socket area.

A *distal or mesial exposure* will supplement the orthoradial exposure in localizing the impacted canine in relation to adjacent teeth. In this regard the rule should be observed that teeth close to the film (i.e., palatal impaction) will move mesially with a mesial shift of the central beam. Labial impactions will move in the opposite direction.

Fig. 6.5. Radiographic visualization of an ectopic maxillary canine. A, B, and C. Distoeccentric, orthoradial, and mesioeccentric exposures respectively. Note shift of the cusp of the canine in relation to the lateral incisor, indicating the palatal position of the canine.

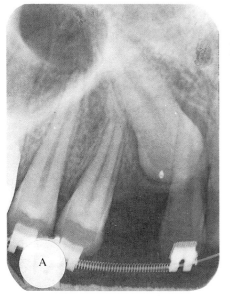
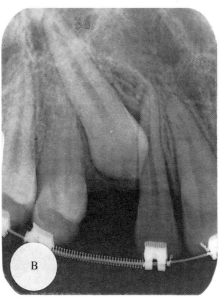
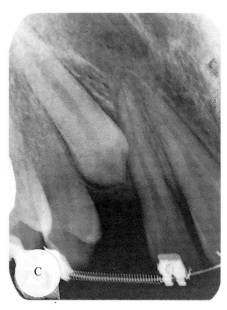

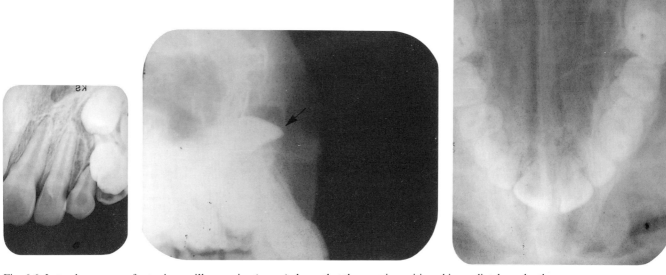

Fig. 6.6. Lateral exposure of ectopic maxillary canine (arrow) shows that the cusp is positioned immediately under the mucosa.

An intraoral axial exposure through the frontal bone is sometimes indicated in order to define the position of the crown in relation to the buccal and palatal alveolar bone surface and the adjacent roots as well as the axis of the root (Fig. 6.6). This information could be of importance deciding whether a palatal or a buccal surgical approach should be chosen (see later). In case of doubt the axial exposure can be supplemented with an oblique lateral exposure which provides detailed information about the relation between the impacted canine and the labial alveolar bone surface (Fig. 6.6).

Mandibular impactions

A panoramic exposure gives information about the depth of impaction and the position of the crown and the apex of the impacted mandibular canine (Fig. 6.7).

Fig. 6.7. The combined information from panoramic, lateral, and axial radiographs of two ectopic mandibular canines used in determining the exact location of the impacted teeth.

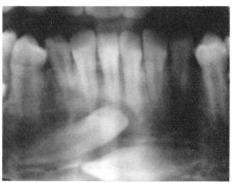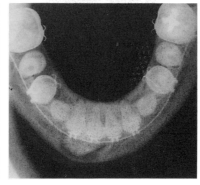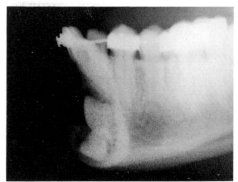

A *distal or mesial exposure* will supplement radial exposures in revealing the same relationship to adjacent teeth as described for maxillary canines. The axial view of the mandible with a projection angle parallel to the apices of the incisors gives important information about the relationship between the buccal and lingual alveolar bone surface as well as the position of the crown in relation to the apices of adjacent teeth. However, this projection should be a true axial projection in relation to the incisors otherwise the exposure will give false information about the position of the impacted tooth (Fig. 6.8). This exposure can be supplemented with a *lateral exposure* which provides a detailed view of the relation between the impacted canine and the labial bone surface (Fig. 6.7).[19,22,29] An orthoradial exposure of the canine region will reveal details of the relationship between the crown and adjacent teeth and the mesiodistal and apicocoronal space conditions in the recipient region.

Surgical procedure

The surgical procedure differs according to the site of impaction:

Maxillary canines in labial deviation

Before a surgical approach is made it is essential that a radiographic examination has revealed the labial position of the crown and that an analysis of the graft and the recipient site dimensions has shown compatibility. The general principle of the surgical procedure is to create a flap which gives good surgical access to both the graft and the recipient region, allows versatility of the procedure (i.e., possibility of simultaneous bone grafting), and ensures optimal gingival healing of the graft. Furthermore the surgical procedure should ensure atraumatic graft removal and socket preparation. In Fig. 6.9 such a procedure is shown for a labially ectopic maxillary canine.

Maxillary canines in palatal deviation

Again, this approach depends entirely upon a valid radiographic demonstration of the location of the graft. The surgical removal of the graft is, especially in older individuals, considerably more difficult compared to canines in a labial position, the reason being the more difficult approach due to the close proximity between the crown of the canine and the roots of the central or the lateral incisor. The surgical procedure is shown in Fig. 6.10.

Mandibular canines

These teeth are almost exclusively displaced labially. In the very rare cases of lingual positioning, the surgical approach to the graft is so difficult that transplantation is not advisable. In some cases where the ectopic canine has migrated a long distance the graft can be removed via a separate flap raised over the crown of the graft. However, in most cases a common flap for both the graft and the recipient site is to be preferred (Fig. 6.11).

Fig. 6.8. Incorrect axial exposure of mandibular canine region (B) gives the wrong impression that the impacted tooth deviates lingually. In a correct exposure (C), the incisors appear in a true axial view. This projection correctly reveals the labial position.

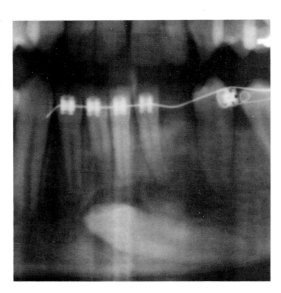

A

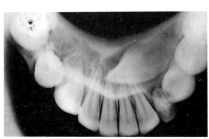

B

C

Fig. 6.9. Maxillary canine transplantation with labial position

Transplantation of an ectopic labially located canine.

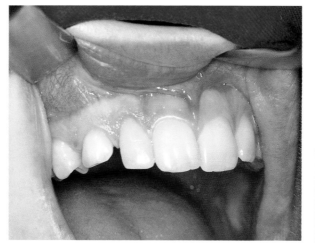

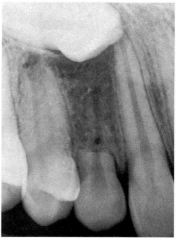

Space evaluation

In this case, space evaluation can be made directly with a sliding caliper (see Appendix 7, p. 296) by comparing the width at the recipient site with the mesiodistal dimension of the erupted contralateral canine.

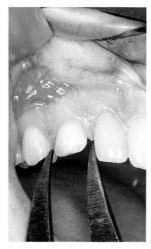

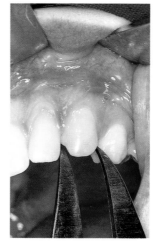

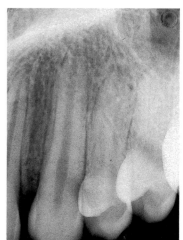

Incision and elevation of flap

A trapezoidal incision is made which ensures intact mesial, distal, and palatal gingiva at the graft site. Elevation of the flap begins at the loosely bound alveolar mucosa.

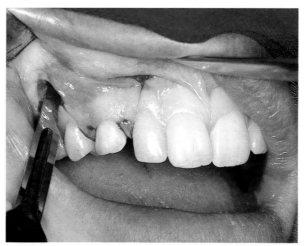

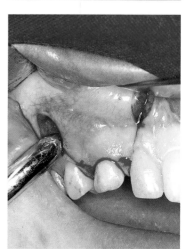

Location of the crown

A bulge in the labial bone discloses the site of the canine. All bone surrounding the maximum circumference of the crown must be removed.

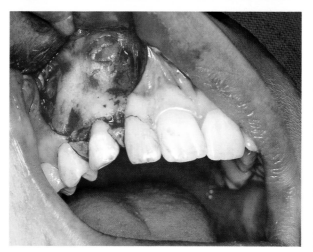

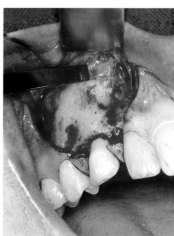

Fig. 6.9. Continued.

Exposure of the crown
The crown of the ectopic canine is exposed either with chisels or with a surgical bur while the crown and the follicle are shielded by a narrow periosteal elevator.

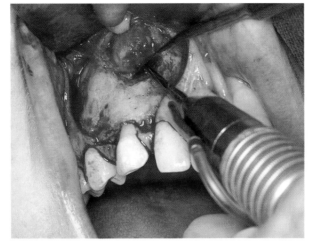 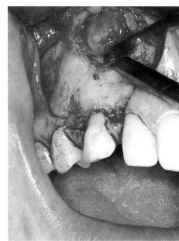

Separation of the follicle
Cervical separation of the follicle from the bone is ensured with an amalgam carver. The tooth is loosened with a periosteal elevator. It is important that the instrument contacts only the crown and not the root surface.

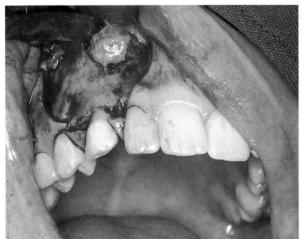 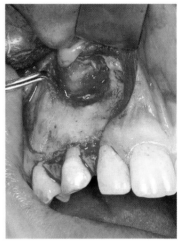

Removal of the graft
The tooth is removed with forceps and placed in saline.

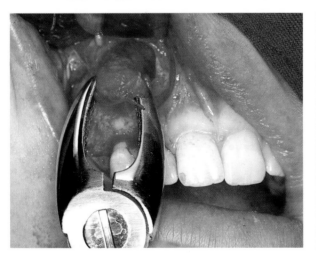 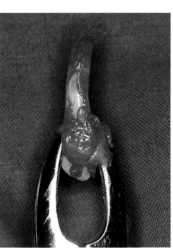

Preparation of a new socket
The primary incisor is extracted. Care should be taken not to fracture the thin labial bone. The socket is enlarged using a bur with internal cooling (see Appendix 7, p. 296).

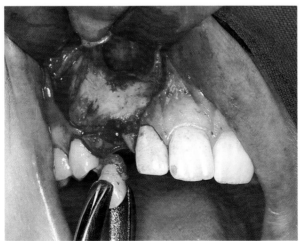 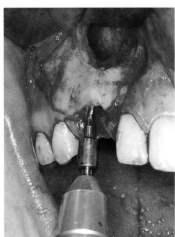

Fig. 6.9. Continued.

Testing the fit of the transplant

The fit of the transplant is tested. A loose fit is to be achieved, where there are no pressure zones on the root of the transplant.

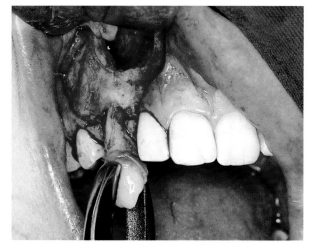
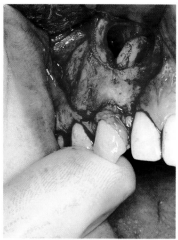

Elongation of the flap and suturing

The labial flap is elongated by sectioning the periosteum at the base of the flap. The flap is then repositioned and should now adapt itself without tension to the cervical region of the graft. Two sutures are placed interdentally followed by sutures along the mesial and distal aspects of the incision.

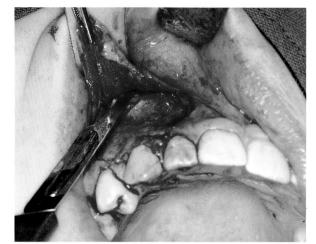
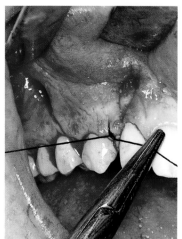

Splinting

To prevent extrusion of the transplant, a ligature-acid-etch splint can be used. In this case a 0.2 mm wire was ligated around the cusp of the transplant and two adjacent teeth and the position of the ligatures was secured with etching and application of composite. Splinting should be maintained for 3-4 weeks.

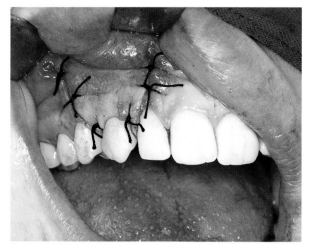
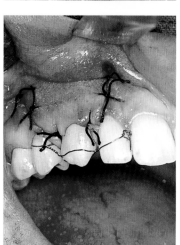

Follow-up

At follow-up one year after transplantation, complete bone regeneration has occurred around the graft.

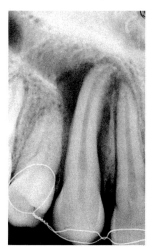
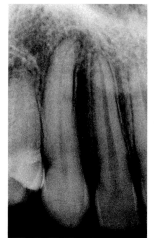
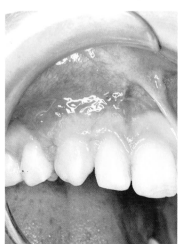

Fig. 6.10. Maxillary canine transplantation with palatal position

Transplantation of an ectopic palatally located canine in a 17-year-old girl.

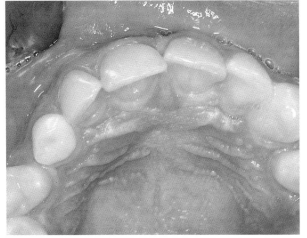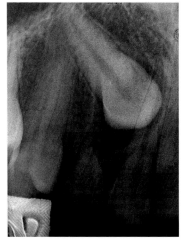

Flap raising

A marginal flap is raised from the first molar to the opposite canine region. The interdental papillae should be left undisturbed in order not to interfere with vascularization in this critical area.

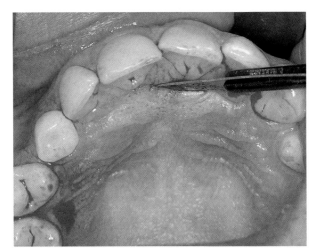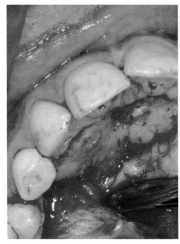

Bone removal

If the position of the graft allows removal in a strict axial direction, it is only necessary to remove bone surrounding the crown and the neck of the tooth.

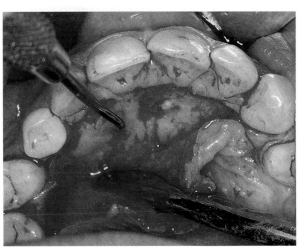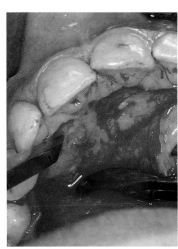

Root exposure

Usually the tooth has to be removed in a palatal direction, which necessitates removal of most of the bone covering the root. This is best achieved by making two osteotomy cuts parallel to the estimated root location and removing the overlying bone with chisels. All fragments of bone should be stored in saline in case they are needed as bone transplants.

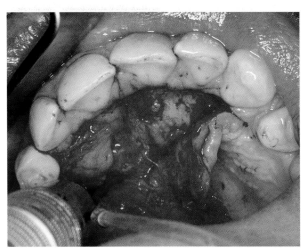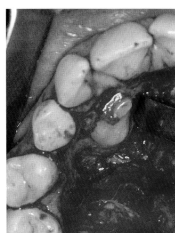

Fig. 6.10. Continued.

Graft removal

Cervical separation of the follicle is ensured with an amalgam carver. The tooth is then luxated slightly with an elevator which is placed along the labial aspect of the follicle covering the crown, i.e., opposite where bone has been removed. The tooth is then grasped by the crown with forceps and removed. Before it is placed in saline, it is inspected for damage to the follicle and the root apex.

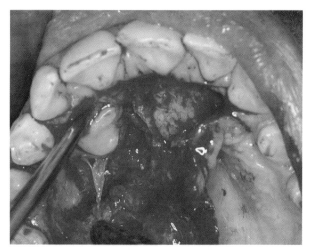
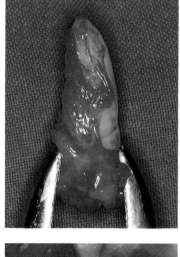

Preparation of a new socket

The new socket is prepared using a bur with internal cooling (see Appendix 7, p. 296). It is essential that adequate space is created so that the transplant can be positioned without pressure on the root surface and with the graft in slight infraocclusion.

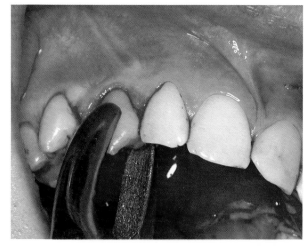
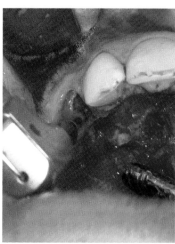

Bone transplantation and suturing

The exposed palatal aspect of the root is covered with the removed bone fragments. The palatal flap is then repositioned and interdental sutures placed.

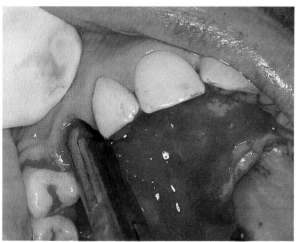
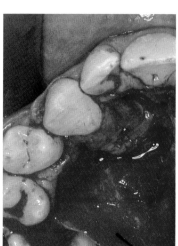

Splinting

An acid-etch splint or a 0.2 mm wire is used to prevent extrusion and premature occlusion. Splinting is maintained for 3-4 weeks.

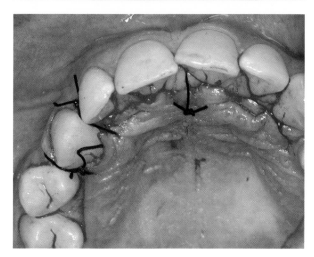
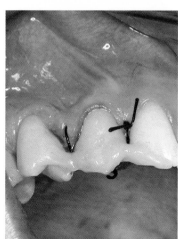

Fig. 6.11. Transplantation of a mandibular canine
An ectopically located mandibular canine.

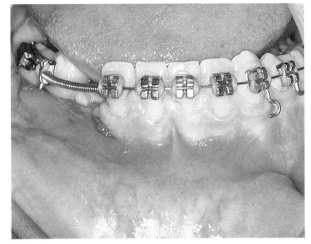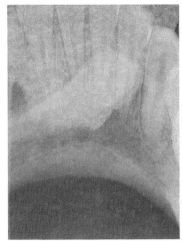

Incision and flap elevation
A flap has been raised which respects the interdental papillae in the canine region.

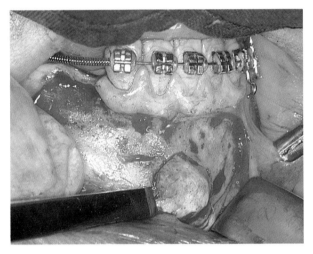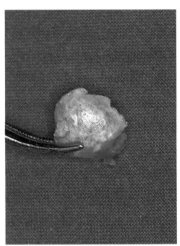

Exposure of the crown
A bulge on the alveolar bone surface indicates the position of the crown. The crown is exposed using chisels or burs.

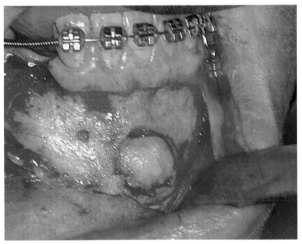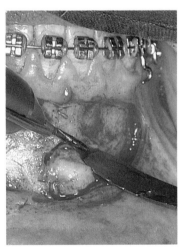

Removing the graft
The tooth is then loosened with an elevator and removed with forceps.

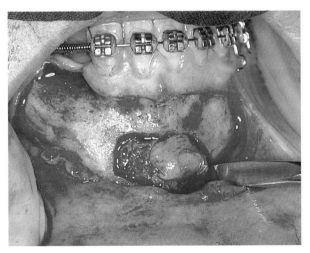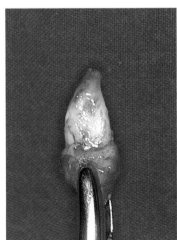

Fig. 6.11. Continued.

Osteotomy to the socket area
An osteostomy cut is made through the labial bone plate according to the size of the future alveolus. Thereafter the bone plate is removed with a chisel.

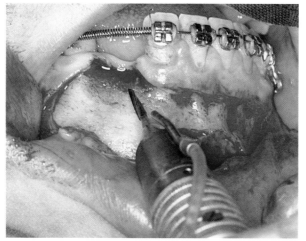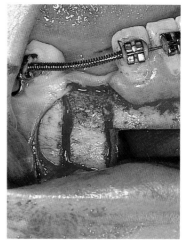

Socket preparation
Because of the labio-lingual atrophy of the alveolar process the labial bone plate is removed with burs and a chisel.

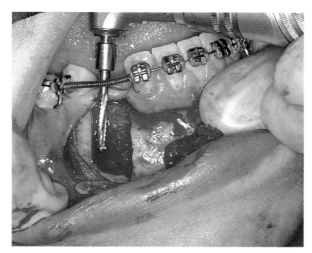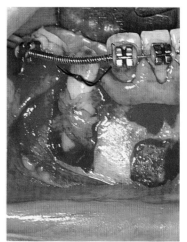

Transplanting the graft
After preparation of the socket the canine is grafted and splinted with a suture in semierupted position. To ensure proper soft tissue coverage of the graft, a horizontal incision is made at the base of the flap. Thereafter the labial bone plate is replaced after cutting it lengthwise in 2 mm wide sections.

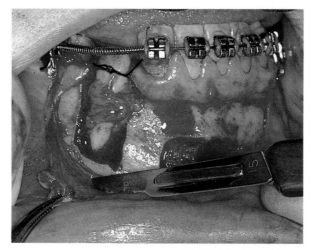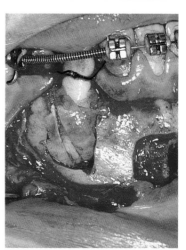

Condition after transplantation
The flap is sutured and a radiograph shows the semierupted graft.

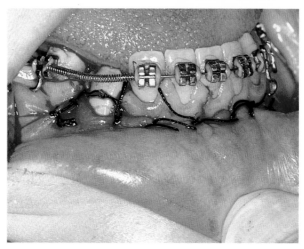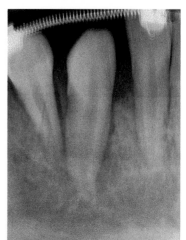

Special cases
Lack of space at the recipient site
Mesiodistal dimension

In many cases a preoperative analysis of the space conditions will reveal that there is a lack of space mesiodistally. In these cases the best solution is orthodontic enlargement of the space. If such a solution is not possible, the following treatment alternatives exist: If the mesiodistal dimension of the recipient site is only slightly too small, slight rotation of the canine can be a solution. This rotation will often make room for the tooth. Furthermore, it should be considered that a mesial rotation of the canine gives a more esthetic appearance than a distal rotation, which exposes the palatal surface.[35] When the space deficiency is greater, the proximal surfaces of the graft can be reduced about 0.5 mm mesially and distally with a diamond under a copious flow of water (Fig. 6.12).

Another way of dealing with insufficient *mesiodistal* space conditions is to position the graft in a labial and semierupted position (Figs. 6.11 and 6.13c). In these cases, a labial marginal flap is raised from the first premolar to the lateral incisor using trapezoidal incision lines. The canine is now exposed and removed as described previously. The labial bone plate is removed corresponding to the potentional new socket area. Bone removal is begun with two vertical cuts through the labial bone plate and a horizontal apical stop-cut. The labial bone plate is removed with a chisel, cut in half lengthwise with heavy scissors, and then stored in saline. The socket is prepared for the canine and the tooth is tested in its new position. When the proper position has been found, the tooth is held in position with a suture cervically and the flap is tried for proper coverage. If there is any tension, the periosteum is incised so that the flap can be repositioned and sutured without tension. However, before suturing the two bone fragments are placed over the root with the cortical surface facing the root. Finally the tooth is splinted as described above. It should be mentioned that this technique is accompanied by a risk of gingival retraction.

Fig. 6.12. Frontal section through a maxillary canine. The enamel is approximately 1 mm thick interproximally. If both proximal surfaces are reduced to about half thickness, the mesiodistal dimension of the graft can be reduced about 1 mm.

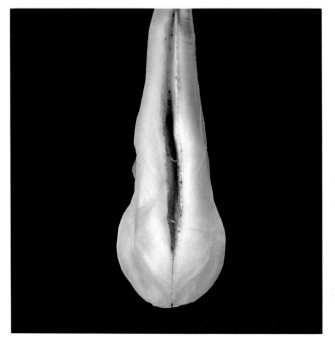
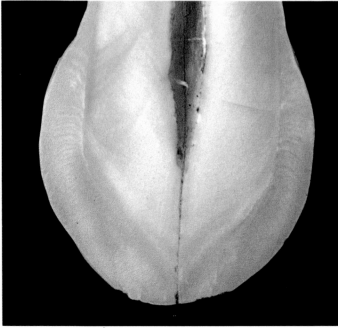

Labiolingual dimension

The palatally impacted maxillary canine often leads to a concavity of the labial bone plate so that there is inadequate space labiolingually, which makes it impossible to accommodate the transplant in its correct orientation.[36,37] Creation of a new socket from the palatal aspect which respects the flat labial bone plate often results in positioning the canine too far palatally, where occlusion will normally not allow positioning of the transplant. One solution is to create a socket and then to fracture the labial bone plate in order to make room for the transplant (Fig. 6.13b). This can be done by making two parallel osteotomy cuts from the palatal aspect through the labial bone plate while taking care not to injure the mucoperiosteum. During the osteotomy procedure a finger should be placed against the labial alveolar mucosa, to feel as the bur penetrates bone. An instrument with a shape comparable to a canine root (e.g., a needle holder or an elevator) is placed as deep as possible in the socket, whereafter the labial bone is used as a fulcrum for labial movement. In this way the labial socket wall can be fractured. The tooth is kept in position with a cervical suture and the palatal flap is repositioned and sutured. The canine is then splinted with an acid-etch splint. As there is a great tendency for the stretched labial mucoperiosteum to displace the tooth palatally, it is necessary to hold the tooth in place while the splinting material sets.

In the mandible a lack of labial eminence can necessitate rotating the graft 90°. Because of the anatomy of mandibular canines such a rotation will usually allow positioning the graft within the confines of the alveolar process. Alternatively, the graft can be placed in a semierupted position in either the maxilla or the mandible.

Fig 6.13a. Transplantation of a canine to a labial semierupted position
The graft is removed as well as the labial bone plate. The socket is then prepared.

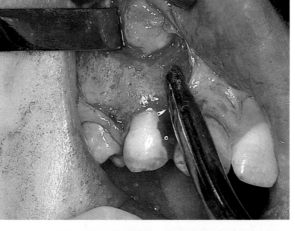
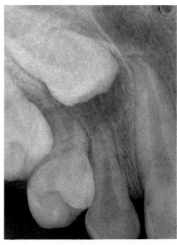

Placing the graft
The graft is then placed in a semierupted position and covered with the removed labial bone plate, which has been transected to improve revascularization.

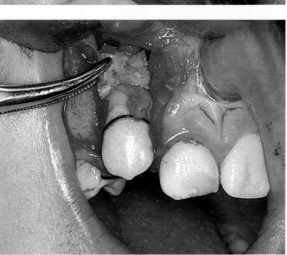
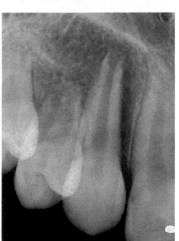

192

Fig. 6.13b. Intentional fracture of labial bone wall
Two parallel osteotomy cuts are placed in the labial bone wall from the palatal aspect of the alveolus whereafter the bone wall is fractured with an elevator or needle holder.

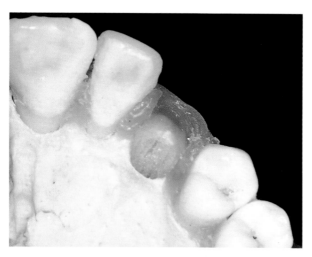 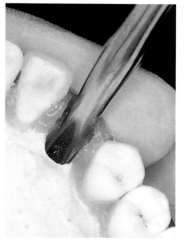

Fig. 6.13c. Rotating a mandibular canine in a case of labial bone atrophy
The graft is rotated 90° in order to be placed within the socket area.

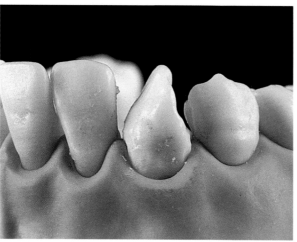 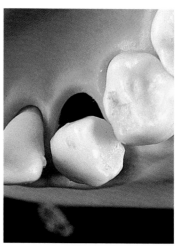

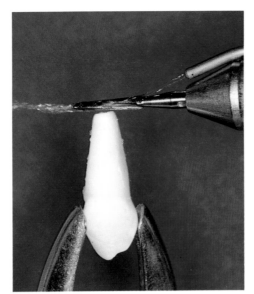
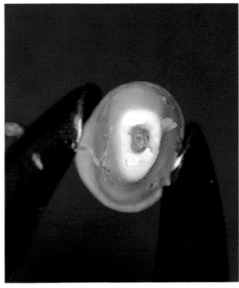

Fig. 6.14. Apex resection of a canine with apical root deflection
The apex is resected with a surgical bur using a copious flow of saline to cool the bur. The resection has created a relatively large pulpal opening.

Root apex deviation

Rather frequently, the root apex is seen to deviate labially. In these cases apicoectomy after graft removal has been suggested, first to facilitate adaptation of the tooth to its new socket, and second to enhance pulpal revascularization (Fig. 6.14). Regarding transplantation, Kallioniemi & Oksala[40] (1977) found evidence of pulpal revascularization in 13% of canines with completed root formation where the apex had been removed accidentally or deliberately, in contrast to a control group of mature teeth without apex resection which showed pulpal revascularization in 21%. In a similar study by Janson & al.[41] (1978), apical resection resulted in pulpal revascularization in 39% of patients up to 25 years of age, whereas no teeth showed pulp survival in older age groups. However, no control group was used in this study. In light of the abovementioned clinical studies, improvement of pulp survival appears to be questionable after apical resection. Therefore, this procedure should be used mainly for the purpose of facilitating the adaptation of the transplant to its new socket and facilitating later endodontic treatment if necessary (Fig. 6.15).

Redressement forcé

The technique of redressement forcé, or surgical repositioning of canines with incomplete root formation, has been described by various authors.[42-47] In this technique a buccal or lingual flap is raised. The crown of the canine is exposed and with burs or chisels a path is made in the bone which allows the tooth to be rotated into the correct position, while the apex is kept in its original position. In this way trauma to the apical blood vessels should be kept to a minimum. However, illustrations from the studies cited indicate that maintenance of the apex in its original location is seldom achieved. Concerning the long-term prognosis of canines treated by surgical repositioning, one report claims that 300 teeth have been treated but no information is given on failure rates.[42-43] In a study reported by Kay[46] (1961), this technique was used in 16 cases with 10 maintaining vitality after repositioning and not exhibiting root resorption. However, in the author´s opinion this technique cannot be recommended until more results pertaining to its use have been reported.

0 days   0 days   1 year

Fig. 6.15. Apex resection performed in a maxillary canine with apex deflection
The tooth reacts normally to sensibility testing at later follow-up.

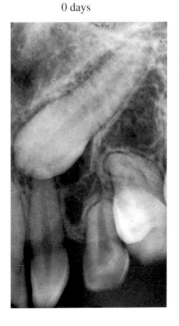
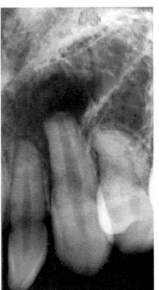
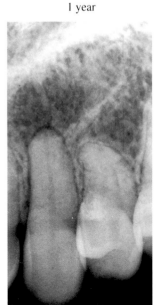

Two-stage procedure with interim graft storage

During the planning of a canine transplantation, it is often found that restricted mesiodistal dimensions in the recipient region make satisfactory graft placement impossible, or that removal of enough bone palatally or labially in order to ensure an atraumatic removal of the transplant leaves the graft with insufficient support. Thus situations like these have led to the development of two-stage transplantation procedures. The first phase is the removal of the potential transplant, followed by storage of this tooth either in the soft tissues of the oral vestibule,[48,50,112-114] in tissue culture medium,[51,53,110] or by cryopreservation (see Chapter 9, p. 242). During the storage period several goals can be achieved. Adequate space can be created orthodontically in the recipient region. Furthermore, bone repair will take place in the donor site, or bone can be transplanted to the region, as in cleft palate cases.[55] Finally it has been suggested, but not proven, that damage to the PDL of the transplant may be repaired by in vivo or in vitro storage.[56,57] Clinical experience has shown that all three methods of long-term storage can be used successfully, although unsuccessful cases have also been reported.[110,112] However, very little is known about the long-term results of these treatment procedures, nor are there any studies where these techniques have been compared. With respect to the biologic background of these methods and the technical procedures involved, the reader is referred to Chapter 9.

Intra-alveolar transplantation

In the case of canines with crown-root fractures, deep cervical caries, or root resorption, intra-alveolar transplantation is sometimes possible, whereby the root is repositioned more superficially, thereby facilitating crown restoration. These procedures are further described in Chapter 7.

Postoperative follow-up

The patient is seen 1 week after treatment, when sutures are removed. At this stage, it is too early to remove the splint, as there is still a tendency towards dislocation. A fixation period of 3-4 weeks is generally necessary to consolidate graft position.

PDL healing

PDL healing evidenced by the presence of a lamina dura is normally seen after 3-6 months.[59,102]

Pulpal healing

Pulpal healing as revealed by a positive sensibility reaction has been found as early as 3 months postoperatively, with the number of reacting teeth increasing with longer observation periods.[60,102,108]

Pulp canal obliteration

Pulp canal obliteration is usually seen after 6 months and also increases with increasing observation periods.[60,102]

Root resorption

The first type of root resorption which can be diagnosed, *inflammatory root resorption*, is usually manifest 4-8 weeks after transplantation, whereas *replacement resorption* (ankylosis) is usually first seen 6 months to 1 year after transplantation. In canine transplants where pulpal revascularization is expected, a close clinical and radiographic follow-up is necessary using the follow-up periods described in Appendix 2, p. 290. If an apical radiolucency, inflammatory root resorption, or internal resorption develops, endodontic treatment should be instituted immediately.

Fig. 6.16. Endodontic treatment of a transplanted maxillary canine. The pulp was extirpated 4 weeks after transplantation and an interim dressing of calcium hydroxide placed in the root canal. After 1 year the endodontic treatment was completed with a gutta-percha root filling. At the final control, there is no sign of root resorption.

0 days	0 days	1 month	2 years

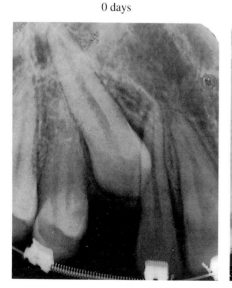 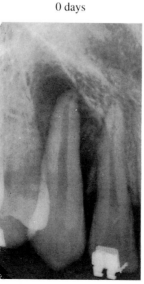 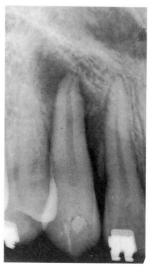 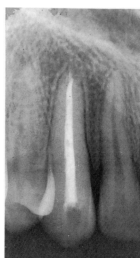

Endodontic treatment

In cases where pulpal revascularization is unlike to occur (see p. 197) or signs of pulp necrosis are present (e.g., periapical radiolucency and/or inflammatory root resorption), the patient should be scheduled for endodontic therapy (Fig. 6.16). At the first visit, the pulp is extirpated and the root canal filled with calcium hydroxide.[107] After another 4 weeks this treatment is repeated. Thereafter the patient is seen again 6 months after transplantation, when a radiographic examination is made. If there are signs of periapical healing, including closure of the apical foramen, formation of a lamina dura, and arrest of eventual root resorption cavities, the patient is scheduled for another control 6 months later and at that time definitive root filling with gutta-percha and a sealer is undertaken and radiographic and clinical examinations are carried out (Fig. 6.16). Details of the endodontic procedure are further described in Chapter 2, p. 62. After 1 year the first long-term prognosis can be determined. Thereafter the tooth should be controlled at 5-year intervals.

Prognosis

The results of canine transplantations have been documented in a number of survey articles[36,37,44,61-64], and case reports[65-79,115-117] as well as in larger clinical studies.[38,39,43,53,54,80-111] In Table 6.1 the results of follow-up studies are shown where the documentation allows evaluation of one or more possible transplantation complications. It appears that there is a wide range of long-term results, a finding related primarily to case selection and also to differences in healing assessment, observation periods, and the surgical techniques used. In the following, the frequency and etiology of the various complications will be discussed.

Tooth survival

It appears from Table 6.1 that tooth survival after transplantation ranges from 86% to 100%. An important factor in tooth survival assessment is naturally the length of the observation period. Furthermore the stage of root development at the time of transplantation is also of importance (Fig. 6.19).

Table 6.1. Long-term results of autotransplantation of canines

	Observation period yr. (mean)	Age of patients yr. (mean)	Number of teeth	Tooth survival %	PDL healing* %	Pulp healing Sensibility %	Pulp healing Canal obliteration %	Gingival healing %
Thonner, 1971[87]	(5)		51	98	69		18	
Cook, 1972[49]	0.5-4	13-27	27	96	67	30		
Reade & al., 1973[59]	0.3-5	12-50	50	100	56	8		88
Lovius & al., 1974[81]	min. 1.5	10-27 (16)	35	97	49	43	49	89
Moss, 1975[84]	1-10		100	100	72	41	36	85
Oksala & Kallioniemi, 1977[92]	4-7	13-43	60	88	25	13	34	
Altonen & al, 1978[90]	0.5-2 (1.5)	13-47 (25.2)	28	86	25	11	14	75
Hardy, 1982[35]	1-9	13-30	81	91	61			88
Reade & Hall, 1982[99] Hall & Reade, 1983[100]	0.5-9	13-43 (20)	131	90	34			
Ahlberg & al., 1983[98]	(6)	16-56 (27.5)	33	88	25	13	14	100
Lownie & al., 1986[102]	0.5-4	12-28	35	88	81	18		
Fagade & Gillbe, 1988[111]	0.2-16	11-35 (17)	200		24			

* PDL healing without any sign of root resorption

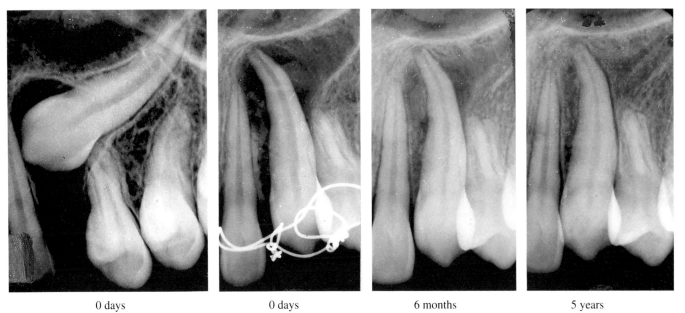

| 0 days | 0 days | 6 months | 5 years |

Fig. 6.17. Pulpal revascularization of an autotransplanted maxillary canine with completed root formation at the time of surgery. Note initial pulpal obliteration, 6 months after transplantation.

Pulpal healing and pulp necrosis

The clinical diagnosis of pulp necrosis depends primarily on the results of sensibility testing and radiographic examination. Thus, signs of pulpal revascularization include a positive response to sensibility testing and gradual obliteration of the pulp canal (Fig. 6.17). However, in this context it should be borne in mind that cases have been reported where teeth have demonstrated pulp canal obliteration and at the same time have not responded to sensibility testing.[81,90,92,96] If, however, pulpal revascularization is estimated based on the results of positive sensibility response, it appears that between 11% to 43% of transplanted canines regain vitality. A strong relationship between a positive sensibility response and root development has been shown by Oksala & Kallioniemi[92] (1977).Thus 31% of canines transplanted with open apices later reacted positively compared to 7% with closed apices.

Besides the effect of root development upon later sensibility testing an age factor is possibly also in operation. Thus, in studies reported by Altonen & al.[90] (1978) and Hasselgren & al.[93] (1977), no canines transplanted in patients above 20 years of age became revascularized. In the evaluation of sensibility testing as an indicator for pulpal revascularization, it is of importance to consider that with prolonged observation periods some teeth previously negative to sensibility testing will become positive (Fig. 6.18). Furthermore teeth which have previously shown a positive sensibility response may later lose this response.[92]

Fig. 6.18. Late return of pulpal sensibility after transplantation of an ectopic mandibular canine with completed root formation at the time of surgery. Two years after transplantation, the tooth reacts to sensibility testing.

| 0 days | 0 days | 1 year | 2 years |

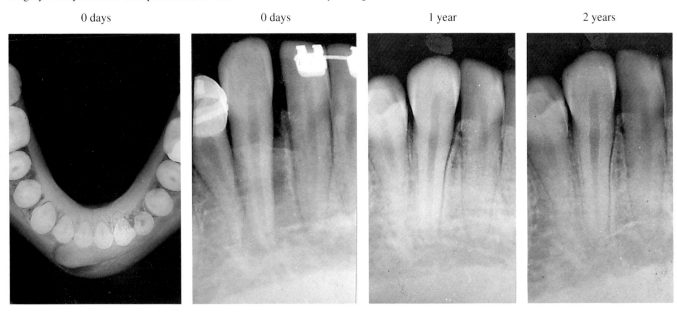

Fig. 6.19. Tooth survival of 48 autotransplanted canines with incomplete and complete root formation at the time of surgery.

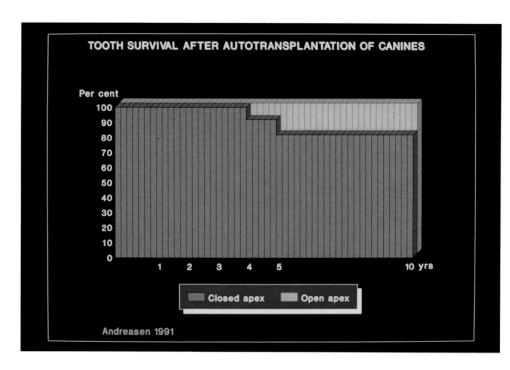

If pulp canal obliteration is considered to be the decisive factor for evaluating pulpal revascularization this results in a slightly larger number of vital pulps (Table 6.1).[40,90,96] Like sensibility testing, pulp canal obliteration has been found to be strongly related to root development (Fig. 6.20) and an age factor might also operate.[83,96]

Several studies have reported pulp canal obliteration indicating pulp vitality after transplantation of canines with completed root formation (Fig. 6.17)[40,87,96] and a few studies have reported figures of 36% to 49%[81,84]. With figures that high the indication for preventive endodontics becomes doubtful. On the basis of the data from the cited studies it appears reasonable to expect pulpal revascularization in patients under 20 years of age. Endodontic treatment should only be performed when obvious signs of pulp necrosis, such as periapical rarefaction or inflammatory root resorption, appear. If these signs are not present, it has been suggested that pulp necrosis is only likely when no change in the pulp canal can be seen and a negative sensibility reaction persists at least 1 year after treatment. In patients above 20 years of age, the likelihood of pulpal revascularization appears to be very limited, and preventive endodontics should then be considered to limit the risk of inflammatory root resorption.

PDL healing and root resorption

It appears from Table 6.1 that the prevalence of PDL healing without root resorption varies considerably. The most important explanation for this could be a difference in definitions of root resorption and variations in observation periods. If materials are selected where the healing criteria are similar, the reported frequencies of PDL healing do not differ greatly, ranging from 25% to 39%.[34,90,92,99-102] However, a few studies have reported remarkably high frequencies of resorption, centering around 70%.[35,49,84,87] Case selection, especially in relation to stage of tooth development and age undoubtedly has had a great influence upon the PDL healing result (see later). One factor which should also be considered in the assessment of PDL healing is that cases which initially are diagnosed as surface resorption ("superficial" or "limited resorption") have been reported to develop into progressive resorption (ankylosis) with increasing observation period.[92,109] An explanation for this could be an initial incorrect diagnosis of ankylosis as surface resorption. For that reason, the frequency of PDL healing without root resorption presented in Table 6.1 includes surface resorption and/or ankylosis and inflammatory resorption.

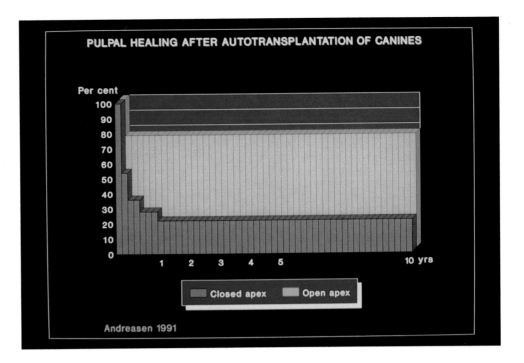

Fig. 6.20. Pulpal healing of 48 autotransplanted canines with incomplete and complete root formation at the time of surgery. From Andreasen 1991.[117]

Concerning the location of root resorption, a common finding has been that resorption usually affects the distal root surface more frequently than the mesial surface,[59,92,99,111] a phenomenon which might be explained by the fact that the distal surface often acts as a fulcrum during elevation of the tooth.[84,111] Furthermore the cervical region appears to be the first surface affected,[60,100,111] but later root resorption is found evenly distributed over the root surface (Fig. 6.21). Inflammatory resorption and replacement resorption often occur simultaneously, indicating similar etiologies.[60,100] In several studies attempts have been made to examine which clinical factors are related to root resorption. In the following, a survey of these factors will be given.

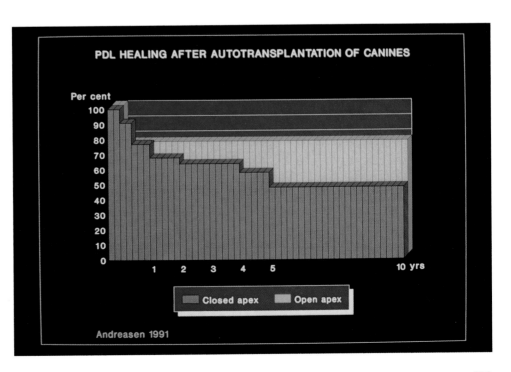

Fig. 6.21. PDL healing of 48 autotransplanted canines with incomplete and complete root formation at the time of surgery. From Andreasen 1991.[117]

Observation period

It has been found that most cases of resorption can be diagnosed within the first year;[100] however, with increasing observation periods significantly more resorptions are found (Fig. 6.21).[84,92] Most cases of progressive resorption will be diagnosed within the first 3 years after transplantation.[84,99] It should be mentioned, however, that later occurrence of root resorption has been found, 5-8 years after transplantation.[92,96]

Stages of root development

When root development was divided into complete and incomplete (see p. 199) Oksala and Kallioniemi found that incomplete root development resulted in a significantly lower frequency of root resorption (38% versus 90%). In this author's material the corresponding figures are 48% versus 76% (Fig. 6.21).[101] This observation parallels the findings for transplantation of premolars and molars (see p. 125 and 164).

Age at time of surgery

The effect of age at the time of surgery is most likely explained by the stage of root development, but no studies to date have attempted to distinguish between these two factors. In one study patients who underwent transplantation before 20 years of age showed significantly less progressive resorption than did older patients (56% versus 93%).[92]

Surgical technique

The use of forceps or heavy elevation has been found to be related to the extent of root resorption.[111]

Endodontic treatment

In studies where *extra-alveolar* endodontic treatment was performed extraorally, it was found that this procedure significantly increased the occurrence of progressive root resorption.[87,95,110]

On the other hand *postponed* endodontic treatment compared to *no* endodontic treatment in cases with complete root formation can significantly decrease the occurrence of inflammatory resorption, whereas the prevalence of replacement resorption is not influenced.[106]

In conclusion, the frequency and extent of root resorption after canine transplantation seem to follow the pattern of premolar and molar transplantation, where the most important factor appears to be the selection of donor teeth with incomplete root development. Furthermore, when teeth with mature formation are transplanted, either postponed endodontic treatment is carried out or revascularization is aimed for.

Root development and developmental disturbances

To date, no data exist on this complication. This is presumably due to the fact that relatively few canines are transplanted before completion of root development. However, completion of root formation can occur following transplantation of canines in early stages of root development (Fig. 6.23).

Fig. 6.22. Radiographic sign of ankylosis (arrows) 2 years after transplantation of a maxillary canine.

| 0 day | 0 day | 2 years | 3 years |

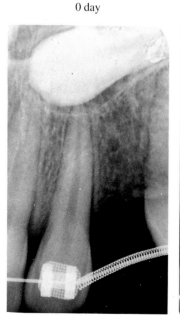 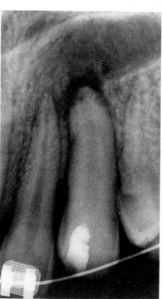 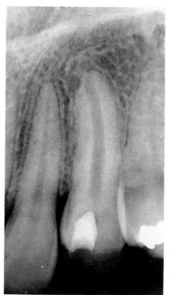 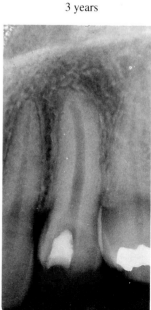

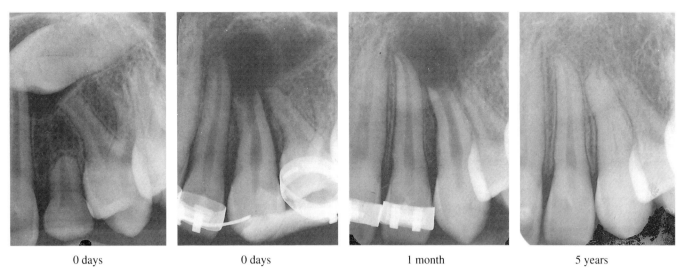

| 0 days | 0 days | 1 month | 5 years |

Fig. 6.23. Completion of root formation after transplantation of a maxillary canine.

Gingival healing and loss of marginal attachment

The reported frequency of loss of marginal support varies considerably in the various studies (Table 6.1). An average loss of attachment has been found to be 1.1 mm with observation periods ranging from 1 to 3 years and this progresses slightly by 0.4 mm over an additional 3.5 years.[92] Loss of attachment has been found equally distributed on the mesial, distal, and lingual surfaces, while the labial surface is affected least.[60] Furthermore, loss of attachment has been found to be related to root development, being considerably less frequent in teeth with incomplete root formation (0.4 mm) than in teeth with completed root formation (2.0 mm).[92] Loosening of the transplanted teeth is an uncommon finding, being found in only 8% to 17% of the cases.[59,84,85,92] Lack of marginal bone repair has also been found to be related to root development, occurring in only 13% of the teeth with incomplete root formation compared to 52% with completed root formation, and is possibly also related to an age factor, as it is uncommon before 20 years of age and affects one-third to one-half of patients above that age (Fig. 6.24).[85,90]

Fig. 6.24. Loss of marginal bone support and replacement resorption. Extensive root resorption exposing the pulp of the lateral incisor necessitated removal of that tooth, whereby mesial bone support in the transplant region was lacking.

| 0 days | 2 months | 1 year | 2 years | 2 years |

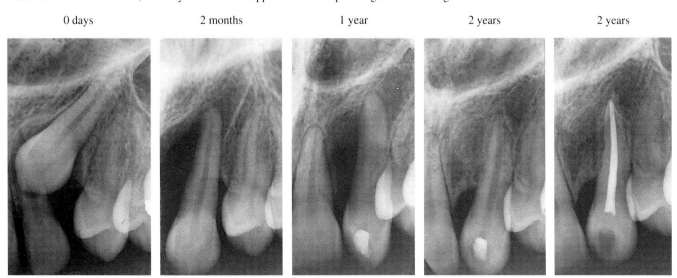

Healing related to graft selection

A synopsis of the various healing parameters and their relation to the stage of root formation at the time of transplantation is shown in Fig. 6.25. It appears that transplantation at stage 4 is optimal (i.e., full root formation and apex wide open).[109]

Fig. 6.25. Graft selection
Pulpal and periodontal healing and root growth after transplantation related to stage of root development at the time of grafting. It appears that full root length with open apices offers optimal healing results when all healing parameters have been considered.[120]

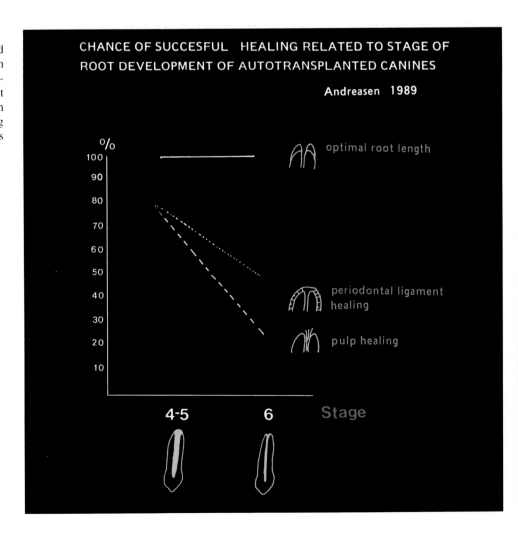

Essentials

Indications

Ectopically positioned canines where surgical exposure and subsequent orthodontic realignment cannot be performed. Ectopically positioned canines eliciting root resorption of adjacent teeth.

Treatment planning

Preoperative radiographs including three-dimensional location of the canine. Space evaluation of the recipient site comprising mesiodistal, apicocoronal and labiolingual dimensions.

Surgical procedure (Figs. 6.9-6.11)

1. Administer local anesthesia and antibiotic therapy
2. Remove the canine from a labial or lingual approach according to its location
3. Prepare the socket
4. Position the transplant in the socket in slight infraocclusion
5. Splint the canine with an acid-etch splint or a wire splint and maintain splinting for 3-4 weeks
6. Take a postoperative radiograph

Special cases

Lack of space at the recipient site
      Grinding of the transplant
      Rotation of the transplant
      Semierupted position of the transplant (Fig. 6.13a)
Labiolingual direction
      Fracture of the labial bone plate (Fig. 6.13b)
      Rotation of the transplant (Fig. 6.13c)
      Semierupted position of the transplant
Root apex deviation
      Resection of the apex (Fig. 6.14)
Two-stage procedure

Follow-up

(See Appendix 2, p. 290)

Prognosis

Tooth survival (5 years)

Incomplete root formation	100%
Complete root formation	82%

Pulpal healing (5 years)

Incomplete root formation	76%
Complete root formation	22%

PDL healing (5 years)

Incomplete root formation	76%
Complete root formation	48%

References

1. Widman L. Om transplantation af retinerede tänder. Svensk Tandläkar Tidskr 1917; 10: 29-40.

2. Widman L. Om transplantationens betydelse. Svensk Tandläkar Tidskr 1918; 11: 25-43, 323-46.

3. Dewel BF. The upper cuspid: Its development and impaction. Angle Orthod 1949; 19: 79-90.

4. Thilander B, Jacobsson SO. Local factors in impaction of maxillary canines. Acta Odontol Scand 1968; 26: 145-68.

5. Jacoby H. The etiology of maxillary canine impactions. Am J Orthod 1983; 84: 125-32.

6. Röhrer A. Displaced and impacted canines. Int J Orthod Oral Surg 1929; 15: 1003-20.

7. Adler-Hradecky C, Polczer MG. Der Geschlechtunterschied in der Frequenz der Dystopie des oberen Eckzähnen. Dtsch Zahnärztl Z 1960; 15: 732-36.

8. Dachi SF, Howell FV. A survey of 3,874 routine full-mouth radiographs. II. A study of impacted teeth. Oral Surg Oral Med Oral Pathol 1061; 15: 1165-69.

9. Sinkovits V, Polczer MG. Die Häufigkeit retinierter Zähne. Dtsch Zahnärztl Z 1969; 19: 389-96.

10. Rayne J. The unerupted maxillary canine. Dent Practit 1969; 19: 194-203.

11. Tränkmann J. Haufigkeit retinierter Zähne der zweiten Dentition. Dtsch Zahnärztl Z 1973; 28: 415-20.

12. Shah RM, Boyd MA, Vakil TF. Studies of permanent tooth anomalies in 7,386 Canadian individuals. I. Impacted teeth. J Can Dent Assoc 1978; 44: 262-64.

13. Paatero YV, Kiminki A. Further study of the palatolabial position of retained upper canines. Finska Tandläkar Forhandlingar 1962; 58: 294-300.

14. Nordenram RÅ, Strömberg C. Positional variations of the impacted upper canine. A clinical and radiologic study. Oral Surg Oral Med Oral Pathol 1966; 22: 711-14.

15. Bass TB. Observations on the misplaced upper canine tooth. Dental Practit 1967; 18: 25-33.

16. Aitasalo K, Lehtinen R, Oksala E. An orthopantomographic study of prevalence of impacted teeth. Int J Oral Surg 1972; 1: 117-20.

17. Mead SV. Incidence of impacted teeth. Int J Orthod Oral Surg Radiograph 1930; 16: 885-93.

18. Hagerström L. Storleksbestämning av icke frambrutna hörntänder och premolarer. En metod studie. Odontol Rev 1966; 1: 50-54.

19. Ostrofsky MK. Localization of impacted canines with Status-X radiography. Oral Surg Oral Med Oral Pathol 1976; 42: 529-33.

20. Hitchin AD. The impacted maxillary canine. Br Dent J 1956; 100: 1-14 .

21. Salman L. The surgical exposure of the impacted and unerupted tooth as an aid to orthodontics . NY Stat Dent J 1961; 27: 273-82.

22. Seward GR. Radiology in general dental practice. Br Dent J 1963; 115: 85-92.

23. Richardson A, McKay C. The unerupted maxillary canine. The clinical level after surgical repositioning. Br Dent J 1965; 118: 123-26.

24. Schmuth GPF, Clar E. Die röntgenologische Lokalisation verlagerter Zähne mit dem Panorexverfahren. Dtsch Zahnärzteblatt 1971; 25: 159-62.

25. Howard RD. The displaced maxillary canine: positional variations associated with incisor resorption. Dent Pract Dent Rec 1972; 22: 279-87 .

26. Langlais RP, Langland OE, Morris CR. Radiographic localization technics. Dent Radiogr Photogr 1979; 52: 69-77.

27. Hunter SB. The radiographic assessment of the unerupted maxillary canine. Br Dent J 1981; 150: 151-55.

28. Matteson SR, Sanders SS, Hill C. Localization of objects in the anterior areas with a single Panorex radiograph. Oral Surg Oral Med Oral Pathol 1976; 42: 847-50.

29. Adam M. Ergebnisse von 50 Fällen mit Variationen der Verlagerung von Eckzähnen nach chirurgisch orthopädischer Behandlung. Fortschr Kieferorthop 1970; 31: 65-71.

30. Rohlin M, Rundquist L. Apical root anatomy of impacted maxillary canines. A clinical and radiographic study. Oral Surg Oral Med Oral Pathol 1984; 58: 141-47.

31. Boyne PJ. Use of freeze-dried homogenous bone grafts in the surgical positioning of teeth. J Oral Surg 1957; 15: 231-37.

32. Boyne PJ. Tooth transplantation procedures utilizing bone graft materials. J Oral Surg 1961; 19: 47-53.

33. Mavaddat I. Tooth transplantation by separation and moving of the adjacent alveolar bone. Oral Surg Oral Med Oral Pathol 1971; 32: 367-70.

34. Rud J. Transplantation of canines. Tandlægebladet 1985; 89: 399-417.

35. Hardy P. The autogenous transplantation of maxillary canines. Br Dent J 1982; 153: 183-86.

36. Shulman LB. Impacted and unerupted teeth: Donors for transplant tooth replacement. Dent Clin North Am 1979; 23: 369-83.

37. Guralnick WC, Shulman LB. Tooth transplantation. Dent Clin North Am 1962; July: 499-511.

38. Flath I. Klinische Beobachtungen bei der echten Transplantation von retinierten Zähnen. Dtsch Stomatol 1963; 13: 562-74.

39. Schmidt-Flath I. Nachuntersuchungen transplantierter Zähne. Stomatol DDR 1974; 24: 596-601.

40. Kallioniemi H. Oksala E. Significance of an open apex or fracture of the root tip for the prognosis of vital maxillary canine autotransplantation. Proc Finn Dcnt Soc 1977 ; 73 : 136-32.

41. Janson M, Janson I, Herforth A. Die Zahntransplantation mit partieller Apektomie. (Eine klinische und histologische Studie). Dtsch Zahnärztl Z 1978; 33: 657-664.

42. Holland DJ. A technique of surgical orthodontics. Am J Orthodont 1955; 41: 27-44.

43. Holland DJ. The surgical positioning of unerupted, impacted teeth (surgical orthodontics). Oral Surg Oral Med Oral Pathol 1956; 9; 130-40.

44. Baden E. Surgical management of unerupted canines and premolars. Oral Surg Oral Med Oral Pathol 1956; 9: 141-92.

45. Williamson JJ. Surgical positioning of maxillary canines. Report of a case. Oral Surg Oral Med Oral Pathol 1964; 17: 289-95.

46. McKay C. Surgical orthodontics applied to the unerupted maxillary canine. Br Dent J 1961; 110: 231-33.

47. Cowan A, Keith JE. Surgical positioning of unerupted maxillary canines. A preliminary report. Dent Pract 1961; 11: 341-50.

48. Briggs CP, Burland JG. A two stage canine transplantation. Br J Orthod 1974; 1: 213-16.

49. Cook RM. The current status of autogenous transplantation as applied to the maxillary canine. Int Dent J 1972; 22: 286-300.

50. Grung B. 1986; Personal communication.

51. Söder P-Ö, Lundquist G. Autotransplantation of teeth with use of cell cultivation technique. Int Dent J 1972; 22: 327-40.

52. Kristerson L, Söder P-Ö, Otteskog P. Transport and storage of human teeth in vitro for autotransplantation and replantation. J Oral Surg 1976; 34: 13-18.

53. Thomsson M, Blomlöf L, Otteskog P, Hammarström L. A clinical and radiographic evaluation of cultivated and autotransplanted human teeth. Int J Oral Surg 1984; 13: 211-20.

54. Schwartz O, Bergmann P, Klausen B. Autotransplantation of human teeth. A life-table analysis of prognostic factors. Int J Oral Surg 1985; 14: 245-58.

55. Hillerup S, Hjørting-Hansen E, Schwartz O. Rekonstruktion af processus alveolaris ved læbe-kæbe-ganespalte. Tandlægebladet 1985; 89: 511- 513

56. Reinholdt J, Andreasen JO, Söder P-Ö, Otteskog P, Dybdahl R, Riis I. Cultivation of periodontal ligament fibroblasts on extracted monkey incisors. A histologic study of three culturing methods. Int J Oral Surg 1977; 7: 215-52.

57. Andreasen JO. Delayed replantation after submucosal storage in order to prevent root resorption after replantation. An experimental study in monkeys. Int J Oral Surg 1980; 9: 394-403.

58. Hillerup S, Dahl E, Schwartz O, Hjörting-Hansen E. Tooth transplantation to bone graft in cleft alveolus. Cleft Palate J 1987; 24: 137-41.

59. Reade P, Monsour A, Bowker P. A clinical study of the autotransplantation of unerupted maxillary canines. Aust Dent J 1973; 18: 273-80.

60. Oksala E. Autotransplantation of vital maxillary canines. A clinical and radiographic study. Proc Finn Dent Soc 1974; 70: Suppl 1.

61. Kominek J, Kominkova O. Transplantation of teeth and dental germs. Cesk Stomatol 1958; 58: 372-84.

62. Cavaillon JP. Applications chirurgicales des greffes d'os heterogene anorganique aux transplantations d'organes dentaires. Rev Franc Odontostomatol 1961; 8: 861-74.

63. Petit H. Suggestion pour ameliorer les réimplantations et les transplantations. Actual Odontostomatol (Paris) 1961; 55: 357-76.

64. Müller EE. Transplantation of impacted teeth. J Am Dent Assoc 1964; 69: 55-63.

65. Ehricke A. Über die Transplantation verlagerter Eckzähne. Dtsch Monatsschr Zahnheilk 1921; 39: 203-09.

66. Turgel OI. Zur Frage der Verwendung retinierter Zähne zur Wiederherstellung des Zahnbogens. Z Stomatol 1932; 30: 26-33.

67. Henry CB. Examples of reimplantation of teeth in young subjects. Proc R Soc Med 1955; 48: 1013-15.

68. Schwenzer N. Die Verflanzung oberer, verlagerter Eckzähne. ZWR 1957; 3: 65-67.

69. Snijman PC. Transplantation of teeth in man. Tydskr Tandheelkd Ver S Afr 1961; 16: 44-47.

70. Nordenram Å. Autoplastic tooth transplantation: its clinical applicability. Oral Surg Oral Med Oral Pathol 1962; 15: 1489-94.

71. Nordenram Å. Tandtransplantationer. Svensk Tandläkar Tidsk 1964; 57: 55-72.

72. Nordenram Å. The unerupted, partially erupted or erupted tooth. A potential autograft. Swed Dent J 1971; 64: 293-309.

73. Fordyce GL. Surgical problems of orthodontic interest. Dent Pract 1965; 15: 388 -96.

74. de Rysky S, Nidoli G, Caprioglio D. Trapianti e reimpianti dentali. Contributo personale. Riv Ital Stomatol 1966; 21: 3-15.

75. Bertolini AG. Auto-trapianto di dente vivente con una tecnica personale. Inf Odontostomtol 1970; 6: 9-12.

76. Frenkel G, Stellmach R. Clinical and therapeutic aspects of impacted teeth. Transplantation of impacted canines. Quintessence Int 1973; 9: 132-35.

77. Wreakes G, Cooke MS. The transplantation of canines using direct bonded orthodontic bracket fixation: An improved technique. Br J Orthod 1979; 6: 5-9.

78. Gombos F, Caruso F, Preteroti AM. Gli insuccessi negli autotrapianti e nei reimpianti dentari. Arch Stomat (Napoli) 1979; 20: 21-35.

79. Murganic Z, Murganic-Vasiljevic M. Transplantation retinierter Eckzähne bei jugendlichen (1). Quintessenz Int 1984; 1: 23-29.

80. Simpson W. The reimplanted maxillary canine. Br J Oral Surg 1966; 4: 150-54.

81. Lovius BBJ, Atherton JD, Wynne THM, Finch LD. Autogenous tooth transplantation: a clinical and histological investigation. Br J Orthod 1974; 1: 27-33 .

82. Heslop IH. Autogenous replantation of the maxillary canine. Br J Oral Surg 1967; 5: 135-40.

83. Moss JP. Autogenous transplantation of maxillary canines. J Oral Surg 1968; 26: 775-83.

84. Moss JP. The indications for the transplantation of maxillary canines in the light of 100 cases. Br J Oral Surg 1975; 12: 268-74.

85. Hovinga J. Autotransplantation of maxillary canines: a long-term evaluation. J Oral Surg 1969; 27: 701-808.

86. Thonner K-E, Meijer M. Autotransplantation of impacted upper canines a clinical and histological investigation. Odontol Tidskr 1969; 77: 113-19.

87. Thonner KE. Autogenous transplantation of unerupted maxillary canines: A clinical and histological investigation over five years. Dent Pract 1971; 21: 251-56.

88. Bolton R. Autogenous transplantation and replantation of teeth: report on 60 treated patients. Br J Oral Surg 1974; 12: 147-65.

89. Luhr H-G, Hammer U, Bull H-G. Indikation, Technik und Ergebnisse der autologen Eckzahntransplantation. Fortschr Kiefer Gesichtschir 198; 20: 129-32.

90. Altonen M, Haavikko K, Malmström M. Evaluation of autotransplantations of completely developed maxillary canines. Int J Oral Surg 1978; 7: 434-41.

91. Reitzik M. Autogenous tooth transplantation: A modified surgical technique based upon histological evidence. J Dent Assoc S Afr 1976; 31; 631-36.

92. Oksala E, Kallioniemi H. A longitudinal clinical and radiographic study of autotransplantation of the maxillary canine. Proc Finn Dent Soc 1977; 73: 117-25.

93. Hasselgren G, Larsson A, Rundquist L. Pulpal status after autogenous transplantation of fully developed maxillary canines. Oral Surg Oral Med Oral Pathol 1977; 44: 106-12.

94. Azaz B, Zilberman Y, Hackak T. Clinical roentgenographic evaluation of thirty-seven autotransplanted impacted maxillary canines. Oral Surg Oral Med Oral Pathol 1978; 45: 8-16.

95. Gardiner GT. The autogenous transplantation of maxillary canine teeth. A review of 100 consecutive cases. Br Dent J 1979; 146: 382-85.

96. Urbanska DK, Mumford JM. Autogenous transplantation of non-root-filled maxillary canines: a long-term follow-up. Int Endod J 1980; 13: 156-60.

97. Kristerson L, Kvint S. Autotransplantation av tänder - 10 års erfarenheter. Tandläkartidningen 1981; 73: 598-606

98. Ahlberg K, Bystedt H, Eliasson S, Odenrick L. Long-term evaluation of autotransplanted maxillary canines with completed root formation. Acta Odontol Scand 1983; 41: 23-31.

99. Reade PC, Hall GH. A clinical study of the autotransplantation of maxillary canine teeth. In: Riviere GR, Hildeman WH, eds. Oral immunogenetics and tissue transplantation. New York, Amsterdam, Oxford: Elsevier/North Holland, 1982: 291-300.

100. Hall GM, Reade PC. Root resorption associated with autotransplanted maxillary canine teeth. Br J Oral Surg 1983; 21: 179-91.

101. Andreasen JO. Long-term prognosis of autotransplanted permanent canines. 1990; In preparation.

102. Lownie JF, Cleaton-Jones PE, Fatti P, Lownie MA. Autotransplantation of maxillary canine teeth. A follow-up of 35 cases up to 4 years. Int J Oral Maxillofac Surg 1986; 15: 282-87.

103. Sagne S, Lennartson B, Thilander B. Transalveolar transplantation of maxillary canines. Am J Orthod 1986; 90: 149-57.

104. Kahnberg KE. Autotransplantation of teeth. (I) Indications for transplantation with a follow-up of 51 cases. Int J Oral Maxillofac Surg 1987; 16: 577-85.

105. Pogrel MA. Evaluation of over 400 autogenous tooth transplants. J Oral Maxillofac Surg 1987; 42: 205-11.

106. Chambers IG, Reade PC, Poker ID. Early post-operative endodontic therapy limits inflammatory root resorption of autotransplanted maxillary canine teeth. Br J Oral Maxillofac Surg 1988; 26: 364-69.

107. Edmunds SH, Beck C. Root resorption in autotransplanted maxillary canine teeth. Int Endod J 1989; 22: 29-38.

108. Robinson PP. A comparision of monopolar and bipolar electrical stimuli and thermal stimuli in determining the vitality of autotransplanted human teeth. Archs Oral Biol 1987; 32: 191-94.

109. Forssell H, Oksala E. A 10-year follow-up of maxillary canine transplantation. Proc Finn Dent Soc 1986; 82: 209-12.

110. Schulz S. Zur Prognose autogener Zahntransplantationen bei der kieferorthopadischen Behandlungsplanung. Fortschr Kieferorthop 1989; 50: 186-95.

111. Fagade OO, Gillbe GV. Radiographic pattern of root resorption in autotransplanted maxillary canines. J Dent 1988; 16: 80-84.

112. Cobley D, Roberts WR. Tooth resorption in the two-stage transplantation technique: a case report. Br J Orthod 1987; 14: 91-93.

113. McBride JL, Rudge SJ. Two-stage maxillary canine transplantation. Br J Orthod 1982; 9: 48-50.

114. Jones ML, Aldred MJ, Hardy P. Tooth resorption in the two-stage transplantation technique - a case report. Br J Orthod 1983; 10: 157-58.

115. da Silveira JOL, Cauduro FS, Wagner JE, Farina JA. Autogenous transplantation of impacted maxillary canines. Oral Surg Oral Med Oral Pathol 1989; 68: 697-700.

116. Lownie JF. Autotransplantation of teeth; a review of current thoughts. Int J Orthod 1987; 25: 4-7.

117. Andreasen JO. Ectopic eruption of permanent canines eliciting resorption of incisors: treatment by autotransplantation of the canine. Tandlægebladet 1987; 91: 487-92.

118. Stoll P, Härle F, Schilli W. Transplantation eines Weisheitzahnes in ein autologes Beckenkammtransplantat am Unterkiefer. Dtsch Zahn-Mund-Kiefer Gesichtschir 1987; 11: 5-7.

119. Stenvik A, Semb G, Bergland O et al. Experimental transplantation of teeth to simulated maxillary alveolar clefts. Scand J Plast Reconstr Surg 1989; 23: 105-08.

117. Andreasen JO. Autotransplantation of canines. Study in progress, 1991.

Chapter 7
Autotransplantation of incisors

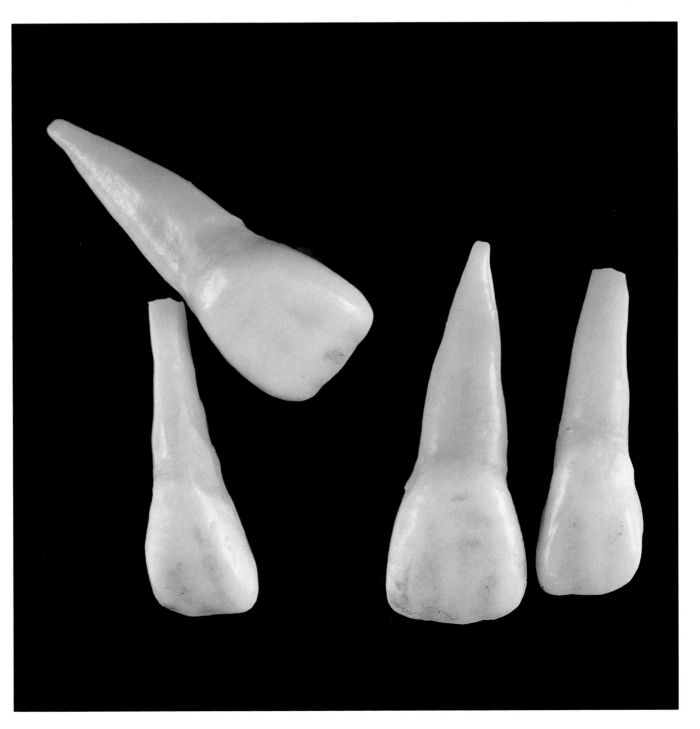

Indications

Autotransplantation of incisors can sometimes be of considerable value in the treatment of various pathologic conditions in the anterior region (Fig. 7.1). Thus, in cases where a cyst or other pathologic condition (e.g., cleft palate)[31] has caused *displacement* or *impaction* of a permanent tooth, autotransplantation can correct the situation.[1-3] In a congenital condition, such as cleidocranial dysostosis, multiple impactions are often seen and transplantation of incisors or other teeth can then be indicated.[4,5] Other indications for transplantation include incisors where malformation of the crown or root (crown or root dilaceration) prevents normal eruption. Futhermore cases with *aplasia* or *accidental loss* of maxillary incisors can be corrected by transplanting supernumerary teeth[7,8,37] or by transplantation of permanent mandibular incisors.[8,9]

Intra-alveolar transplantation of incisors has been developed as a method for treating teeth which have been severely damaged by crown-root fracture, deep cervical caries, or external cervical root resorption. In these cases transplantation of the root to a more coronal site facilitates fabrication of a crown restoration.[10-12,32-36,39]

Fig. 7.1. Various indications for incisor transplantation
A. Single or multiple impactions, e.g.,cleidocranial dysplasia and crown or root malformation. B. Follicle cysts. C and D. Crown-root fractures, cervical caries, or cervical root resorption.

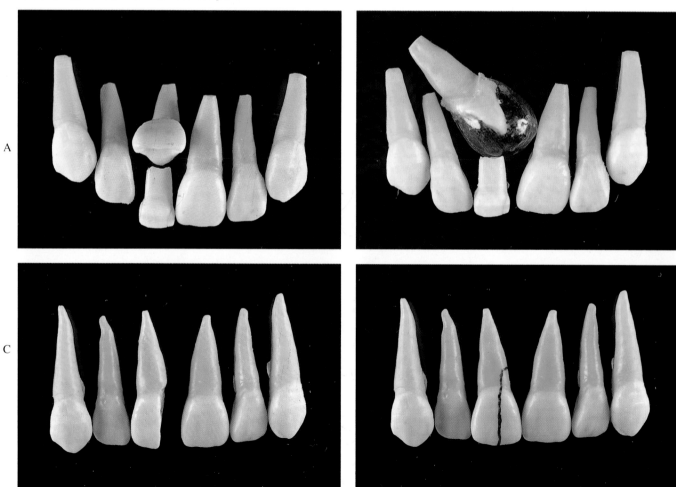

Treatment planning and surgical procedures

In the following, the treatment procedures for each of these conditions will be described.

Impactions

In this context, the preoperative clinical and radiographic evaluation follows the guidelines for canine transplantations (see Chapter 6, p. 180).

When the location of the permanent tooth graft and its space requirements have been determined and it has been ascertained that there is enough space in the recipient site for the transplant, the tooth is removed as atraumatically as possible using the flap, osteotomy, and splinting techniques described for canines (Fig. 7.2).

When crown or root malformations indicate transplantation, it is important to consider whether the crown anatomy has been altered. In cases with *root angulation*, crown anatomy is usually normal. In these cases a deviating socket is prepared which will allow the crown to be positioned normally. In cases with *crown dilaceration*, the crown is usually so severely deformed that it needs considerable restoration.[6] In such cases the root is transplanted to a normal position. The dilacerated crown is later reduced (i.e., 3 months after transplantation) to allow recontouring.

Fig. 7.2. Transplantation of a central incisor displaced by a cyst
Condition at 7 years of age. A dentigerous cyst has developed around the supernumerary incisor, possibly elicited as a sequel to a trauma to the primary incisors. The supernumerary tooth was removed and the cyst fenestrated. One year later, there is no sign of eruption of the central incisor. The displaced incisor was then transplanted into an upright position. At follow-up 2 years later root development is complete.

0 days	1 year	0 days	2 years

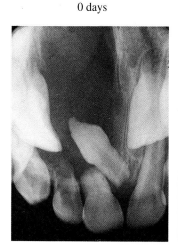 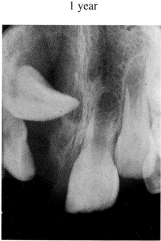 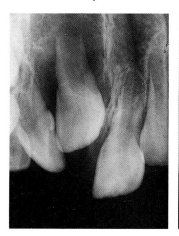 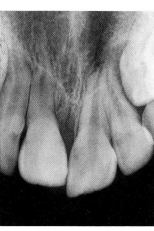

Recently transplantation of impacted incisors into a bone graft site in cleft palate cases has been developed (Fig. 7.3).[31]

Cleidocranial dysplasia

The name of the condition designates that it is a cranial malformation combined with aplasia or hypoplasia of the clavicles. However, several studies have indicated that it is a generalized skeletal dysplasia.[39-41]

The underlying pathogenetic mechanism appears to be a defect in bone remodeling primarily affecting bone resorption.[13,38,40] Thus, histologic examination of alveolar bone has shown dense bone without evidence of apposition or resorption.[14] The dental anomalies consist of multiple supernumerary permanent teeth, delayed resorption of primary teeth, multiple impacted permanent teeth, abnormalities of crown and root morphology of permanent teeth, and cyst formation especially around impacted molars. The supernumerary impacted teeth may be found in all regions but are most frequently observed in the incisor and premolar regions.[15,39]

The general mechanism behind these dental abnormalities has recently been suggested to be (a) persistence of the dental lamina leading to formation of supernumerary teeth and (b) lack of eruption of these teeth owing to a defect in bone and dentin resorption capacity.[16-19,39]

The primary teeth and the first permanent molars erupt spontaneously in nearly all cases, probably because there is very little bone covering the incisal edges or the occlusal surface of these teeth in comparison to the remaining permanent and supernumerary teeth.

Characteristically apices of the supernumerary teeth are malformed.[17,18] It has been suggested that the pathogenesis for this is root formation into the lumina of vascular canals in the apical area due to inadequate bone resorption.[17,18] Histologic examination of unerupted, extracted teeth has generally shown lack of cellular cementum.[16,18] This finding could be related to the nonfunctional status of the teeth. When erupted teeth are examined, cellular cementum is found.[18]

Fig. 7.3. Cleft palate patient treated with an iliac bone graft and subsequent incisor transplantation
Condition after closure of the cleft and secondary bone grafting in the right maxillary incisor region. The left lateral incisor is semi-impacted (arrow). From Hillerup & al., 1987.[31]

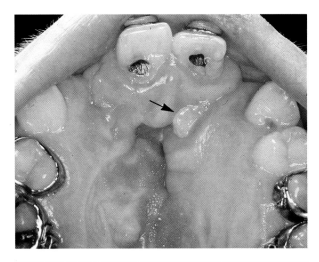

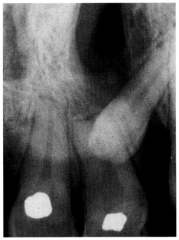

Follow-up
Condition after transplantation of the left semi-impacted incisor into the bone graft on the right side.

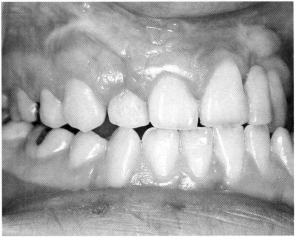

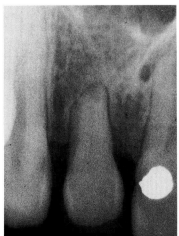

Various treatment procedures have been attempted. It has been found that extraction of primary teeth alone does not aid in the eruption of the permanent successors. Surgical exposure of the impacted teeth has been attempted.[18,23-27] However, it should be mentioned that this is not always successful and supplementary orthodontic therapy can therefore be necessary.[15,26] In these cases the treatment period is usually long and severely strains the anchoring teeth. If patients are left untreated there is a risk of cyst formation around the impacted teeth.[29,30] These cysts may later become infected, leading to multiple sinus tracts along the alveolar ridge. In 1967 Müller[4] demonstrated the use of transplantation for the realignment of impacted teeth, a procedure which has since been used successfully in several cases (Fig. 7.4).[5]

The goal of the surgical technique is to assist the retained permanent teeth in normal eruption. This includes removal of primary and supernumerary teeth. As the situation is usually rather complex, it is helpful to use a panoramic radiographic technique to reveal the number and location of the impacted teeth. A drawing is made over this radiograph, indicating the number of impacted teeth, which teeth are to be removed, and their sequence of removal (Fig. 7.5). In this regard it should be kept in mind that a minimum of bone should be removed.

The following technique has been used in a case with 29 impacted teeth (Fig. 7.5). The operation was performed in four sessions in order not to overload healing. A labial marginal flap was raised from the first molar to the central incisor region. Primary teeth were extracted gently in order not to damage supporting bone. Thereafter permanent teeth were removed in an order which ensured maximum preservation of

supporting bone. Normally, removal of one tooth will give access of the next impacted tooth. As a minimum, lingual and interdental bone should be preserved. Each removed tooth is placed in saline. After removal of all impacted teeth, those are selected which can be transplanted. The teeth to be transplanted are selected according to root formation (incomplete root formation is to be preferred), the amount of macroscopic periodontal ligament (PDL) on the root surface, and the length of the root. Sockets are prepared for these teeth. Teeth with incomplete root formation are placed with their incisal edges or occlusal surfaces at the gingival level whereas teeth with completed root formation are placed in a half or completely erupted position. Transplanted teeth are splinted using suture splints (see Chapter 5, p. 160). All teeth which cannot be used for transplantation are cryopreserved for later transplantation (see Chapter 9, p. 242).

In the case of permanent teeth with incomplete root formation and normal orientation in the alveolar process where the presence of supernumerary teeth has prevented eruption, removal of the supernumerary teeth and the bony covering may be all that is necessary to allow spontaneous eruption.

Fig. 7.5. Autotransplantation in an 18-year-old boy with cleidocranial dysplasia. (Page 212)

A. Only central incisors and some permanent molars have erupted spontaneously; 36 permanent teeth are impacted. B. A tracing is made on the radiograph indicating the position of the impacted teeth. The sequence of their removal is determined in order to ensure minimum sacrifice of alveolar bone. C. Follow-up 9 years after transplantation of 14 teeth; supernumerary teeth which were not transplanted were cryopreserved for later use (see Fig. 9.5, p. 245). From Jensen & al., 1991.[42]

Fig. 7.4. Transplantation of impacted teeth in a patient with cleidocranial dysplasia

In this case transplantation of 14 teeth was performed in an 18-year-old girl suffering from cleidocranial dysostosis. The status before transplantation is shown. From Oksala & Fagerström, 1971.[5]

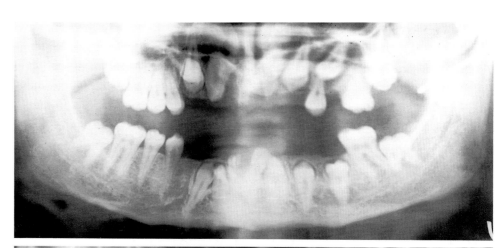

Follow-up
Condition at 3-year follow-up.

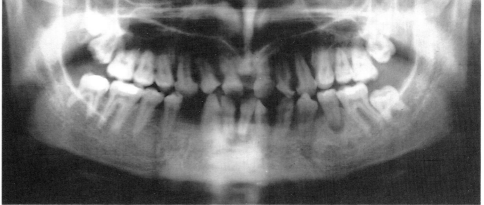

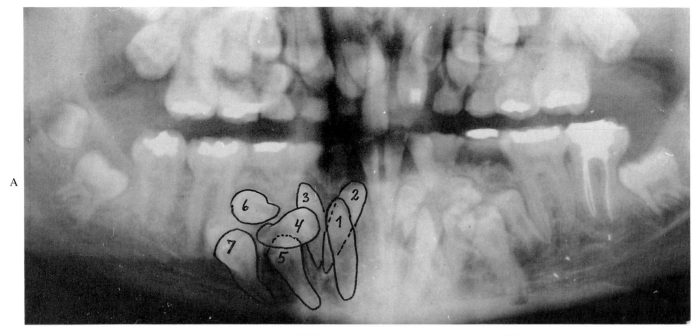

A

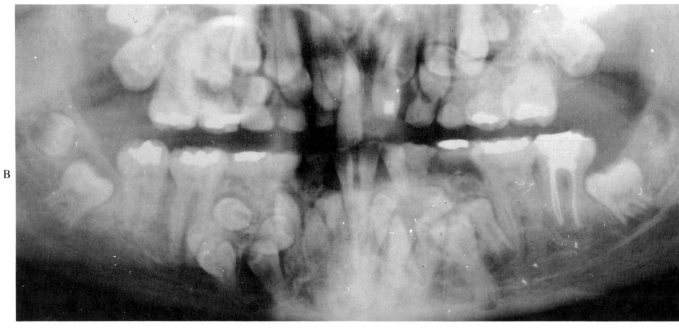

B

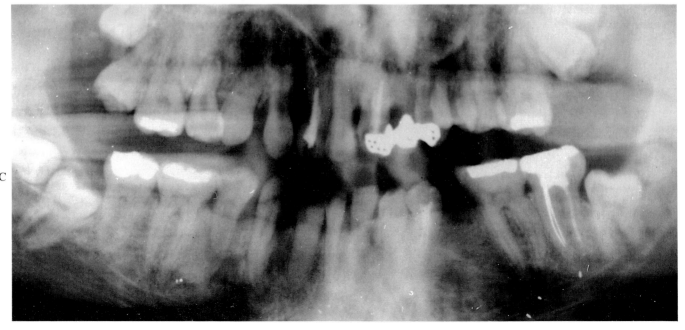

C

Fig. 7.6. Autotransplantation of a supernumerary incisor as a replacement for a geminated central incisor

This 8-year-old boy has a geminated right central incisor and an ectopic supernumerary incisor placed palatal to the right central incisor.

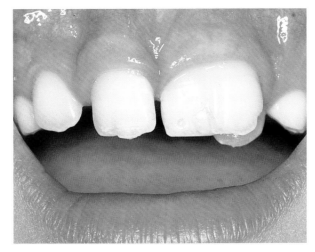 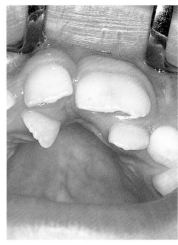

Extracting the geminated incisor

The treatment plan is to extract the geminated incisor and allow the large socket to partially heal before autotransplanting the supernumerary incisor.

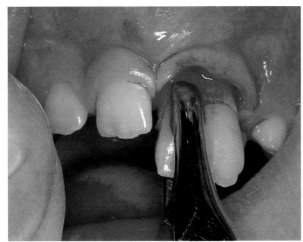 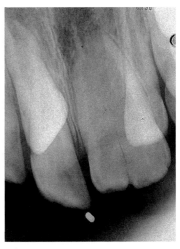

Status of extraction

Gemination of the root is also apparent after extraction.

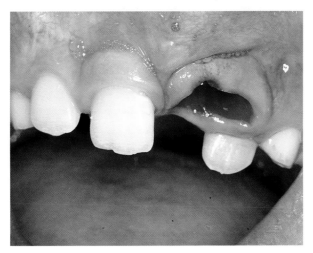 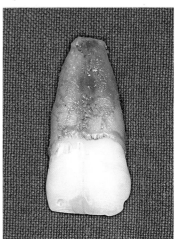

3 weeks later

Autotransplantation is planned, as the major part of the alveolus is now filled out with granulation tissue and osteoid. The future alveolus is created with a bur with internal cooling, whereafter the supernumerary tooth is extracted after incision of the PDL with a narrow scalpel blade. (see Appendix 7, p. 296)

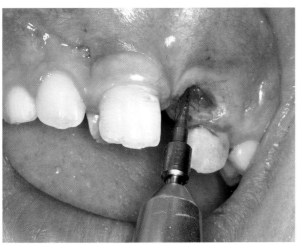 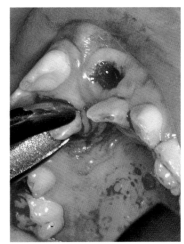

Fig. 7.6. Continued

**Condition after transplanta-
tion**
The supernumerary incisor fits into
the newly created socket.

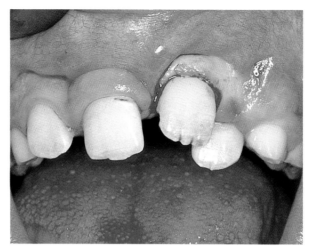 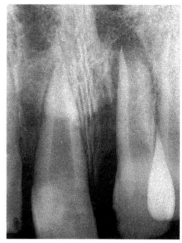

The sutures are removed 1 week after transplantation. The radiographic and clinical follow-up follows the outline given for other transplanted teeth (see Appendix 2, p. 290).

Due to the small number of cases treated by autotransplantation very little can be said at the present time about the long-term prognosis (Fig. 7.5).

Aplasia or loss of incisors

The transplantation of supernumerary incisors should be carried out at a stage of development which is optimal for PDL and pulpal healing. No studies have yet examined the optimal stage for transplantation of incisors, but it seems logical to assume that the guidelines used for premolars (i.e., 2/3-3/4 root formation) can also be applied to incisors. The possible donor teeth could be supernumerary teeth and in special circumstances mandibular lateral incisors (Fig. 7.6).

Intra-alveolar transplantation

This type of transplantation has recently been developed by Tegsjö & al.[10] (1978), Kahnberg & al.[11,12] (1982, 1985), and Bühler[35,36] (1984,1987), and is indicated in cases of crown-root fractures, teeth with cervical caries, or root resorption where enough root substance is left to support a post-retained crown restoration.

Two surgical approaches have been described for intra-alveolar transplantation. The first consists of an apical approach, where pressure is applied to the apex to extrude the tooth out of its socket.[10,38] In a simplified version described by Kahnberg et al.[11,12] (1982, 1985) the apical approach is omitted and mobilization is achieved by simple extraction. As the latter procedure seems to significantly reduce apical root resorption (i.e., surface resorption), the description of intra-alveolar transplantation will be based on this technique (Figs. 7.7 and 7.8).

As intra-alveolar transplantation is generally employed only in teeth with completed root formation, endodontic treatment is an integral part of the transplantation procedure. If the root canal is accessible, the pulp can be extirpated at this time and the root canal filled with gutta-percha and a sealer preoperatively. If a permanent root filling cannot be performed satisfactorily before transplantation, an alternative approach is to seal the root canal with a zinc oxide-eugenol cement. In this case the pulp is extirpated 3-4 weeks after transplantation and the root canal filled with calcium hydroxide as an interim dressing.[33] A gutta-percha root filling is made after 6 months where an apical hard tissue barrier has been performed. At this time the definitive restoration can be carried out. This technique appears to lead to an increased periapical healing rate.[39] In the case of initial root filling with gutta-percha a permanent restoration can be completed after 2 months (Fig. 7.7).

Fig. 7.7. Intra-alveolar transplantation of a crown-root fractured incisor with 180° rotation

The fracture extends 5 mm below the bone margin palatally.

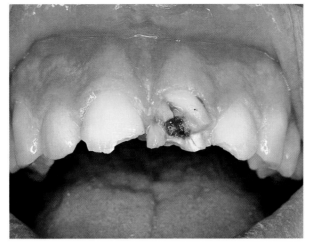

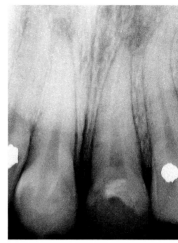

Endodontic treatment

The crown fragments are temporarily united with composite. Pulp extirpation and root filling with gutta-percha and a sealer is carried out.

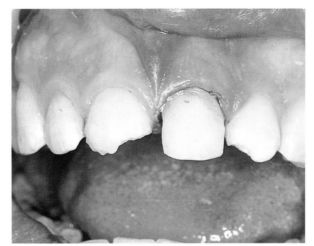

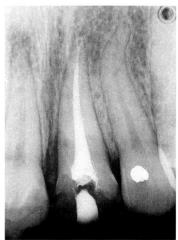

Incision of PDL and luxation

The PDL is incised as far apically as possible with a modified surgical blade (see Appendix 7, p. 296) around the entire circumference of the root. The tooth is then luxated using an elevator placed at the mesiolingual and the distolingual corners of the root, allowing a minimum of contact between the elevator and the root surface. Antibiotics are administered 1 hour before surgery and maintained for 4 days postoperatively.

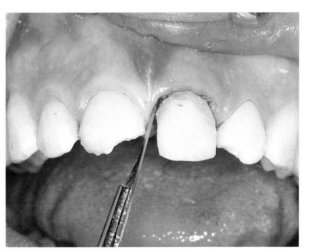

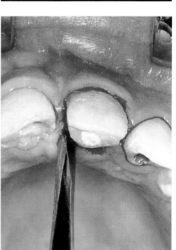

Tooth removal

The tooth is removed with forceps using slight rotation movements. The fracture extends deep on the palatal aspect of the root. At this time it is important to examine whether there are any incomplete fractures which could prevent healing.

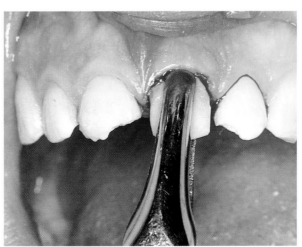

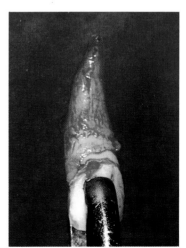

Fig. 7.7. Continued

Rotation of the root

Rotation of the root minimizes the intra-alveolar fracture extension. On this model is shown a crown-root fracture which extends 4 mm below the gingival margin.

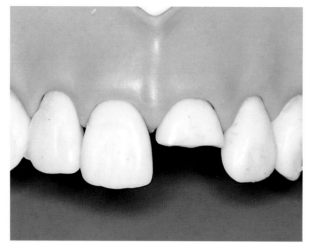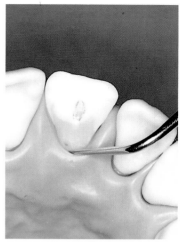

Status after rotation

The palatal part of the root is now placed labially, whereby the fracture surface has now an extra-alveolar location.

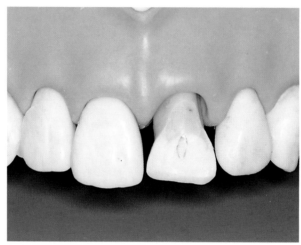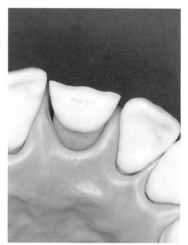

Intra-alveolar transplantation

The tooth is then transplanted to the desired position. It is important that the entire periphery of the line of fracture is placed at least 1 mm above the crest of the alveolar process.

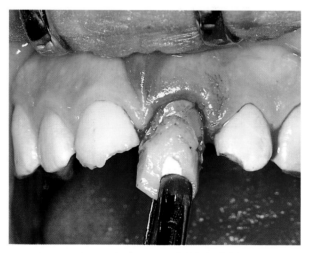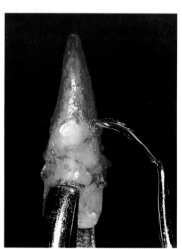

Splinting

After repositioning, the transplant is united with the adjacent incisors using an acid-etch splint. 2 months later the tooth can be restored.

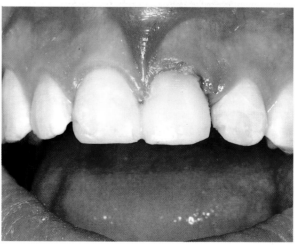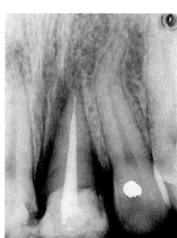

Fig. 7.8. Intra-alveolar transplantation of a crown-root fractured incisor with 90° rotation

The fracture extends 5 mm below the bone margin distally.

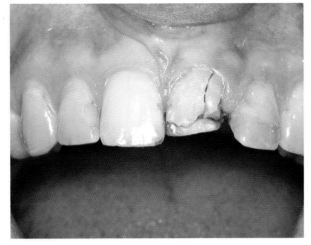 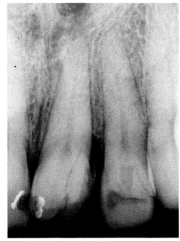

Incision of the PDL

The gingival and cervical fibers are incised with a modified surgical blade (see Appendix 7, p. 296). Thereafter the root is loosened with a narrow elevator.

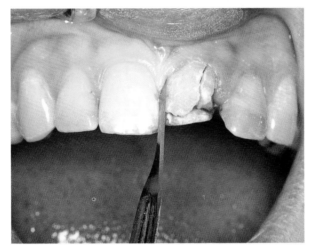 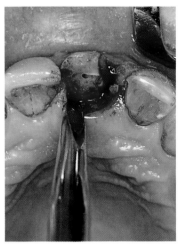

Tooth removal

The tooth is removed with a forceps.

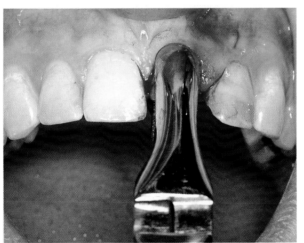 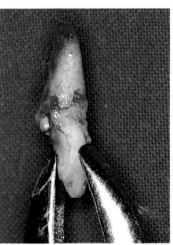

Repositioning and splinting

The tooth is rotated 90°, whereby the entire fracture surface is exposed.

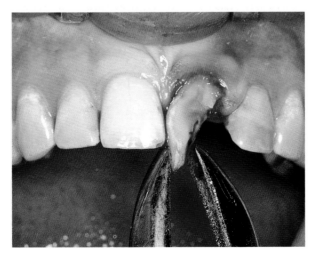 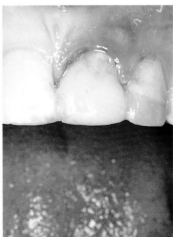

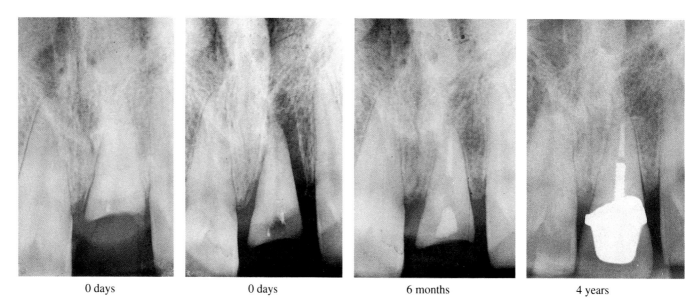

| 0 days | 0 days | 6 months | 4 years |

Fig. 7.9. Intra-alveolar transplantation of a crown-root fractured central incisor. No sign of root resorption is seen 4 years after transplantation. From Kahnberg, 1985.[12]

Prognosis

In the reported series of patients treated by intra-alveolar transplantation, either no root resorption was reported (Figs. 7.9 and 7.10) or there was surface resorption located only apically and resulting in a slight shortening of the root.[32] The latter resorption was found to be markedly reduced when a coronal instead of an apical approach was used for root removal (Table 7.1).[32] The long-term prognosis of these procedures as illustrated by Figs. 7.11 and 7.12, which appear to reveal good long-term results. The resorptions recorded in Fig. 7.12 have in all cases been found to be surface resorption and not progressive.[32,34]

Table 7.1. Long-term results of intra-alveolar transplantation of anterior teeth

	Observation period yr. (mean)	Age of patients yr. (mean)	Number of teeth	Tooth survival %	PDL healing %	Periapical healing %	Gingival healing %
Tegsjö & al., 1987[38]	4 (4.0)	9-33 (15.0)	56	91	88	98	
Kahnberg & al., 1988[33]	(5.5)	13-75 (31.0)	17*	100	65***	94	100
	(2.4)	13-75 (31.0)	41**	100	74***	95	100

*   Transplant performed via apical exposure
**   Transplant performed via coronal approach
*** Including cases with surface resorption that resulted only in slight shortening of the roots.

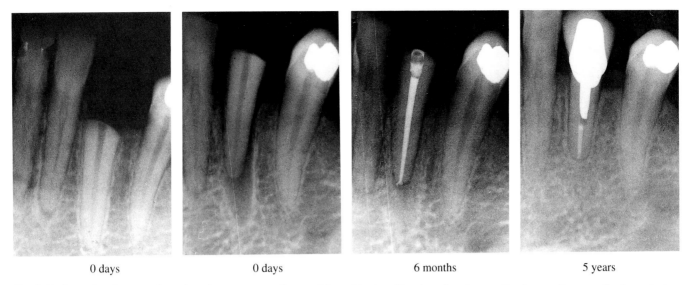

| 0 days | 0 days | 6 months | 5 years |

Fig. 7.10. Intra-alveolar transplantation of a crown-root fractured lateral incisor. No sign of root resorption is seen 5 years after transplantation. From Kahnberg, 1985.[12]

Fig. 7.11. Tooth survival of 68 intraalveolar transplanted anterior teeth with completed root formation at time of surgery. From Kahnberg 1990.[34]

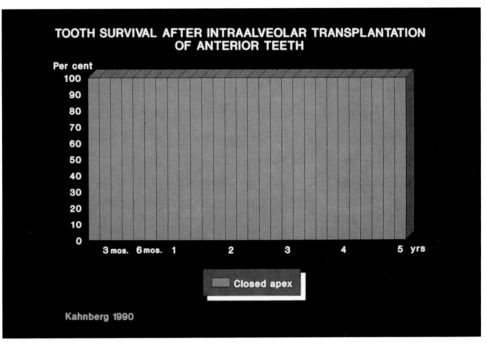

Fig. 7.12. PDL healing of 68 intraalveolar transplanted anterior teeth with completed root formation at time of surgery. From Kahnberg 1990.[34]

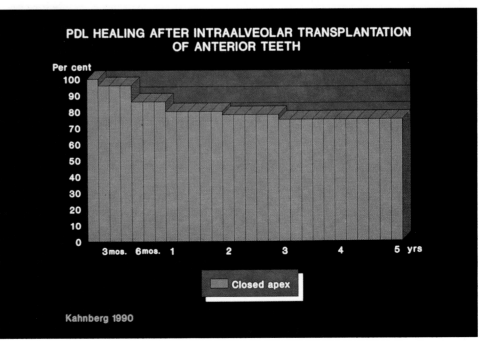

Essentials

Indications

Impacted incisors
Congenital or accidental loss of incisors
Crown-root fractured incisors
Cervical caries or root resorption extending below the alveolar crest

Treatment planning

Preoperative radiographs
Space evaluation

Impaction of incisors

1. Administer antibiotics and local anesthesia
2. Remove the impacted incisor as atraumatically as possible
3. Prepare the socket
4. Place the transplant in its new socket slightly in infraocclusion
5. Splint the tooth, preferably with sutures
6. Take a postoperative radiograph

Congenital or accidental loss of incisors

1. Administer antibiotics and local anesthesia
2. Prepare the socket
3. Remove the donor tooth atraumatically by incision of the PDL
4. Place the transplant in its new socket, slightly in infraocclusion
5. Splint the tooth, preferably only with a suture
6. Take a postoperative radiograph
7. If necessary the crown anatomy of the transplant can be altered by grinding and using an acid-etch/composite technique 3 months postoperatively (see Chapter 11, p. 220)

Crown-root fractured incisors and teeth with cervical caries or root resorption (Figs. 7.7 and 7.8)

1. Administer antibiotics and local anesthesia
2. The pulp should be extirpated and the root canal filled with gutta-percha and a sealer prior to intra-alveolar transplantation. Alternatively the root canal entrance is sealed with zinc oxide-eugenol cement
3. The PDL is incised using a long narrow scalpel blade. Thereafter, the tooth is luxated with an elevator placed in the PDL at the distolingual and mesiolingual corners. The tooth is then extracted with forceps
4. The root surface is inspected for incomplete root fractures, which would contraindicate transplantation.
5. The root is repositioned at a level 1 mm coronal to the alveolar creast. If desirable, the root can be rotated to achieve a maximum periodontal surface area within the socket
6. The tooth is stabilized using interproximal sutures
7. Take a postoperative radiograph
8. After 3 to 4 weeks, the transplant is usually firm. If the root canal has not been filled, calcium hydroxide is used as a dressing in the root canal. A temporary restoration can now be made
9. After 6 months, a permanent root filling as well as a definitive crown restoration can be undertaken
10. If a gutta-percha root filling has been made before transplantation, the tooth can be restored after 2 months

Follow-up

(See Appendix 2, p. 290)

Prognosis

Tooth survival (5 years)   100%
PDL healing (5 years)   75%

References

1. Ködel G. Über die Transplantation traumatisch verlagerter Frontzähne mit unvollendetem Wurzelwachstum. Dtsch Zahnärztl Z 1965; 20: 1151-56.

2. Perl P, Perl T, Goldman M. Surgical and orthodontic treatment of an unerupted, undeveloped, inverted central incisor. Tydskr Tandheelkd Ver S Afr 1966; 21: 152-54.

3. Hillerup S, Hjørting-Hansen E, Schwartz O. Rekonstruktion af processus alveolaris ved læbe-kæbe-ganesplate. Tandlægebladet 1985; 89: 511-13.

4. Müller EE. Transplantation of teeth in cleidocranial dysostosis. In; Husted E, Hjørting-Hansen E, eds. Oral Surg, Transact. 2nd cong. Int Assoc Oral Surg. Copenhagen: Munksgaard. 1967: 375-79.

5. Oksala E, Fagerström G. A two-stage autotransplantation of 14 teeth in a patient with cleidocranial dysostosis. Suom Hammaslääk 1971; 67: 333-338.

6. Andreasen JO. Traumatic injuries of the teeth. 2nd ed. Copenhagen: Munksgaard, 1981: 314

7. Kvam E, Bjercke B. Dentes confusi - en kasusrapport og et behandlingsalternativ. Nor Tandlægeforen Tid 1976; 86: 305-08.

8. Bjercke B. Autotransplantasjon av tenner på børn. In: Hjørting-Hansen E, ed. Odontologi. Copenhagen: Munksgaard, 1979: 7-25.

9. Henry CB. Examples of reimplantation of teeth in young subjects. Proc R Soc Med 1955; 48: 35-44.

10. Tegsjö U, Valerius-Olsson H, Olgart K. Intra-alveolar transplantation of teeth with cervikal root fractures. Swed Dent J 1978; 2: 73-82.

11. Kahnberg K-E, Warfvinge J, Birgersson B. Intraalveolar transplantation (I). The use of autologous bone transplants in the periapical region. Int J Oral Surg 1982; 11: 372-379.

12. Kahnberg K-E. Intraalveolar transplantation of teeth with crown-root fractures. J Oral Surg 1985; 43; 38-42.

13. Kreiborg S, Leth Jensen B, Björk A, Skieller V. Abnormalities of the cranial base in cleidocranial dysostosis. Am J Orthod 1981; 75: 549-58.

14. Fleicher-Peters A. Zur Pathohistologie des Alveolarknochens bei Dysostosis Cleidocranialis. Stoma 1970; 23: 212-15.

15. Kalliala E, Taskinen P. Cleidocranial dysostosis. Report of six typical cases and one atypical case. Oral Surg Oral Med Oral Pathol 1962; 15: 808-02

16. Rushton MA. The failure of eruption in cleido-cranial dysostosis. Br Dent J 1967; 63: 641-45 .

17. Hitchin AD, Fairley JM. Dental management in cleido-cranial dysostosis. Br J Oral Surg 1974; 12: 46-55.

18. Hitchin AD. Cementum and other root abnormalities of permanent teeth in cleido-cranial dysostosis. Br Dent J 1975; 139: 313-18.

19. Migliorisi JA, Blenkinsopp PT. Oral surgical management of cleidocranial dysostosis. Br J Oral Surg 1980; 18: 212-20.

20. Winther GR. Dental condition in cleidocranial dysostosis. Am J Orthod 1943; 29: 61-89.

21. Gorlin R, Pindborg JJ. Cleidocranial dysostosis (Scheuer-Marie-Sainton syndrome mutational dysostosis). In: Syndromes of the head and neck. New York: Mc Graw-Hill, 1964: 138-45.

22. Rushton MA, An anomaly of cementum in cleido-cranial dysostosis. Br Dent J 1956; 100: 81-85.

23. Kjellgren B. Bite conditions and treatment in cases of cleidocranial dysostosis. Int Dent J 1952-53; 3: 83-85.

24. Ascher F. Zur Lösung des zahnärztlichen Problems bei Dysostosis Cleidocranialis. Dtsch Zahn-Mund-Kieferheilk 1958; 29: 27-32.

25. Fleischer-Peters A. Therapeutische Möglichkeiten bei der Dysostosis cleidocranialis. Dtsch Zahnärztl Z 1967; 22: 80-88.

26. Smylski PT, Woodside DG Harnett BE. Surgical and orthodontic treatment of cleidocranial dysostosis. Int J Oral Surg 1974; 3: 380-85.

27. Hutton CE, Bixler D, Garuer LD. Cleidocranial dysplasia-treatment of dental problems: report of case. J Dent Child 1981; 48: 456-62.

28. Elomaa E, Elomaa M. Orthodontic treatment of a case of cleidocranial dysostosis. Suom Hammasläk 1967; 63: 139-151.

29. Koch PE, Hammer WB. Cleidocranial dysostosis: Review of the literature and report of cases. J Oral Surg 1978; 36: 539-42.

30. Oatis GW Robertson GR. Sugg WE. Firtell DN. Cleidocranial dysostosis with mandibular cyst. Report of a case. Oral Surg Oral Med Oral Pathol 1975; 40: 62-67.

31. Hillerup S, Dahl E, Schwartz O, Hjørting-Hansen E. Tooth transplantation to bone grafts in cleft alveolus. Cleft Palate J 1987; 24: 137-41.

32. Kahnberg KE. Surgical extrusion of root-fractured teeth - a follow-up study of two surgical methods. Endod Dent Traumatol 1988; 4: 85-89.

33. Warfvinge J, Kahnberg KE. Intraalveolar transplantation of teeth. IV. Endodontic considerations. Swed Dent J 1989; 13: 229-233.

34. Kahnberg KE. 1990. Personal communication.

35. Bühler H. Nachuntersuchung wurzelseparierter Zähne. (Eine röntgenologische Langzeitstudie). Quintessenz Int 1984; 35: 1825-37.

36. Bühler H. Intraalveoläre Transplantation von Einzelwurzeln. Quintessenz Int 1987; 38: 1963-70.

37. Jensen BL, Kreiborg S. Development of the dentition in cleidocranial dysplasia. J Oral Pathol Med 1990; 19: 89-93.

38. Spuller RL, Harrington M. Gemination of a maxillary permanent central incisor treated by autogenous transplantation of a supernumerary incisor: case report. Pediatr Dent 1986; 8: 299-302.

39. Tegsjö U, Valerius-Olsson H, Frykholm A, Olgart K. Clinical evaluation of intra-alveolar transplantation of teeth with cervical root fractures. Swed Dent J 1987; 11: 235-50.

40. Kreiborg S, Jensen BL, Björk A, Skieller V. Abnormalities of the cranial base in cleidocranial dysostosis. Am J Orthod 1981; 79: 549-57.

41. Jensen BL. Somatic development in cleidocranial dysplasia. Am J Med Gen 1990; 35: 69-74.

42. Jensen BL, Kreiborg S, Schwartz O, Andreasen JO. Management of dental problems in cleidocranial dysplasia. In preparation 1991.

Chapter 8
Allotransplantation of human teeth

O. Schwartz

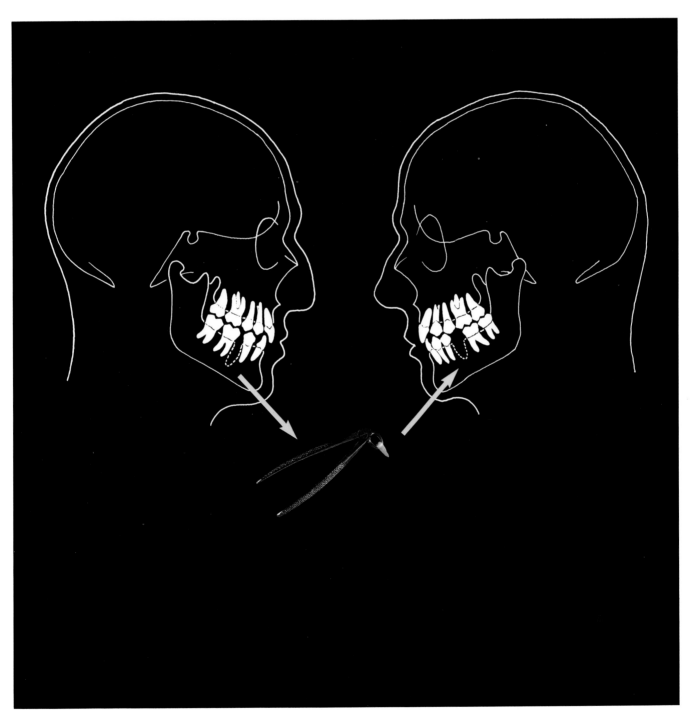

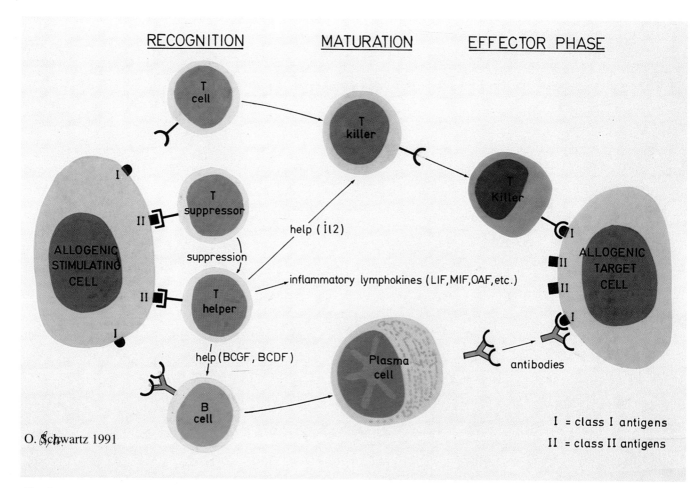

O. Schwartz 1991

I = class I antigens

II = class II antigens

Fig. 8.1. Immune reactions to transplantation of allogenic cells
Donor cells (gray) equipped with histocompatibility (H) antigens on the cell surface membrane trigger specific populations of recipient lymphocytes. When these immunocompetent cells recognize the foreign HLA class I or II antigens of the graft, specific clones of T- and B-cells are maturing into effector cells. The donor cells are then attacked by the cell-mediated (CMI) and the humoral-mediated (HMI) immune responses. Homeostasis of the immune reaction is maintained by a series of interactions among the lymphocyte subpopulations.

Transplantation immunology

When living tissues are transplanted to genetically different individuals of the same species (allotransplantation), immunologically characteristic reactions will influence the healing of the allograft. When a tooth is autotransplanted, no genetic challenge exists, and the tooth graft is accepted with normal periodontal and pulp healing, provided appropriate surgical techniques are employed and acceptable anatomic conditions are ensured with respect to the graft and recipient site.

When teeth are allotransplanted, the tooth graft elicits immune reactions in the host that will impair healing. The reactions aimed at rejection of the allograft are due to the immunologic barrier by which the recipient organism seeks to separate "self"-tissues that are equipped with own tissue type or histocompatibility (H-) antigens, from "nonself" tissues of the graft.

Consequently allotransplantation of a tooth from a donor mismatched for H- antigens of the recipient can trigger a population of the recipient's immunocompetent cells to a series of cell-mediated and humoral rejection mechanisms specifically directed against the donor cells of the graft carrying the mismatched H- antigens (Fig. 8.1).

In contrast to autotransplanted teeth, the usual healing event after allotransplantation is the formation of an ankylosis which gradually resorbs the root. This resorption may take a very protracted course, permitting clinical function of allotransplanted teeth for 32 years after transplantation.[1] Within the last decade the development of long-term implants which also heal by the formation of an "ankylosis" (osseointegration) but without resorption has influenced the indication for allotransplantation. A further factor which has influenced allotransplantation policy is the concern about the theoretical possibility of transmission of viruses such as HIV and hepatitis virus by way of organ transplantation. The use of tested cryopreserved donor teeth can, however, eliminate this possibility (see Chapter 9).

As tooth allotransplantation shows interesting biologic and clinical features with respect to pulpal and periodontal healing, this chapter will present a review of the clinical results obtained to date.

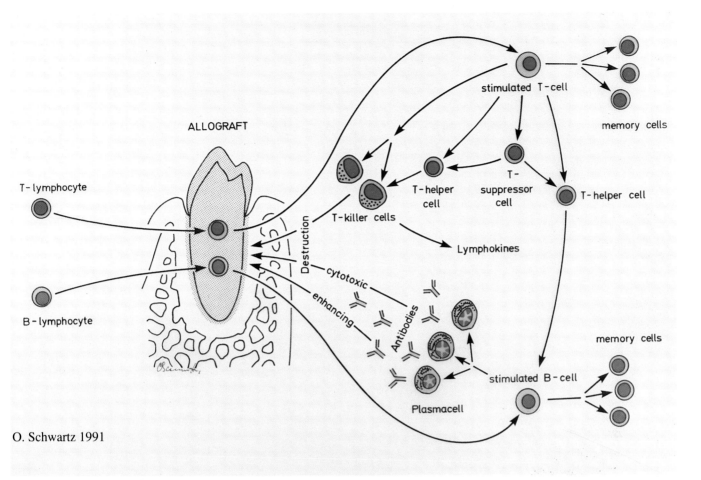

ALLOGRAPH

T-lymphocyte

B-lymphocyte

stimulated T-cell

memory cells

T-killer cells

T-helper cell

T-suppressor cell

T-helper cell

Destruction

Lymphokines

cytotoxic

enhancing

Antibodies

Plasmacell

stimulated B-cell

memory cells

O. Schwartz 1991

Fig. 8.2. Cell-mediated and humoral immune reactions leading to graft rejection
When the specific immunocompetent cells recognize the foreign H- antigens on the tooth allograft, T- and B- cell clones multiply and mature into effector cells. Ultimately, the specific attack on the donor cells is initiated by T- killer cells and specific antibodies directed against the donor tissue. Lymphokines, intercellular mediators of the immune system, modify the immune response among the lymphocyte subpopulations. Lymphokines also recruit inflammatory cells into a nonspecific attack on the graft.[9] The local inflammatory response leads to destruction of the donor tissue and resorption of the hard tissues of the tooth allograft.

Ultimately, these reactions can lead to destruction of the transplanted cells and resorption of the hard tissue of the tooth allograft (Fig. 8.2).[1] The alloimmune reactions involved in the rejection of a tooth graft include:

-**sensibilization** of the recipient by the foreign histocompatibility antigen by

-**activating** specific immunocompetent **T cells** and forming specific **antibodies**, which in turn will induce

-**local specific and nonspecific inflammation**, including cell damage and resorption of the foreign grafted tissues and

-**future memory** towards the specific donor antigen.

Prevention of allograft rejection leading to healing and long-term survival of an allograft thus requires circumvention of one or more components of the alloimmune reaction. This could theoretically be accomplished by:

HLA–SYSTEM

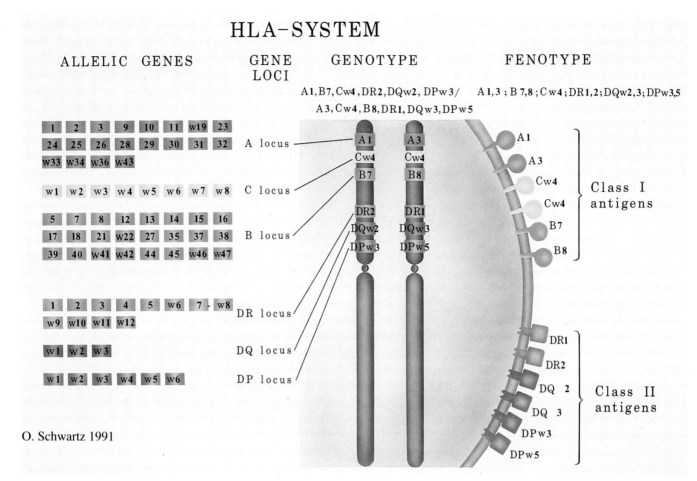

ALLELIC GENES	GENE LOCI	GENOTYPE	FENOTYPE

A1,B7,Cw4,DR2,DQw2,DPw3/   A1,3 ; B7,8 ; Cw4 ; DR1,2 ; DQw2,3 ; DPw3,5
A3,Cw4,B8,DR1,DQw3,DPw5

A locus

C locus

B locus

DR locus

DQ locus

DP locus

Class I antigens

Class II antigens

O. Schwartz 1991

Fig. 8.3. The HLA system
Schematic drawing of the major histocompatibility (HLA) system of man. The HLA complex contains *genes* located on chromosome pair no. 6, encoding for phenotypic *antigen* specificities of classes I and II, located on the cell surface. The HLA antigens are identically expressed on most cells of each individual. At each of the six known HLA loci on the two chromosomes in pair no. 6, there are a series of different *alleles* (alternative genes), only one of which can be found on any of the two chromosomes. Thus any individual will be equipped with one A allele on each A locus of each chromosome, and hence present a total of at most two different HLA-A antigenic specificities. Each HLA phenotype is individually very rare, for which reason it is difficult to find unrelated individuals having identical HLA phenotypes.

1. Histocompatibility matching of the donor and recipient according to a sufficient number of H- antigens, so that the graft could be accepted as "self" tissue.

2. Specific or nonspecific immunosuppression of the recipient immunocompetent cells. However, drugs presently used for this purpose in organ allotransplantation, such as cyclosporin A and steroids, have in therapeutic doses such severe general side-effects as to preclude their use in clinical allotransplantation of teeth at present.

3. Depression or removal of the graft antigenicity, so that the graft is not recognized as foreign. Hitherto this has not been possible without removing all living tissues of the allograft, leaving an "allostatic" implant of nonvital hard tissue. This type of implant falls outside the scope of the present chapter.

In humans, the histocompatibility antigens causing the most vigorous allograft rejection reactions are called the HLA antigens (Fig. 8.3). Matching of donor and recipient for the strong HLA antigens has been shown to lead to prolonged survival of organ allografts such as kidneys[2] as well as tooth allografts.[3] Details concerning transplantation immunology and its implications in *experimental* tooth allotransplantation are presented elsewhere.

Indications

Allotransplantation of teeth has been in clinical use since the late 1950's especially in Scandinavia where long-term survival and clinical function of these grafts have been demonstrated (Table 8.1).[1,3-5,7-10] Despite the fact that gingival or supraalveolar healing of allografts often resembles autografts with long-standing clinically normal marginal conditions, the intraalveolar healing usually takes place in the form of an ankylosis between the intraosseous part of the graft and adjacent bone.[1,8,11-14] Consequently, a gradual replacement of the root with bone will ultimately lead to loss of the graft. However, due to the normally protracted course of replacement resorption, especially in older individuals, a relatively long survival period can usually be expected.[1] Furthermore, when the graft is finally lost, there is generally very little alveolar bone loss in the graft region (Fig. 8.4). This is in contrast to the situation after loss of, for example an implant. Thus, the bone-maintaining nature of replacement resorption of the graft often leaves the region with sufficient alveolar bone for subsequent retransplantation or alternative treatment.

Allotransplantation has thus been used in selected cases as temporary replacement for nonrestorable teeth or in partially edentulous areas where preservation of the alveolar bone and integrity of adjacent teeth was of importance, and where alternative treatment was ruled out. With this in mind allotransplantation has been indicated in the following clinical situations.[1,8,10]

For single or multiple tooth replacements in cases of aplasia or loss of teeth where autotransplantation was not indicated, obviating or deferring conventional removable or fixed prostheses or implants. In these situations allotransplantation could be performed at the time of surgical removal of the tooth to be replaced. Transplantation at a later time could be performed under the premise that no severe bone loss had occurred, as in contrast to autotransplants, only limited new bone induction can be expected.

In single edentulous sites where the integrity of intact adjacent teeth has been of high priority. Allotransplantation might be indicated in the maxillary anterior region after traumatic avulsion. It is important to consider that ankylosis will develop subsequent to allografting. Thus, transplantation should await termination of vertical growth of the alveolar process; otherwise the transplanted tooth may gradually move into infraposition. In general, the recipient must therefore be over 20 years of age.

Treatment planning

The following guidelines have been applied in the allotransplantation of teeth in Copenhagen.

Recipients

Prior to surgery, a clinical and radiographic examination of the recipient region is made to ascertain available space and status of the supporting bone (Fig. 8.4).

Sufficient bone support implies that at least half the root length of the allograft can be placed within a bony socket. In order to avoid bone resorption, if a tooth is present at the recipient site, removal is postponed until the time of transplantation. In contrast to autotransplantation, firm splinting has been found necessary for uneventful healing. It is therefore preferable if adjacent teeth allow application of an acid- etch splint, arch bar, or an acrylic bar.

Donors

Potential donors are healthy children or young adults with an indication for extraction of premolars in connection with orthodontic treatment. Any history of previous or present malignant or infectious diseases or treatment with blood products excludes the patient as a donor. The donor should furthermore permit the collection of a blood sample (approximately 50 ml) 3 months after tooth extraction for tissue typing and medical tests including *HIV* and *hepatitis tests* (HBsAg, Anti Bc and anti-HCV). Although the potential donor population is a low-risk group for such infections - 10- to 12-years-old children with no history of risk behavior [male homosexuality, intravenous drug abuse, residence in high risk areas, or treatment with blood products], it is mandatory to ensure a negative test for both HIV and hepatitis virus. To further increase the safety of the procedure, cryopreserved donor teeth are used, as this technique permits blood testing of the donor at least 3 months after tooth extraction and cryopreservation of the potential donor teeth, thereby excluding possible seroconversion of the donor in the postextraction period. These procedures reduce the risk transmission of HIV via tooth allotransplantation to virtually below the value of clinical relevance.

Donor tooth

A clinical and radiographic examination of the potential graft reveals the mesiodistal and apicocoronal dimensions, stage of root formation, and number of root canals of the donor tooth. For endodontic reasons, single rooted fully developed grafts have been chosen. Alternatively, teeth with immature root formation have been used, which allows ingrowth of new connective tissue in the pulp cavity; however, no pulp canal obliteration can be expected (Fig. 8.4). Mandibular premolars are particularly well-suited donor teeth. Although crown morphology is unacceptable in the anterior region, the crown can easily be transformed to simulate both canines and incisors (Fig. 8.4) (see also Chapter 11, p. 280).

Tissue typing and matching

Blood samples (50 ml) from the recipient and potential donor are tested for blood groups (AB0 and Rh), and major histocompatibility types, including HLA-ABC and -DR (Fig. 8.3). Tissue matching is the goal. Close collaboration with a tissue typing laboratory is necessary for this purpose.

HLA matching

Previous clinical studies seem to indicate that HLA matching is of major importance for prolonged tooth graft survival.[3] Because of the close linkage of HLA genes (Fig. 8.3), the probability of a good match or even HLA identity is high among siblings. Child-to-parent transplantation will at least share half of the HLA antigens. Thus, selection and matching of donor and recipient is primarily sought within the family whenever possible. However, as teeth from related donors are seldom available, the actual graft choice is usually made from nonrelated donors. In these cases, there is an overwhelming probability of HLA mismatch. To obtain 50% or more HLA class I match among nonrelated donor-recipient pairs in the first study of HLA in tooth transplantation, Ivanyi & Kominek[3] 1977 used the tissue typing capacity from a pool of up to 90 different potential donors for each recipient. Even such partially good matches, however, showed significantly longer survival than poorer matches (see Fig. 8.14). In a recent and more limited clinical study with only a few alternative donors available for each recipient, a low number of good matches was achieved and thus the effect of HLA matching in that study was not conclusive.[9]

AB0 blood group

AB0 blood group compatibility has not yet been shown to be of any clear prognostic importance in allotransplantation of teeth. However, in view of the rigid transplantation policy concerning AB0 match in organ allotransplantation,[2] this has been preferred.[9]

Rhesus (D)

Rhesus (D) compatibility is only of importance when Rh (D)-negative fertile female recipients are considered. Rh (D)-positive donors are excluded to prevent the theoretical possibility of rhesus sensitization of the recipient.[9]

Donor teeth from a tooth bank

To obtain better HLA class I and class II antigen compatibility, a tooth bank has proved helpful[10] (see Chapter 9). Briefly, teeth (preferably premolars) are cryopreserved with viable periodontal ligament (PDL) at -196^0C for unlimited periods. The donors are HLA tissue typed and HIV tested from a blood sample collected at least 3 months after tooth extraction. From the banked teeth of known tissue type, the most optimal match is easily selected for each potential recipient. This technique has been used clinically over a period of 8 years, resulting in better HLA matches and improved graft survival.[10]

Fig. 8.4. Allotransplantation of immature premolars from related donor

This 22-year-old man had suffered avulsion of two incisors in a traffic accident. His 12-year-old sister, who is HLA-identical, served as a donor, as four premolars had to be extracted for orthodontic purposes.

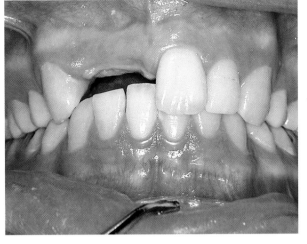 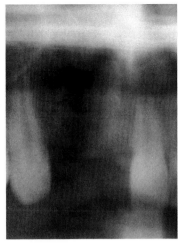

Preparing the new socket

Considerable alveolar bone was lost with the avulsed teeth. Adjacent teeth were intact. A circular incision was made corresponding to the circumference of the tooth at the cementoenamel junction, whereafter the socket was prepared with surgical burs as described for autotransplantation.

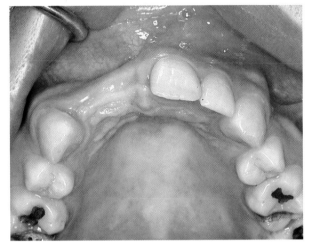 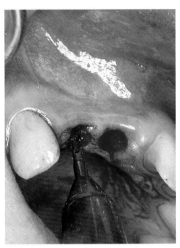

Status after transplantation

The tooth grafts were positioned in near-occlusion, ensuring maximum bony coverage of the root. An acid-etch acrylic splint was applied to the adjacent teeth to ensure correct orientation during healing.

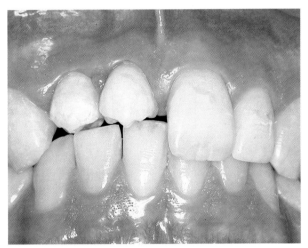 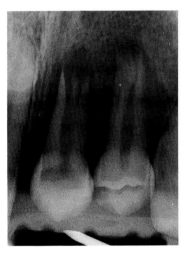

Final restoration of the grafts

The crowns of the two mandibular premolars were restored with composite resin to simulate incisors. Note the normal gingival conditions 6 years after transplantation. Radiographically, an ankylosis of both grafts is seen. No pulp canal obliteration or further root formation is seen.

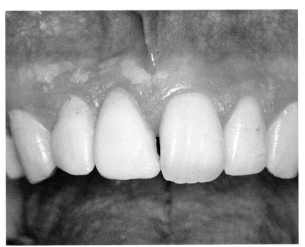 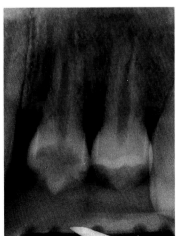

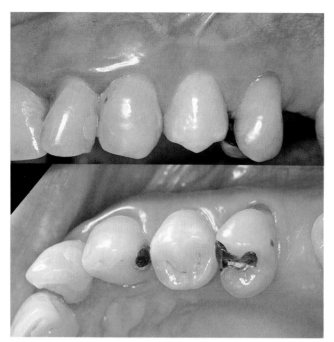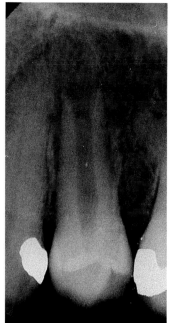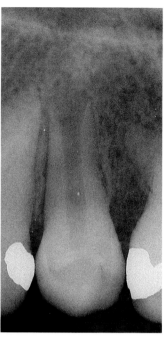

Fig. 8.5. Allotransplantation to the premolar region from a related donor
Allograft to the first maxillary premolar in position 5 years after transplantation. The donor of the first mandibular premolar was the daughter of the recipient (50 % HLA identity). Radiographs show formation of a PDL-like structure that later turns into ankylosis.

Surgical procedure

When the desired graft was available, e.g., in tissue culture medium after thawing from the tooth bank (see Chapter 9) or after fresh extraction from a family donor (provided a negative HIV test and a HLA and AB0-test), the clinical and surgical procedures essentially followed those outlined in the previous chapters for autotransplantation of the given tooth type (see Figs. 8.4 and 8.5). In teeth with complete root formation, endodontic treatment should be performed either extra-orally or after 3-4 weeks. A post-operative radiograph is then taken.

Postoperative follow-up

This is in principle similar to that of autografts. Sutures are removed after 1 week. If the tooth is not root filled extra-orally, pulp extirpation and calcium hydroxide dressing of the canal is made after 3-4 weeks. The splint is removed 6 weeks after transplantation, when the graft is usually firm (see Appendix 3, p. 291).

Parallel to these findings immunologic monitoring of the cell-mediated and humoral antidonor response will demonstrate antibodies and T- cell reactions within the first 6 months, which, however, later disappear.[9,27]

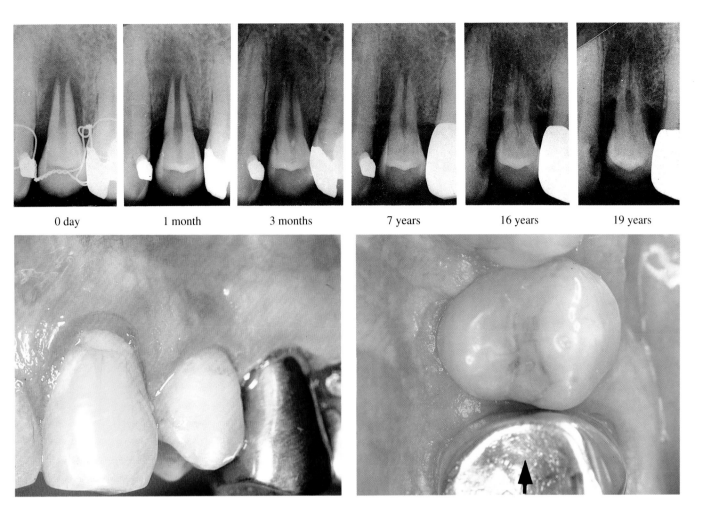

| 0 day | 1 month | 3 months | 7 years | 16 years | 19 years |

Fig. 8.6. Slow progression of replacement resorption
In this 48-year-old recipient long-term survival of an allograft from an unmatched and unrelated donor is seen. Only moderate progression replacement resorption is seen. Normal gingival condition is shown after 19 years.

PDL healing

What appears radiographically to be a PDL space, often broader than normal, can sometimes be seen as early as 6-8 weeks after transplantation (Fig. 8.4). The percussion sound is, however, usually a high, metallic ankylosis tone after some months.

The clinical and radiographic signs of *ankylosis* are usually seen 6 to 12 months after transplantation.[1,10] This type of root resorption is seen in nearly all allotransplanted teeth, and eventually leads to final graft loss (Figs. 8.6 and 8.7). There is no treatment for this condition at present; however, this process can take several years, in some cases 30 years or more. The crown of the graft will ultimately break off at the gingival crest, leaving the alveolar bone with only limited atrophy.

Inflammatory resorption

Inflammatory resorption can be diagnosed 4 to 6 weeks post-operatively and if left untreated will lead to rapid loss of the graft.[1,8] The treatment of this type of resorption is similar to treatment in autografts; that is, pulpal extirpation and canal dressing of calcium hydroxide.[1,9,13,15] Once PDL healing has been confirmed, a final root filling with gutta-percha and a sealer can be made (Fig. 8.11).

Pulpal healing

In teeth with incomplete root formation signs of pulpal re-vascularization and further root formation do not take place due to immunologic rejection of the soft tissues.[1,8,11,13,17,18] However, a gradual replacement of the content of root canal with bone is sometimes found (Figs. 8.5 and 8.6).[1] Mature grafts will develop pulp necrosis similar to autografts. Thus endodontic treatment of such grafts is necessary, either before, during - or after transplantation (Figs. 8.10 and 8.11).[1,10,13]

Gingival healing

In most cases gingival conditions are found to be similar to those in respect of autografts throughout the control period (Fig. 8.8).[1,10] This has been corroborated by the experimental finding of nearly normal PDL in allografts in the supra-alveolar cervical area in light and electron microscopic studies (Fig. 8.9).[13,14,16] Lack of gingival healing or loss of marginal attachment was the cause of loss of only 3% of 75 grafts over a period of 28 years.[1]

Fig. 8.7. Ankylosis after allotransplantation

Ankylosis, appearing after 6 months, was present in almost all 85 allografts. Replacement resorption gradually replaces the hard tissues of the root of the graft with alveolar bone. Finally when the crown is lost alveolar bone remains for retransplantation or alternative treatment. From Schwartz, 1987.[10]

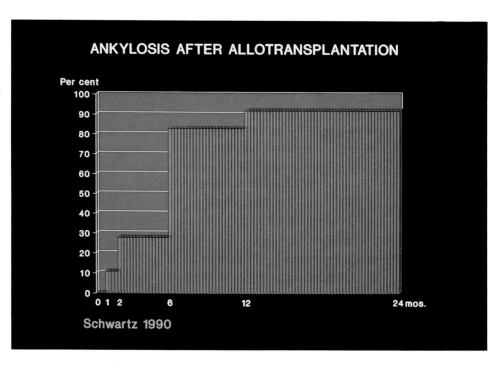

Fig. 8.8. Gingival healing of cryopreserved allograft from tooth bank
Considerable bone loss at the recipient region due to a root fracture of the premolar to be replaced. The tooth graft has no vestibular alveolar wall. Although ankylosis is present, healing shows no pathologic periodontal pocket and only limited retraction of gingiva 5 years postoperatively.

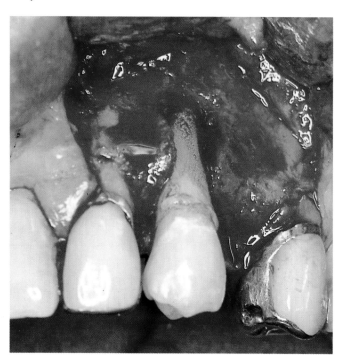
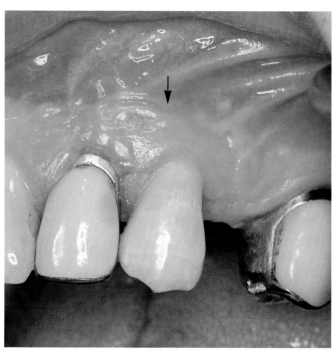

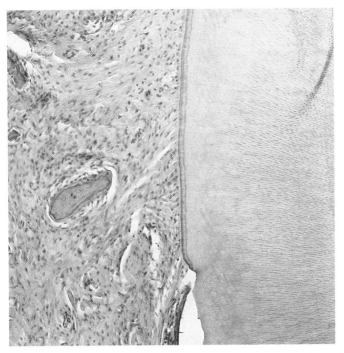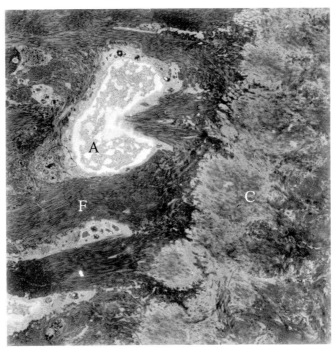

Fig. 8.9. Supra-alveolar healing of tooth allografts. Histologic section of an allografted incisor of an unmatched monkey (*Cercopithecus Aethiops*) 8 weeks after transplantation. Electron microscopy of the interface of root and connective tissue at the supra-alveolar region of allotransplanted tooth in monkeys. A, PDL-cell; C, Cementum; F, PDL-collagen fibers. From Schwartz & al., 1990.[16]

Prognosis

The literature of the last four decades on clinical allotransplantation of teeth comprises numerous case reports and a sparse number of systematically documented clinical trials[1,3-10,18-25,29-54] supplemented by several reviews.[55-61]

Allotransplantation of teeth in man has until the current decade been performed on an immunogenetically empirical basis. Some of the previous literature dealing with this subject is based on surgical techniques where the graft has been stored in different types of media and frozen to, for example -10°C without cryopreservation for 24 hours to several months prior to transplantation, or treated with a great variety of chemical agents.[19-24] The stored or treated transplants in these studies are considered more or less avital "allostatic" implants. Problems concerning these implants will not be discussed here.

Numerous definitions of success of tooth transplantation have been used to describe the prognosis of allotransplanted teeth. "Success" has varied from conditions similar to a successful autotransplant, with continued root formation, normal PDL, and signs of pulpal revascularization to the mere persistence of graft function in the jaw (Table 8.1).[1,3] Between these two concepts lies a wide range of clinical and radiographic signs which have been suggested to distinguish success from failure.[1,3-10,15,25] Consequently, analysis and comparison of the results of the many clinical studies appearing in the literature are very difficult.

Fig. 8.10. Effect of endodontic treatment

Unmatched allografts 20 years after allotransplantation. From the radiograph it appears that inflammatory resorption was present on the apex of the mature allograft (arrow). Endodontic treatment, however, arrested this type of resorption. Ankylosis and replacement resorption thereafter progressively replace the mineralized part of the root by bone. The graft can, however, be expected to function for an extended period of time.

0 days	3 months	6 months	12 years	20 years

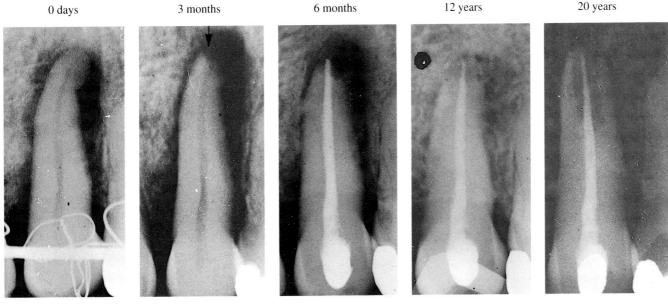

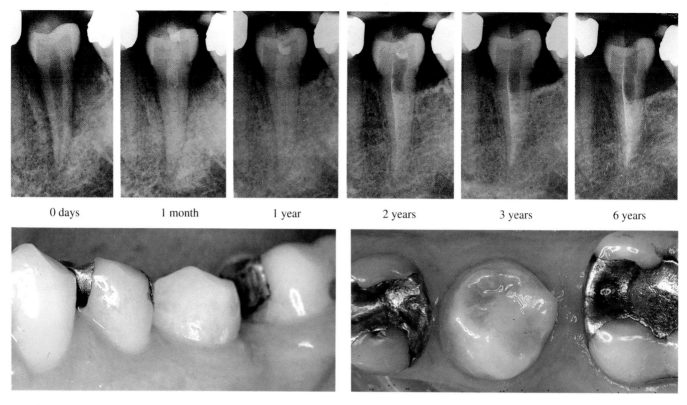

| 0 days | 1 month | 1 year | 2 years | 3 years | 6 years |

Fig. 8.11. Cryopreserved allograft from tooth bank
A good HLA match was achieved by the use of the tooth bank. Endodontic treatment of the mature graft was necessary. The calcium hydroxide root canal dressing was shifted several times during the first year, thereafter once a year. Since replacement resorption could not be prevented, a definitive root canal treatment with gutta-percha was not used in this case. Note the radiographic signs of "normal" PDL in large areas of the PDL after 6 years. At follow-up after 6 years normal gingival conditions are seen with gingival pockets measuring less than 3 mm.

Graft "survival"

Asymptomatic clinical function of the graft is an important parameter (Tables 8.1) In the following this is considered as "survival" of the graft irrespective of the fact that replacement resorption of the root is almost always present.

In a recent retrospective evaluation of a series of allografts, graft loss was especially high during the first 2 years, after which the intensity of loss declined.[1] Mean survival was 6.8 years (Fig. 8.12), with a maximum recorded survival period of 28 years. The calculated survival curve of 291 *autotransplanted* human teeth, transplanted by the same surgeons[20,21] over the same period, showed most autograft losses within the first 2 postoperative years, although the overall graft survival was much higher in autografts than allografts.

Fig. 8.12. Survival of unmatched tooth allografts
Previous surveys of series of unmatched allotransplanted teeth show survival and function of the grafts for a limited number of years. Thus mean survival time ranged from 2.5 years to 6.8 years. From Nordenram, 1982[7] and Schwartz & al., 1987[1].

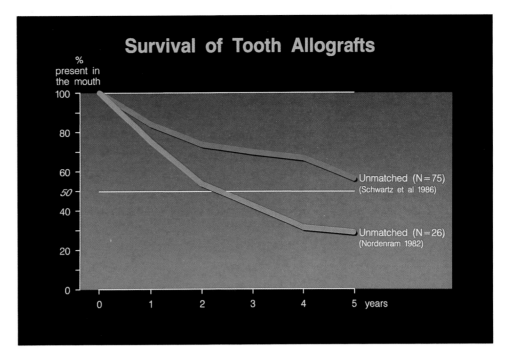

The high number of allografts lost early could, therefore, only in part be due to clinical, technical, or surgical causes. Early loss of in allografts is consequently assumed to be caused by immunologic rejection due to genetic differences between donors and recipients. When teeth from the tooth bank are used and endodontic treatment is performed within the first few months, most early losses seem to be eliminated, thereby increasing the 5-year survival to 81%.[23] This is an improvement of 20% compared to the earlier unmatched series (Fig. 8.15 and Table 8.1).[1,3]

Table 8.1. Long-term results of allotransplantation of teeth

	Observ. period (years)	No. of grafts	Graft stage*	Graft type** P/M	Tissue typing	In vitro response ***	Root resorption %	Graft survival			
								2 yr	5 yr	10 yr	15 yr
Apfel, 1954[4]	?	12	I	M	-	-		0			
Mezrow, 1964[5]	1-3	27	I	P+M	-	HMI	?	100			
Nordenram & Björnsjö,1970[6]	1-3	32	I+C	P+M	NLT*****	-	63	60			
Nordenram, 1982[7]	0-16	23	I+C	P+M	-	-	100	60	40	30	20
Hansen & Fibæk, 1972[8]	1-15	54	I+C	P+M	-	-	89	80	60	33	
Ivanyi & Kominek, 1977[39]	0-3	90	I	M	HLA	-	?		70		
Schwartz et al, 1982[9]	0-1	20	I	P+M	HLA	HMI+CMI	50				
Schwartz et al, 1987[1]	1-28	73	I+C	P+M	-	-	95	82	63	36	
Schwartz, 1987[10]	1-5	85****	C	P	HLA	-	95	91	81		

*   I= incomplete root formation, C= complete root formation
**   M= molars, P= premolars
***   CMI= cell-mediated immune reaction; HMI= humoral (antibody)- mediated immune reaction
**** Allografts from tooth bank
***** NLT= Normal lymphocyte test

Effect of various factors on prognosis

HLA matching

That HLA class I matching has a significant impact on survival of allotransplanted teeth was demonstrated by Ivanyi & Kominek[3] 1977 on 90 HLA-A and HLA-B matched grafts. Due to an available pool of 80-90 different potential but unrelated donors for each transplant recipient, an impressive number of good matches was obtained. When transplantations were divided into two groups, one with 50% Class I match or more, the other with less than 50% Class I match, even the partial HLA class I compatibility showed significantly greater graft survival in a life table analysis (Fig. 8.15).

In the literature, a single case of a full house HLA class I and II match has been described between a girl donating a third molar to her mother. This match resulted in what appeared to be both pulp obliteration and further root development after 3 years, a condition that has not been reported previously in allotransplantation of teeth clinically or experimentally.[25] Other cases have been published where premolars were allotransplanted among HLA class I identical siblings, resulting in ankylosis similar to mismatched transplantations[9] (Fig. 8.4).

In conclusion, although an impressively large number of data support the effect of HLA matching in tooth graft survival, this effect still appears to be a matter of controversy and further clinical proof is required.

Immunosuppressive agents

In a single study, high doses of corticosteroids were administered to 32 tooth allograft recipients during the initial postoperative months. Six grafts displayed long term survival of up to 16 years, and the mean survival time for the entire series of 32 allografts was 2.6 years.[6,7] However, in another study of a comparable group of 72 allografts no immunosuppressive agents were used, and in spite of this a mean survival of 6.8 years was achieved (Fig. 8.12).[1]

In conclusion, no clinical data have yet been presented that indicate the beneficial effect of immunosuppression on clinical tooth allotransplantation. Furthermore, the presently available immunosuppresive drugs used in organ allotransplantation have such severe side effects that their use in clinical allotransplantation of teeth is precluded.

Age of the recipient at the time of surgery

An age factor apparently affects tooth allograft survival. Thus, in two clinical studies it was shown that recipients who were older than 45 years at the time of transplantation displayed greater graft survival than did younger recipients (Figs. 8.13 and 8.14).[1,8] The effect of age upon allotransplant survival can in part be related to reduced immune responsiveness with increased age and in part to a slower remodeling rate of the ankylotic process known to take place in older individuals (Fig. 8.14).

Inflammatory root resorption

Inflammatory root resorption is found to cause rapid allograft loss in humans.[1,9] It appears that allografts were lost more rapidly due to this type of resorption (mean survival period 1.1 years) than were autografts performed at the same center over the same period (mean survival period 6.8 years) (Fig. 8.14). This finding suggests that alloimmune processes are triggering factors in inflammatory root resorption following allotransplantation. This is confirmed by the finding that inflammatory root resorption of human allografts is related to

Fig. 8.13. Effect of age of the recipient on graft survival
Age seems to have a considerable impact on the survival of tooth allografts. Thus the mean survival of unmatched grafts transplanted to recipients over the age of 45 was 9.8 years. From Schwartz & al., 1987.[1]

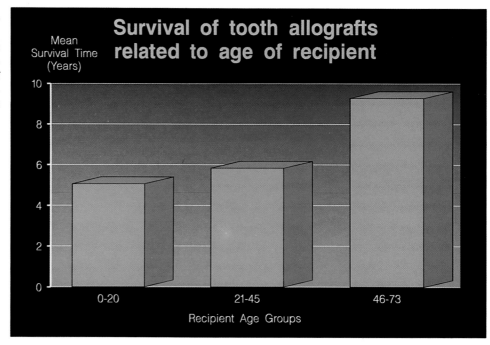

Fig. 8.14. Effect of age of the recipient on resorption of allograft
Especially in the older recipient age group, ankylosis and replacement resorption seem to affect the unmatched allografts. Inflammatory resorption is frequently arrested by endodontic treatment. After Schwartz & al., 1987.[1]

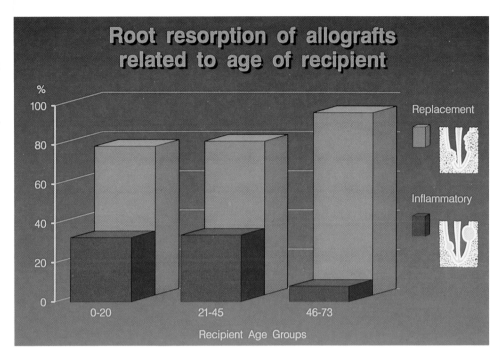

a donor-specific cell-mediated immune response detected within the first 6 months after transplantation.[9] Endodontic treatment is able to reduce inflammatory root resorption dramatically in allografts even on a long-term basis[1,10,13] (Figs. 8.10 and 8.11).

Replacement root resorption (ankylosis)

Replacement root resorption is the major postoperative complication of allotransplantation. Thus, most grafts functioning 1 year after transplantation demonstrate ankylosis.[1-10] The slow but progressive replacement root resorption will eventually lead to graft loss (Fig. 8.7). Resorption of dentin can elicit donor-specific alloimmune reactions in humans, explaining the greater frequency of graft loss due to replacement resorption in allografts than in autografts.[1,26,27]

Since the rejecting tooth allograft can still function satisfactorily clinically despite ankylosis, future clinical research on allotransplantation of teeth could be aimed at reducing the progression of replacement resorption (Fig. 8.15). Various chemical or physical methods of allograft preparation such as fluoride immersion have been suggested.[28] These methods, however, need clinical confirmation before application in human allotransplantation on a larger scale.

Fig. 8.15. Survival of tooth allografts
Even partial HLA class I match has a highly significant impact on tooth allograft survival. Allotransplantation of teeth from a tooth bank shows the hitherto highest survival curve. After Ivanyi & Kominek, 1977[3] Nordenram, 1982[7]and Schwartz, 1987.[10]

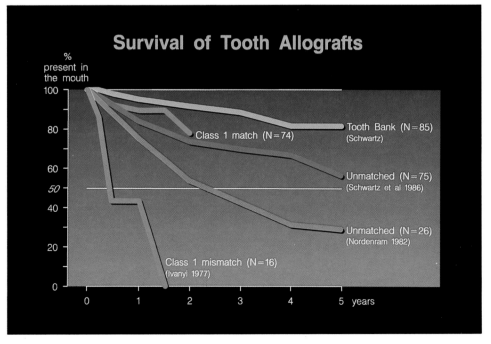

Essentials

Transplantation immunity

Foreign histocompatibility antigens of the donor on an allotransplanted tooth elicit an immune reaction of the recipient, which results in general destruction of the PDL and pulp of the graft. Therefore mature donor teeth should be preferred on the premise that endodontic treatment has to be performed. Furthermore extensive ankylosis can be expected in the intraalveolar part of the root. Gingival healing of the tooth allograft seems to be comparable to autograft healing.

Treatment planning

Donors

Three to six months after cryopreservation of donor teeth in a tooth bank, a blood sample should be tested for HIV and hepatitis infection, and AB0 and HLA tissue typing can be performed.

Matching

HLA tissue type matching has proven valuable; however, the impact of this effect on prognosis is still uncertain.

Surgical procedure (Fig. 8.4)

1. Thaw the selected graft from the tooth bank
2. Extirpate the pulp and perform an extraoral root filling with gutta-percha and a sealer; prevent drying of PDL
3. Administer antibiotic therapy and local anesthesia
4. Prepare the socket
5. Place the graft in the desired position
6. Splint the graft for 6 weeks
7. Take a postoperative radiograph

Follow-up

See Appendix 3, p. 291

Prognosis

Tooth survival (5 years)   81%

Pulpal healing   0%

PDL healing (1 year)   100% ankylosis

The function time on the graft is dependent of the progression of the replacement resorption of the graft, which seems to be slow, especially in older individuals; up to 32 years of function have been recorded.

References

1. Schwartz O, Frederiksen K, Klausen B. Allotransplantation of human teeth. A retrospective study of 73 transplantations over a period of 28 years. Int J Oral Maxillofac Surg 1987; 16: 285-301.

2. Terasaki PI, Mickey MR, Cecka M, Cicciarelli J, Cook D, Iwaki Y, Toyotome A, Wang L. Overview in: Terasaki PI (ed): Clinical transplants 1987, 467-90. UCLA Tissue Typing Laboratory. Los Angeles, CA. USA.

3. Ivanyi D, Kominek J. Tooth allografts in children matched for HLA. Transplantation 1977; 23: 255-60.

4. Apfel H. Transplantation of teeth. Transpl Bull 1954; 1: 209-10.

5. Mezrow RR. Homologous viable tooth transplantation. A clinical, immunological and histological study. Oral Surg Oral Med Oral Pathol 1964; 17: 375-88.

6. Nordenram Å, Björnesjö KB. Allotransplantation of teeth in man on the basis of the normal lymphocyte transfer (NLT) test. Odont Revy 1970; 21: 169-88.

7. Nordenram Å. Allogenic tooth transplantation with an observation time of 16 years. Clinical report of 32 cases. Swed Dent J 1982; 6: 149-56.

8. Hansen J, Fibæk B. Clinical experience of auto- and allotransplantation of teeth. Int Dent J 1972; 22: 270-85.

9. Schwartz O, Donatsky O, Hjörting-Hansen E, Fibæk B. Immunological and clinical aspects of allo-transplantation of HLA-tissue typed teeth. In: GR Riviere, WH Hildemann eds. Oral Immunogenetics and Tissue Transplantation. Elsevier North Holland 1982; 259-73.

10. Schwartz O. Allotransplantation from a bank of cryopreserved teeth. 5 years clinical experience. J Dent Res 1987; 66: 171.

11. Fong C, Berger J, Morris M. Experimental allogenic tooth transplantation in the rhesus monkey. J Dent Res 1968; 47: 351–57.

12. Shulman LB, Kalis PJ. A comparison of autologous and allogenic tooth transplants in rhesus monkeys. J Oral Surg 1970; 28: 168-74.

13. Schwartz O, Andreasen JO. Auto- and allotransplantation of mature teeth in monkeys. Effect of endodontic treatment. J Oral Maxillofac Surg 1988; 46: 672-81.

14. Schwartz O, Andreasen JO. A time related histoquantitative study of allotransplanted mature teeth in monkeys. Endod Dent Traumatol; in press.

15. Schwartz O, Bergman P, Klausen B. Autotransplantation of human teeth. A life table analysis of prognostic factors. Int J Oral Surg 1985; 14: 145-58.

16. Schwartz O, Groisman M, Attström R, Andreasen JO. Transmission electron microscopy of supra-alveolar periodontal healing of auto- and allotransplanted teeth in monkeys. Endod Dent Traumatol; 1990; 6: 26-32.

17. Atkinson ME. A histological study of tooth allografts transplanted to unrelated and immunologically prepared mice. J Oral Pathol 1975; 4: 167-79.

18. Chauvin P, David P, Martin E, Guibert M, Laudenbach P. Témoins indirects et directs de la réparation pulpaire des homogreffes humaines. Rev Stomatol Chir Maxillofac 1980; 81: 164-79.

19. Cserepfalvi MP. Homotransplantation of human teeth with and without pulp tissues. J District Colombia Dent Soc 1976; 11-15.

20. Knochel J F. Remplacements unitaires par homogreffes dentaires. Inform Dent 1975; 12: 5-32.

21. Maksudov MM, Dranovskij GE. Allografting of tooth germs in experimental and clinical practice. Acta Chir Plast 1980; 22: 220-31.

22. Molhant G, Payen J. 25 cas d'homogreffes dentaires. Rev Stomatol 1975; 76: 1-12.

23. Molhant G. Suites des homogreffes dentaires. Rev Stomatol Chir Maxillofac 1984; 85: 151-52.

24. Viener AF. Homotransplantation of cultured teeth: a preliminary report. J Am Dent Assoc 1969; 78: 761-66.

25. Sveen K, Vindenes H, Solheim BG. Selection of allogenic tooth graft using HLA-A, -B, -C and DR typing and the MLC test. Int J Oral Surg 1980; 9: 433-38.

26. Schwartz O, Bergman P, Klausen B. Resorption of autotransplanted human teeth: a retrospective study of 291 transplantations over a period of 25 years. Int Endod J 1985; 18: 119-31.

27. Schwartz O. Cell-mediated and humoral alloimmune reactions after subperiosteal implantation of allogenic demineralized dentin in humans. Int J Oral Surg 1983; 12: 95-105.

28. Mellberg JR, Shulman LB. Treatment of human teeth with fluoride for replantation and allotransplantation. J Dent Res 1974; 53: 844-46.

29. Keresztesi K. Transplantation eines Zahnkeimes. Österr Z Stomatol 1954; 51: 41-44.

30. Apfel H. Transplantation of the unerupted third molar tooth. Oral Surg Oral Med Oral Pathol 1956; 9: 96-97.

31. Pafford EM. Homogenous transplant of preserved frozen teeth. Tooth bank. J Oral Surg 1956; 9: 55-70.

32. Barrelle J, Jacquemin O. Considerations sur les autogreffes et les heterogreffes. Rev Fr Odontostomatol 1960; 5: 1-7.

33. Gripwall B, Tegner G. Fall av homeoplastisk transplantation. Swed Dent J 1961; 54: 325-30.

34. Hühne S. Zahnkeimtransplantationen bei Kindern. Dtsch Stomatol 1961; 11: 304-09.

35. Held A-J, Spirgi M, Pedrinis T. Les homotransplantations dentaires. Sweiz Monatsschr Zahnheilk 1962; 72: 607-20.

36. Mezrow RR, Friedman H. Clinical and immunologic study of homologous tooth transplantation. J Albert Einstein Med Center 1963; 11: 244-53.

37. Cserepfalvi M. Clinical report of homotransplantation. J Am Dent Assoc 1963; 67: 35-40.

38. Urban DE. Case report. Tooth transplant between unrelated patients. Dent Survey 1963; 35: 35.

39. Cserepfalvi M. Experimental homogenous transplantation of human teeth obtained from a human cadaver. J Oral Implant Transplant Surg 1966; 12: 66-72.

40. Collins LR, White RP, Bear SE. A clinical study of tooth transplantation: A preliminary report. W Virginia Dent J 1967; 44: 4-19.

41. Marzola C. Homogenous orthotopic germ tooth transplantation. Arq Cent Est Fac Odont 1969; 6: 161-72.

42. Coletti GDN. A new technique for replants and transplants. J Oral Med 1971; 26: 82-84.

43. Lohbauer R. Zahntransplantationen Kind-Mutter. Chir Zahnheilk 1971; 8: 27-32.

44. Spirescu I. Application of osseus-dental homografts to monkeys and men. In: Goldsmith EI, Moor-Jancowski, eds. Medical Primatology 1972. Karger, Basel 1972: 212:-16.

45. Benqué EP. Autogreffes et homogreffes dentaires (100 cases). Acta Odontostomatol 1973; 27: 515-31.

46. Lindholm K, Westerholm N. Transplantation of endodontically treated third molars. Proc Finn Dent Soc 1973; 69: 17-20.

47. Mostiler TW. Homotransplantation and autotransplantation of teeth in humans. Virg Dent J 1973; 50: 15.

48. Scheffer P, Lerondeau JC, Verdier M. Transplantation des germes dentaires. Rev Stomatol 1976; 77: 469-71.

49. Eskici A. Replantation und Transplantation von Zähnen und Zahnkeimen. Dtsch Zahnärztl Z 1980; 35: 343-45.

50. Baum AT, Hertz RS. Autogeneic and allogeneic tooth transplants in treatment of malocclusion. Am J Orthod 1977; 72: 368-96.

51. Hertz RS, Baum AT. Repeated human tooth allograft after a previous rejection. In: Riviere GR, Hildemann WH, eds. Oral immunogenetics and tissue transplantation. Elsevier North Holland N.Y. 1982: 285-90.

52. David P, Chauvin P, Wearle R, Robain O, Mugnier A. Mise en évidence de la repousse nerveuse des pulpes des homogreffes dentaires humaines. Quintessence Int 1982; 13: 65-73.

53. Sadjak A, Pfragner R, Klingenberg HG, Eskici A, Tilz GP. Antibody determination in homologous tooth transplant. Exp Path 1982; 22: 253-55.

54. Sheb TC. Vital homogenous tooth transplant procedure and solution to possible problems. Oral Implantol 1984; 11: 564-69.

55. Cserepfalvi M. Transplantation of teeth in humans. In: Peer LA, ed. Transplantation of tissues, vol 2. Baltimore: The Williams and Wilkins Co., 1959: 300-09.

56. Hansen J. Auto y homotransplante de dientes. Rev Asoc Odontol Argent 1968; 56: 86-96.

57. Natiella JR, Armitage JE, Greene GW. The replantation and transplantation of teeth. Oral Surg Oral Med Oral Pathol 1970; 29: 397-412.

58. Shulman LB, Hovinga J, Feingold RM. Recent advances in allogenic tooth transplantation. In: Hjörting-Hansen E, Walker RV, eds. Transactions of the Fourth International Conference of Oral Surgery. Baltimore: Williams & Wilkins, 1971: 68-72.

59. Shulman LB. Allogenic tooth transplantation. J Oral Surg 1972; 30: 359-408.

60. Boyne PJ. Implants and transplants: Review of recent research in this area of surgery. J Am Dent Assoc 1973; 87: 1074-80.

61. Marzola C. Transplantes e reimplantes. Pancast editorial. Sao Paolo, Brasil. 1988: 141-62.

Chapter 9

Cryopreservation of teeth before replantation or transplantation

O. Schwartz

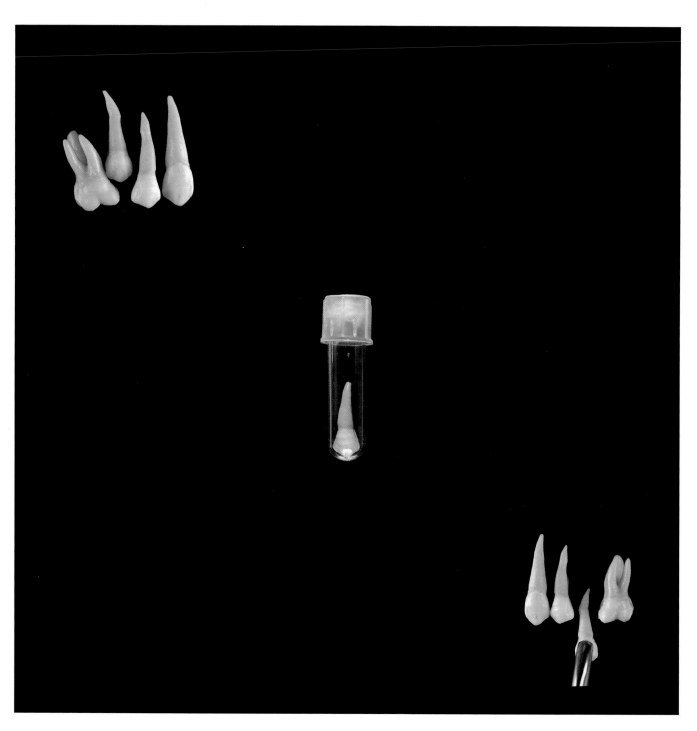

Extraoral storage

Short-term extra-alveolar storage of teeth (i.e., for minutes or a few hours from the time of avulsion or surgical removal of the tooth until reinsertion into the recipient region) is indicated when immediate positioning of the tooth is not possible or advisable. These techniques have been described in Chapters 1 and 2.

Intermediate storage of teeth for days or weeks *in vivo* in a submucosal site or *in vitro* in physiologic saline or a tissue culture medium has also been mentioned previously (Chapter 6).

Long-term storage of teeth for later re- or transplantation is the issue of the present chapter. In this regard, the storage period can range from months to years, during which time it is essential that all biologic functions of the soft tissue of the graft, especially the periodontal ligament (PDL), remain intact. Cryopreservation is the only technique currently available which seems able to achieve this goal.[1-14]

Fig. 9.1. Cryobiology of cells during freezing

Shrinkage of cells during slow freezing is a result of egress of intracellular water, which is essential for the avoidance of cellular injury during the freezing process. The shrunken cell with little or no intracellular ice crystals will be able to resume function once thawed. In contrast, intracellular ice crystals are formed in rapidly frozen cells. Such cells are avital upon thawing. Cryoprotective agents, such as dimethylsulfoxide (DMSO) or glycerol, are effective in countering cellular injury caused by freezing by reducing intracellular ice crystal formation and by reducing osmolarity stresses to cell membranes.

Cryobiology

The aim of cryopreservation of living tissues is the controlled reversibility of the cessation of all biologic functions which is achieved by controlled cooling at temperatures below -150° C. Living cells and tissues exposed to uncontrolled freezing below the crystallization temperature of the extra- and intracellular fluids (i.e., -7° C) will suffer extensively from the effect of freezing (Fig. 9.1). Damage is due to ice crystals formed within the biologic system as well as the physiochemical effects of increasing solute concentrations during water crystallization. A detailed presentation of the effect and control of these factors is beyond the scope of this book, and readers are referred to textbooks on cryobiology.[8-10] The development of a cryoprofile optimal to the specific cell types in question forms the basis for the principles of cell protection from freezing injury. A given cryoprofile describes (a) the *type*; (b) the *concentration*; (c) the *equilibration* and (d) the *dilution* of a *cryoprotective agent* (e.g. DMSO or glycerol); (e) the *freezing rate* and (f) the *thawing conditions* needed for the specific tissue (Fig. 9.2). Such cryoprofiles have been developed for several human cells and tissues, such as embryos and corneas, and enable the cells to function in a biologically similar way to unfrozen cells after storage for extensive periods in liquid nitrogen (-196° C).[1-4] A similar cryoprofile has recently been developed for PDL cells for tooth grafts.[11-14]

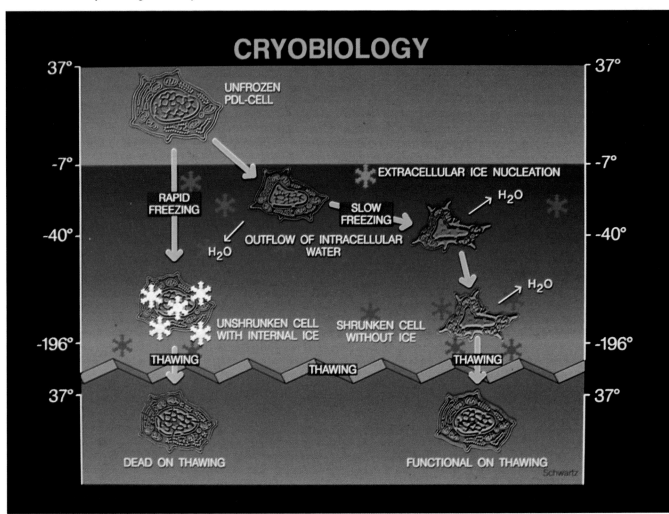

Fig. 9.2. Cryoprofile

A set of conditions for each of the factors which can produce optimal cell survival after cryopreservation. Cryoprofile conditions for PDL cells have proven clinically feasible. Also shown is a plastic tube with transport medium for short-term storage before and after freezing. A freezing tube with screw cap (Nunc) is suitable for the size of a human premolar, canine, or incisor. Schwartz 1991

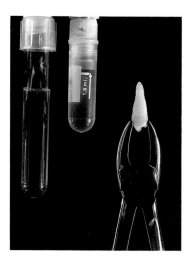

Cryopreservation

- Equilibration of cryoprotective agent
- Cooling rate
- Crystallization
- Freezing rate
- Storage temperature
- Thawing
- De-equilibration of cryoprotective agent

Banking of human teeth

Cryopreservation has been demonstrated to be an acceptable technique for long-term storage of mature teeth in a monkey model.[11,12] The technique has recently been applied to human teeth as well[13,14] (see also Chapter 8, p. 227). Thus, after autotransplantation, cryopreserved human teeth showed clinical and radiographic signs of regeneration of a normal periodontium similar to the healing observed following immediate autotransplantation (Fig. 9.3). The PDL cells of cryopreserved human teeth could survive at least 18 to 54 months´ storage in a frozen state, and after thawing form a normal PDL similar to the healing of unfrozen autografts (Fig. 9.4). An increasing number of teeth are stored in the tooth bank in Copenhagen for possible future autotransplantation according to indications outlined below.

Fig. 9.3. Experimental replantation of cryopreserved teeth

The freezing rate and concentration of a cryoprotective agent was investigated in a monkey model. PDL healing of a replanted cryopreserved incisor (to the right) appear histologically similar to an immediately replanted contralateral incisor (to the left). After Schwartz & Andreasen, 1983.[11]

Control tooth
Cryopreserved tooth

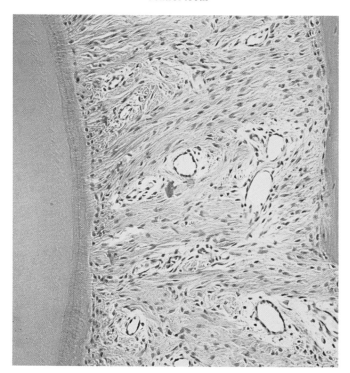
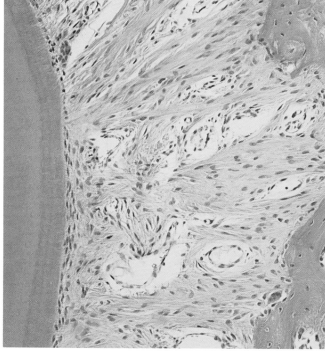

Indications for long-term storage of teeth

Storage of human teeth before replantation or transplantation can be indicated in the following situations where immediate positioning of the graft is not possible or indicated, but where future re- or autotransplantation can be indicated.

Autotransplantation

In cases where premolars are to be extracted for orthodontic reasons and where the prognosis is dubious for traumatized and/or endodontically treated teeth, later autotransplantation of a stored premolar could be indicated to replace the failing teeth ("spare wheel principle") (Fig. 9.4).

In cases where extraction of the donor tooth is necessary in order to allow orthodontic creation of sufficient space at the recipient site (Fig. 9.10).[14] Similar situations may appear in orthognathic surgery where teeth are extracted.

Fig. 9.4. Cryopreserved premolar used in the anterior region
First maxillary premolars were extracted as a part of orthodontic treatment and cryopreserved, as there was doubt about the prognosis of a traumatized incisor. 2.5 years later, a vertical root fracture necessitated extraction of the right central incisor.

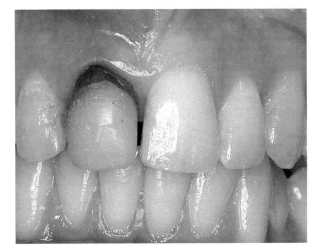
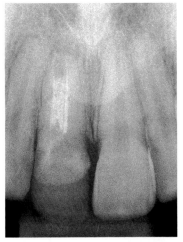

Transplantation of banked tooth
One of the cryopreserved premolars was thawed from the tooth bank after 30 months´ storage and transplanted to the region. Note the mature double root of the graft.

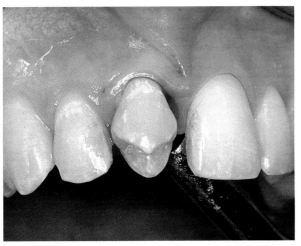
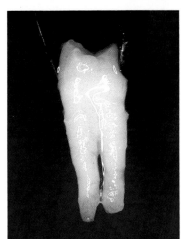

Conditions after transplantation
Endodontic treatment was initiated 2 weeks after transplantation. Two years later, the grafted premolar is seen restored as an incisor.

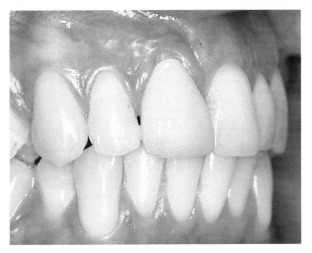
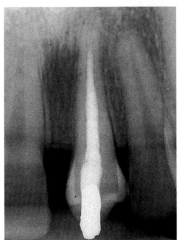

In cases of cleidocranial dysostosis, autotransplantation is used to solve the problem of multiple tooth impaction. In these cases supernumerary teeth which are not initially used can be stored for later transplantation (Fig. 9.5).

In cleft palate patients it is often necessary to extract one or more teeth in the alveolar cleft region before surgical closure of the cleft with a bone graft can be performed. Cryopreservation of these teeth and later transplantation to the healed cleft area can solve important orthodontic and prosthodontic problems (Fig. 9.6).[15]

Fig. 9.5. Cleidocranial dysplasia
Autotransplantation of cryopreserved supernumerary teeth in a patient with cleidocranial dysostosis. Nine of the supernumerary teeth that could not be autotransplanted immediately were cryopreserved for later use (hatched teeth).

Autotransplantaion of cryopreserved tooth
The partially impacted left central incisor did not respond to orthodontic eruption and was cryopreserved for 2 years before autotransplantation to the right lateral incisor area. Endodontic treatment was performed 2 weeks later. Normal PDL is found radiographically 5 years after transplantation.

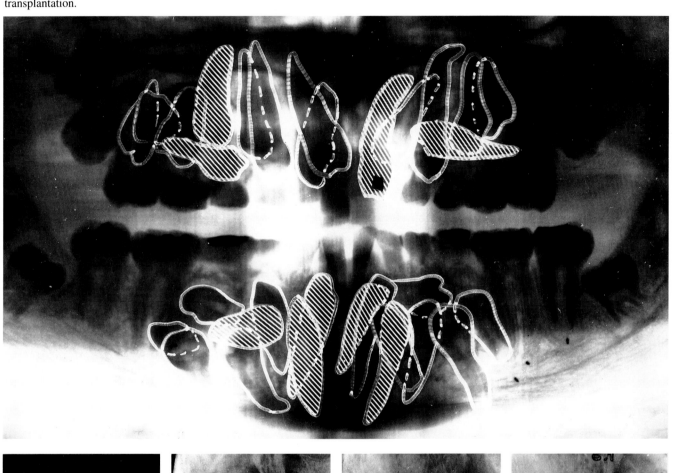

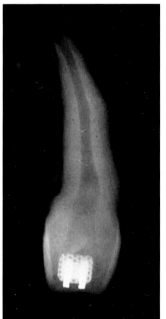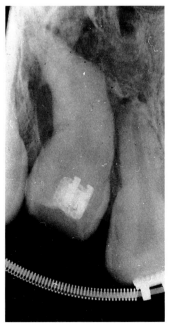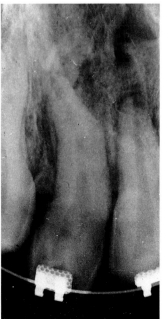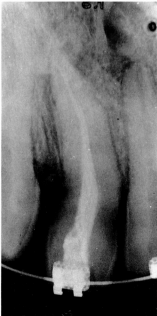

Fig. 9.6. Cryopreserved canine transplanted to a bone graft in the alveolar cleft

Unilateral alveolar cleft with an ectopic canine in the cleft area. The canine was extracted and cryopreserved 2 months prior to bone grafting.

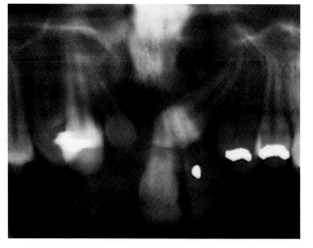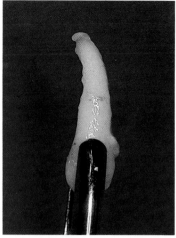

Tooth thawing and transplantation

Condition 6 months after bone grafting to the cleft (8 months after tooth extraction). Healing of the bone graft is sufficient for subsequent tooth grafting. The cryopreserved canine was thawed. A punch biopsy knife is used for the circular incision at the recipient site.

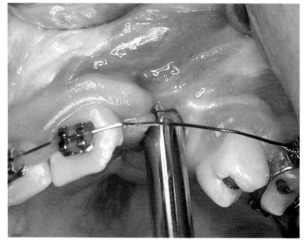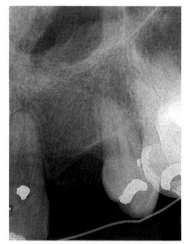

Tooth graft in position

Two weeks after transplantation the pulp was extirpated and the root canal filled with calcium hydroxide. Subsequent conventional root canal treatment was performed 6 months later.

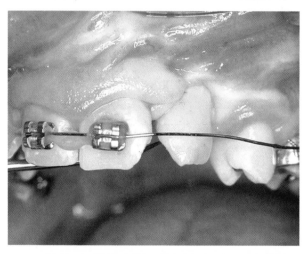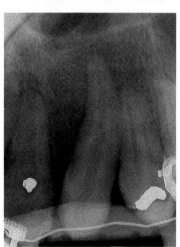

Conditions after 6 months

The position of the graft was adjusted by orthodontic treatment. Radiograph shows normal periodontal healing.

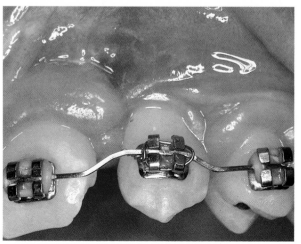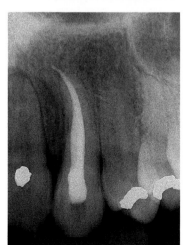

Replantation

Although long-term storage of teeth has a rather limited area of indication, the following examples describe situations where a tooth bank could be used in connection with replantation:

In cases of traumatic avulsion where the contusion of the socket walls needs a period of healing before replantation can be performed.[17]

In the case of a complicated jaw fracture through an alveolus which indicates extraction of the tooth in order to safeguard fracture healing without pulpal and periodontal interference. In these instances the tooth can be stored during the healing period and later replanted.

Allotransplantation

Long-term storage of teeth in a tooth bank is indicated in allotransplantation of teeth where it can solve the logistic problem of ensuring that a suitable donor tooth is available to a recipient at the required time and place (Fig. 9.7 and Chapter 8, p. 227). The tooth bank can considerably reduce the problem of matching the donor and recipient by means of time-consuming techniques for serologic and cellular tissue typing and matching. Furthermore, the tooth bank optimizes conditions for testing donors for viral infections by introducing the possibility of collecting test blood samples months after removal of the donor tooth. By postponing the collection of the test blood sample by at least 3 months after extraction of the cryopreserved teeth, the technique solves the problem of a possible seroconvertion of the donor in the test for HIV and hepatitis virus. Finally, a tooth bank can increase the utilization of a large number of teeth available for allotransplantation by the use of premolars extracted for orthodontic reasons. Thus the policy in allotransplantation of seeking out a donor to suit an available recipient is considerably altered by the use of a tooth bank, as this can provide a suitable tooth for each recipient among a panel of available tissue typed teeth, thereby considerably increasing the probability of a good match for each recipient (see Chapter 8, p. 236).

Fig. 9.7. Cryopreserved allograft to an anterior region with severe bone loss
Extensive bone loss was present around the left central incisor 2 years after replantation of both central incisors after traumatic avulsion. In the bony cavity where almost all of the bony alveolar walls were lost, an allografted lower second premolar was positioned after thawing from the tooth bank. Endodontic treatment was done by calcium hydroxide obliteration of the pulp chamber, and replaced yearly. The allograft is ankylosed and replacement resorption of the graft is slowly progressing. Bone maintenance around the graft is obvious. Four years and 6 months later, there are clinically normal conditions and with gingivtal pockets not exceeding 3 mm.

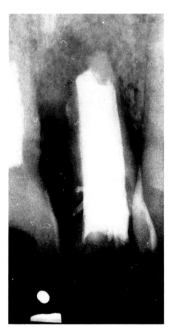
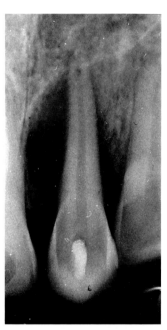
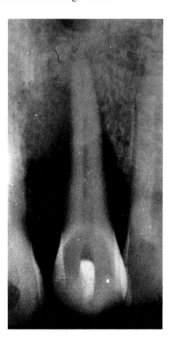
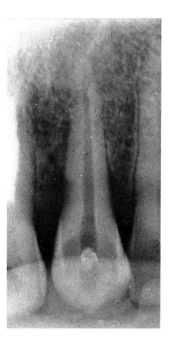

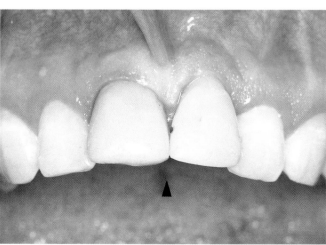
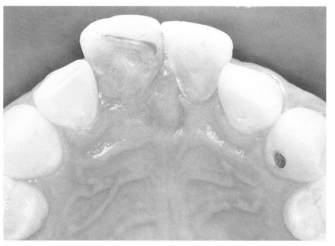

Laboratory and clinical procedures

Experimental and clinical investigations[11,14] have shown the following *laboratory and clinical procedures* to be required for cryopreservation of teeth (Figs. 9.8-9.11):

Extraction

In order to withstand the summation of nonphysiologic stresses associated with cryopreservation, the tooth must be in a reasonably good state before storage. Thus, donor teeth should not be affected by extensive caries or marginal periodontitis. The morphology of the root and the root canal should enable atraumatic extraction and allow adequate root canal therapy. The potential donor teeth are at present limited to incisors, canines, or premolars in order to fit the freezing tubes presently used for cryopreservation (Fig. 9.8).

Donors for *allotransplantation* are usually patients with an orthodontic indication for two or four premolar extractions. HLA tissue typing of the donor has proven efficient (see Chapter 8). Ethically it is necessary that the donor and the parents or relatives are properly informed, and accept tooth donation and are willing to provide a blood sample 3 months after tooth donation for blood tests by informed consent.

Surgical removal of the donor tooth follows the methods described in autotransplantation of the tooth type in question. After removal, the graft is examined carefully for accidental damage before being placed in an upright position with the crown downwards in a tube containing a complete tissue culture medium. After being placed in this medium, radiographs are taken of the faciolingual and proximal aspects of the tooth (Fig. 9.2).

Short-term storage during transport

During equilibration and removal of the cryoprotective agent and during transport to and from the freezing facilities prior to freezing and after thawing prior to transplantation, the teeth are stored in a **complete medium** (Fig. 9.8). One of the currently acceptable tissue culture media is used, such as:

RPMI-1640 supplemented with 10% heat-inactivated and sterile filtrated fetal calf serum (FCS) and 25 mM HEPES buffered to a pH of 7.4 (Gibco Ltd., Scotland) supplemented with antibiotics (penicillin 0.5×10^6 U/l, streptomycin 500 mg/l), heparin 15,000 U/l, and glutamine 1.2 mM. This procedure would adequately meet the requirements needed for the tissue during short-term storage (i.e., up to 12 hours).

Equilibration with cryoprotectant

The aim of this phase is to achieve an appropriate concentration and uniform distribution of the cryoprotective agent DMSO or glycerol throughout the soft tissues and to prevent irreversible toxic damage or severe osmotic shock to the PDL cells. The pulp tissue, however, is not expected to be protected; therefore endodontic treatment should be performed after transplantation. The tooth is transferred, crown downwards, into a small sterile freezing tube with a screw cap containing complete medium with 20% heat-inactivated (56^0C, 30 min.) and sterile filtrated fetal calf serum (FCS) (Fig. 9.8). Equilibration of the highly diffusable cryoprotectant DMSO (dimethylsulfoxide, Merck GmbH, Germany) as described by Schwartz (1986)[13] seems to be appropriately slow, thus avoiding intracellular ice crystal formation during freezing. The four-step procedure involves 5 min in 2.5% DMSO, 5 min in 5% DMSO, 5 min. in 7.5% DMSO, and 5 min in 10% DMSO at room temperature ($18-22^0$C).[13]

Freezing and freezing equipment

The tube containing the tooth in cryoprotectant is transferred to an automatic freezing device (LC 40, L´Air Liquide, France or BV10, Cryozon GmbH, Germany), where controlled cooling and freezing are performed according to a cryoprofile shown in Fig. 9.10. Intracellular ice formation is reduced by slow freezing and a limitation of supercooling before crystallization (Fig. 9.10). Freezing rates are automatically controlled and monitored simultaneously for sample and chamber temperature (Fig. 9.8).

Tooth bank file

The clinical use of a tooth bank could be based on a mechanical or computerized file (Fig. 9.9) which enables matching of the donors for a given recipient to be carried out easily and permits swift localization of the tooth and donor cells in the tooth bank. The file card contains information concerning the donor, the clinical and radiographic recordings of the graft, and data from the blood sample from the donor, including blood (AB0 and Rh) and tissue type (HLA classes I and II). Furthermore, donor lymphocytes are cryopreserved for eventual cross-match or later immunologic monitoring (see Chapter 8, p. 228). Macroscopic recordings concerning the morphology of the crown and root, the appearance of the PDL, and the size of the apical foramen are recorded on the file of each tooth graft in the bank.

Storage

The frozen teeth should be stored in the sealed tubes at -196^0C in a liquid nitrogen container (BT 55, L´Air Liquide, France or BSR, Cryozon GmbH, Germany) (Fig. 9.12). The constant temperature of -196^0C in the container is ensured by a weekly re-filling routine, supplemented with an automatic temperature alarm system (Fig. 9.12).

Fig. 9.8. Cryopreservation of teeth

Extraction of the donor teeth follows the guidelines for extraction of teeth for autotransplantation. Single rooted mature teeth are preferred with subsequent endodontic treatment in mind. The morphology of the root and macroscopic signs of damage to the PDL are recorded on the file card (see Fig. 9.9).

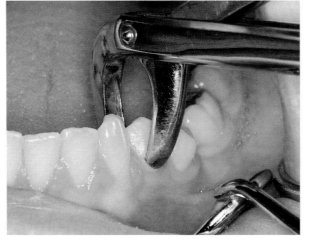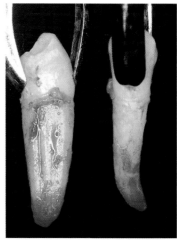

Teeth placed in transport medium

Donor teeth for the tooth bank are collected in 5 ml plastic tubes containing transport medium with antibiotics (see text). In the front a cryotube with a screw cap is shown.

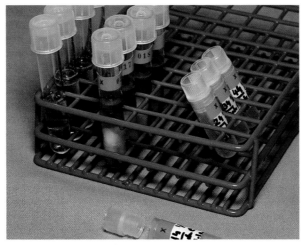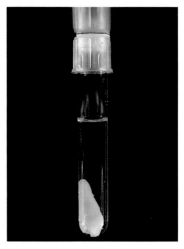

Biologic freezer

A programmable biologic freezer consists of a freezing chamber, connected to a liquid nitrogen supply, and a programmable temperature controller. Liquid nitrogen is used as a refrigerant; it is transferred in a controlled manner into the freezing chamber, and a fan ensures uniform temperature distribution. In the chamber, in a control cryotube, a temperature sensor is connected to the programmer for monitoring the freezing of the teeth according to the planned freezing curve (see Fig. 9.10).

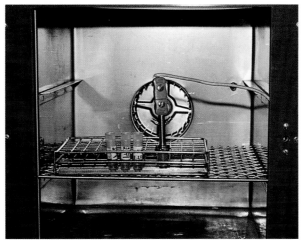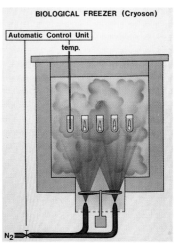

Liquid nitrogen container

Cryotubes are stored in a liquid nitrogen container organized in a drawer system so that the individual tooth is easily found among the approximately 1,000 spaces, which is the capacity of the container (BT 55, L´Air Liquide, France or BSR, Cryozon GmbH, Germany).

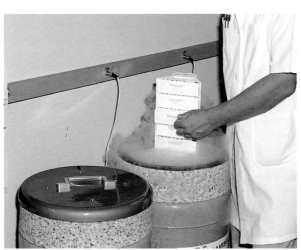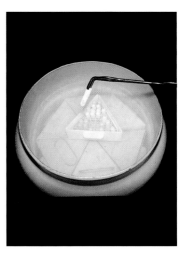

Selection of a donor tooth for allotransplantation

A blood sample (50-80 ml) is collected from the donor at least 3 months after extraction of the teeth in order to allow tissue type analysis including AB0, RhD, and HLA typing (see Chapter 8, p. 228). A prerequisite for donation of teeth is a negative test for HIV and hepatitis virus. Based on the AB0 and HLA tissue type (see Chapter 8), teeth are selected from the file. The punched out holes along the edge of each file card are cut away according to the blood type and HLA-tissue types, tooth type, etc. (Fig. 9.9). This is then used when matching is done mechanically by using a knitting needle for selection of donor teeth for, e.g., for an exact HLA-DR tissue type. If several teeth with similar tissue type match are available, the tooth to be transplanted is selected according to clinical and radiographic recordings to fit into the recipient condititons. The present capacity of the tooth bank in Copenhagen is approximately 400 teeth from HLA-tissue typed donors for allotransplantation and 200 teeth for autotransplantation. The local extraction policy of the cooperating orthodontic clinics means that the donor teeth for the bank are almost exclusively premolars. Mature root formation of the teeth is preferred, with a single root to facilitate the endodontic treatment. Storage time is supposed to be unlimited for these teeth as well as for other tissues stored under similar conditions, provided there is continous addition of liquid nitrogen.[1-14]

Thawing

The tube containing the selected frozen tooth is transferred directly from liquid nitrogen (-196°C) to a water bath at 37°C with continuous agitation. Once the ice nucleus has disappeared (within 2-3 minutes), the tooth in the freezing medium is transferred to a larger tube at 0°C and heated within 10 min to room temperature (18-21°C) (Fig. 9.11). Removal of cryoprotective agent is now initiated by addition of equal aliquots of complete medium with 20% FCS in a four-step procedure 5 min. each step, resulting in the following final concentrations: 10%, 7.5%, 5%, 2.5%, and 0% DMSO. The tooth is then transferred to a plastic tube containing transport medium (Fig. 9.8) and kept there at room temperature until replantation or transplantation can be performed, preferably within a few hours.[13]

Transplantation

The clinical procedures follow the techniques shown in previous chapters, varying in accordance with the type of transplantation and the tooth type in question.

Fig. 9.9. File card. To the *left*: clinical and radiographic data of the donor tooth and cryopreservation. In the *middle*: information about the donor and a radiograph of the tooth. To the *right*: test results of a blood sample collected at least 3 months after extraction in those teeth planned for allotransplantation.

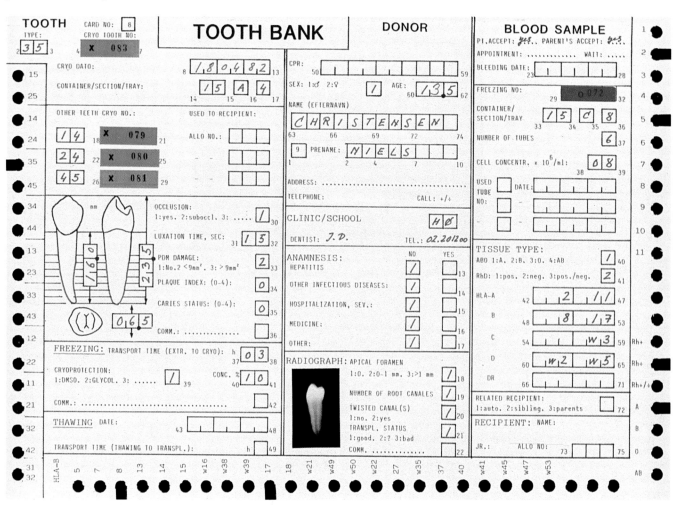

Fig. 9.10. Freezing curve

The freezing curve from room temperature to final temperature before liquid nitrogen storage comprises several stages:

Liquid phase cooling controlled by programmed biologic freezing (Fig. 9.8), 1-2°C/min., to a sample temperature of -7°C.

Crystallization at -7°C, the freezing point of the sample. Automatic injection of liquid nitrogen compensates for the heat by the crystallization of the sample. The controlled burst of cooling induces crystallization and eliminates supercooling of the liquid.

Freezing. Slow solid phase cooling, at a rate of 0.5°C/min, to -40°C. In this interval the slow cooling rate reduces the intracellular ice crystal formation. Thereafter the freezing curve declines rapidly to -100°C, whereafter the tube is plunged into liquid nitrogen for storage.

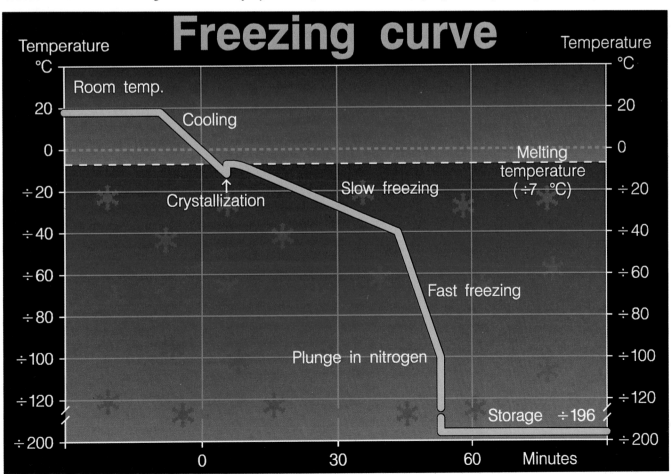

Fig. 9.11. Thawing curve
Thawing of ice crystals in the sample and rehydration of cells is connected to the used freezing curve. Rapid thawing by storage for 1-2 minutes in a 37°C waterbath (Fig. 9.12) results in a thawing rate of approximately 100°C/min. The tube is removed from the waterbath as soon as the last ice nucleous has disappeared, and slowly heated to room temperature for deequilibration of the cryoprotective agent.

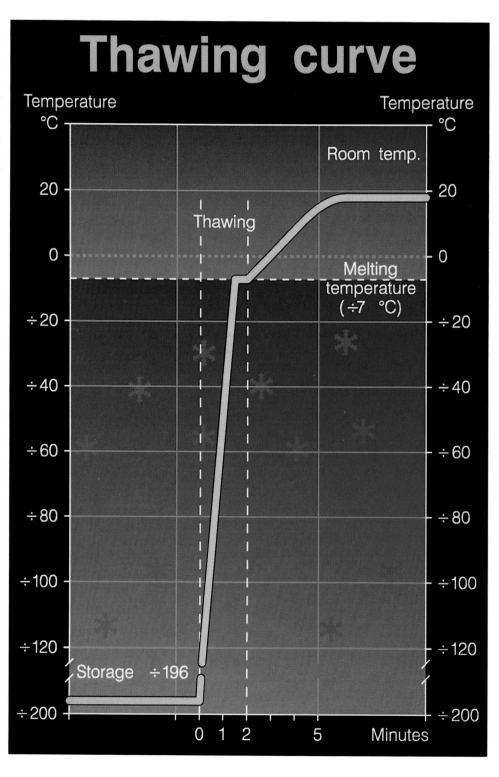

Unilaterally distributed multiple aplasia

When two teeth are missing in one quadrant, and there is a full complement of teeth in another, transplantation may change the situation into one where there is only one premolar missing in each quadrant (Figs. 10.5 and 10.6).[8-10] This would result in a situation which can usually be treated by conventional orthodontics.

Treatment planning in aplasia cases
Aplasia of mandibular second premolar(s)

Before transplantation is considered, a complete case analysis and treatment plan must be made, based on cephalometric radiographs and prediction of growth.[8-10] It is clear that transplantation should not be performed when extraction of premolars would otherwise be part of the orthodontic treatment plan. Potential graft teeth for the premolar region include maxillary premolars and maxillary and mandibular third molars. Due to root anatomy, maxillary first premolars should be avoided as graft teeth. Before transplantation is decided upon, a detailed analysis of space conditions at the recipient site and of the potential graft is necessary (see Chapter 4, p. 114 and Chapter 5, p. 143). The size of mandibular third molars, however, usually prevents them from being used for transplantation to the premolar regions unless the recipient site is expanded. In the case of premolars used as donor teeth, it is usually only necessary and possible to get information about the mesiodistal dimension of the crown and the root length. After an analysis of the recipient region, it must be decided whether transplantation to the recipient site is possible or whether additional space should be created orthodontically.

With respect to crown and root anatomy, premolars from one quadrant generally fit best in the contralateral quadrant of the opposing jaw. Concerning the position of the graft, it is usually necessary to rotate the tooth 45° or 90° distally in order to place it within the relatively narrow alveolar process. This rotation also serves to create interproximal contacts and precludes surgical preparation of the mesiofacial aspect of the socket, which may damage the mental vessels and nerve.

Third molars can also serve as premolar replacements. However, normally only the maxillary molars have a dimension suitable for this purpose (Fig. 10.7). In these cases, it is essential that a three-dimensional evaluation of tooth size is made.

The technique used consists of orthoradial and axial radiographic exposures of the graft (see Chapter 4, p. 114). In this context, it should be remembered that the faciolingual diameter is usually greater than the mesiodistal. This implies 90° mesial rotation of the graft when transplanting to the mandibular arch to fit the space conditions in the recipient site, where the mesiodistal dimension is normally greater than the faciolingual. For a successful surgical procedure, it is essential that the space in the recipient region is equal to or slightly greater than the graft. The optimal time for transplantation is when root formation has reached 2/3-4/4 root length with an open apex (see Chapter 4, p. 133). It is advisable to retain the primary molar until transplantation can be performed, even where the molar demonstrates ankylosis or periapical complications, to avoid undesirable migration of teeth into the recipient site and to prevent atrophy of the alveolar process. Premature tooth loss in the recipient area with resultant loss of space necessitates orthodontic expansion prior to transplantation.

Aplasia of mandibular central incisors or canines

The same treatment principles are generally followed when mandibular central incisors or canines are missing. The purpose is then to shift the edentulous site distally in the dental arch by moving the lateral incisors mesially to replace the central incisors, etc. (Fig. 10.8). In this way, the edentulous area can be moved to a more distal location in the mandible (e.g. canine or premolar region), where the faciolingual dimension of the alveolar process allows premolar transplantation.

Aplasia of two adjacent maxillary premolars

A good treatment alternative when both the first and second premolars in the same maxillary quadrant are absent is to transplant one premolar from the intact segment. This will provide one premolar in each quadrant (Fig. 10.6). The topography of the maxillary sinus must be considered when planning maxillary premolar transplantation. Thus, transplantation must be performed at an early stage of root development; or special surgical techniques should be used where the graft is placed free of the sinus (see Chapter 5, p. 172).

Fig. 10.6. Two maxillary premolar aplasias can be treated by transplantation of the contralateral maxillary second premolar.

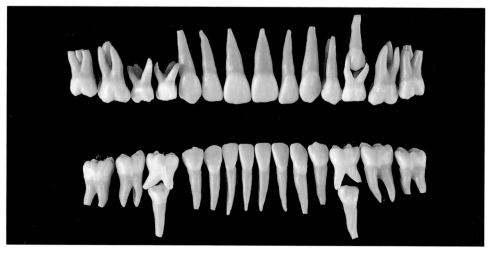

In conclusion, aplasia in the premolar region should be diagnosed as early as possible so that transplantation of premolars can be incorporated into the orthodontic treatment plan. This requires a radiographic examination at the age of 9-10 years when the premolars have not yet erupted.[22] Transplantation of premolars to edentulous areas due to agenesis offers a unique treatment possibility in some cases; but it should be weighed carefully against alternative treatment forms.

The molar region

The need for molar replacements is usually related to the extraction of first or second molars due to caries.[23] However, it may also be related to other causes, such as lack of eruption and juvenile periodontitis.

The treatment possibilities for molar loss are confined to the following:

Orthodontic or spontaneous space closure
Prosthetic replacement
Transplantation of third molars

Fig. 10.7. Transplantation of maxillary third molars as replacements for mandibular second premolar aplasias.

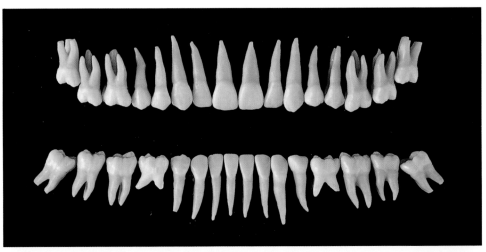

Fig. 10.8. Aplasia of two mandibular central incisors can be treated by forward movement of the lateral segments and transplantation of two maxillary second premolars to the mandibular first or second premolar region.

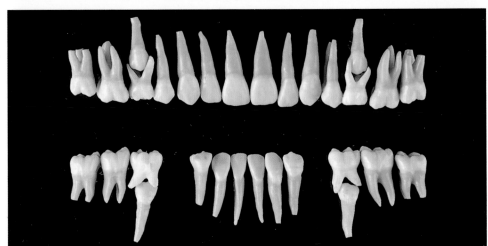

Orthodontic or spontaneous closure

Space closure after extraction of the first (or second) molar may be part of an interceptive treatment plan in geographic areas with high caries incidence and limited dental and orthodontic resources. Spontaneous closure, however, is not as reliable in the mandible as in the maxilla. This is due to less mesial drift and a less favorable axial inclination of the mandibular molars, which will be accentuated by mesial tipping.

Spontaneous closure and an acceptable occlusion may be obtained in some class I cases with slight crowding after extraction of the mandibular molars. Extraction of the maxillary counterpart to the extracted molar may be indicated in order to achieve optimal occlusion. This should be done prior to eruption of the adjacent (second or third) molar and when it has reached about half of its anticipated root length. Extraction of the maxillary molar will then allow the adjacent mandibular molar to erupt in contact with its maxillary counterpart[23,24].

The mandibular first or second molars are not considered the ideal teeth to extract for orthodontic purposes. However, due to high caries susceptibility, the prognosis for these teeth is sometimes poor. If extraction is delayed until after eruption of the adjacent molar, the adjacent molar will tend to tip mesially and rotate mesiolingually; this makes orthodontic alignment difficult and it will usually take several years to complete.[101]

Prosthetic replacement

The prognosis of this form of treatment is described on p. 267.

Fig. 10.9. Transplantation of a third molar from the opposite quadrant as a replacement for a first mandibular molar.

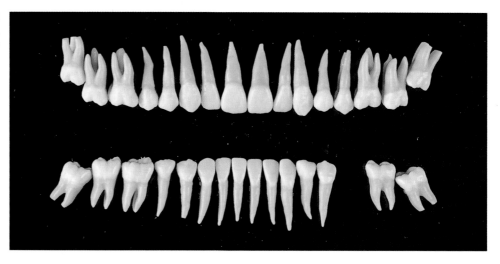

Transplantation of third molars

Before this treatment procedure is adopted, the possibility and feasibility of orthodontic treatment should be considered. In this regard, it is important to consider that transplantation cannot compete with the results obtained after orthodontic movement. On average, about 75% of molar transplants can be considered successful on a long-term basis with proper graft selection (see Chapter 4, p. 133). When transplantation is considered as the treatment of choice, a three-dimensional space analysis of the recipient site and the graft should be made (see Chapter 4, p. 114). Only if this analysis reveals acceptable conditions should transplantation be carried out. With respect to graft preference, extracted molars should preferably be replaced by grafts from other quadrant (Fig. 10.9) or from the opposing arch (Fig. 10.10). This is apart from anatomic considerations due to the fact that if the transplant is made from the same quadrant, and fails, two molars would be missing in that quadrant.

Concerning the development of the potential third molar graft, the following should be considered: The tooth should have reached approximately 3/4 root development. Moreover, in the case of maxillary third molars, the occlusal surface of the graft should have erupted to the cervical level of the adjacent second molar to ensure uncomplicated graft removal[24.]

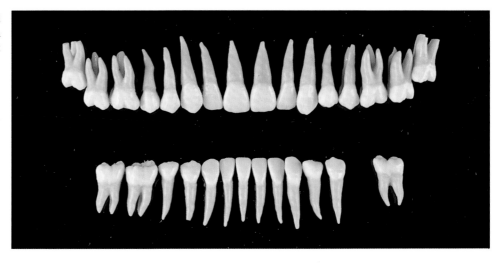

Fig. 10.10. Transplantation of a third molar from the opposing jaw as a replacement for a mandibular first molar.

The canine region

The usual indication for treatment in this region is ectopic positioning of the canine.[25-35] Treatment possibilities are usually confined to the following:

Retention of the primary canine and surgical removal of the permanent canine

Surgical removal of the primary and permanent canines and prosthetic replacement

Orthodontic space closure by mesial movement of posterior teeth after removal of the primary and permanent canines

Surgical exposure of the ectopically placed canine and orthodontic repositioning

Autotransplantation of the ectopically placed canine into correct alignment

In the following, the prognosis of these different treatment modalities will be described. As a general rule, an attempt should be made to save the permanent canine whenever possible due to its superior long-term value.

Retention of the primary canine

To date, no long-term studies have been published on this form of treatment. However, despite occasional exceptions, clinical experience has shown that primary canines seldom last more than 5-10 years beyond the expected time of normal exfoliation.

Prosthetic replacement

The prognosis of this treatment is described on p. 267

Orthodontic movement of posterior teeth into the canine region

In some situations, a premolar can replace a missing or impacted canine, a fact which should be evaluated before transplantation is considered. If this treatment is chosen, it is essential from an esthetic point of view that the premolar is rotated mesially and the lingual cusp reduced slightly.[99]

Surgical exposure of the canine and subsequent orthodontic repositioning

This is usually the treatment of choice in cases of ectopia and normally leads to a predictable and successful result.[26-35] However, it should be mentioned that minor complications can be encountered, such as loss of pulpal sensibility, root resorption, loss of marginal bone support, and gingival retraction.[36-50] Thus, in a detailed study of the long-term prognosis of 49 unilaterally impacted canines which were surgically exposed and later brought into occlusion orthodontically, it was found that the involved canines showed an increased threshold to electrometric pulp testing and in 4% of these cases, no sensibility reaction could be elicited. Furthermore, 23% of the teeth showed initial pulp canal obliteration, and a slight increase in pocket depth (0.7 mm) compared to control teeth (Fig. 10.11).

Clearly, the desire to correct the position of an impacted canine must be weighed against the disadvantages of long-term treatment (approximately 2 years) with fixed appliances.[50]

The prognosis for orthodontic correction depends upon several factors. These include the patient's age, space conditions, and the sagittal and transverse position of the canine crown and root. The optimal age for treatment is adolescence. However, treatment can even be instituted in adults, provided that the position of the impacted tooth is not extreme. It should be remembered that treatment begun at a later age must be performed more slowly than treatment begun at the optimal time. Factors to consider with respect to final prognosis include the following: The more vertical the orientation of the impacted canine the better. An axial inclination which is greater than 45° distally may worsen the prognosis. The closer the crown is to the midline and the root to the midpalatal suture, the poorer the prognosis. Finally, the periodontal ligament space should be visible along the entire root surface and the root apex should not be dilacerated.

Fig. 10.11. Sequelae after surgical exposure and orthodontic readjustment of unilateral ectopic canines. Note the slight shortening of the root length of the orthodontically treated tooth (O) due to surface resorption and marginal bone loss compared to the nontreated homologous canine (C). From Buchhorn, 1985.[50]

C   O   O   C   O   C

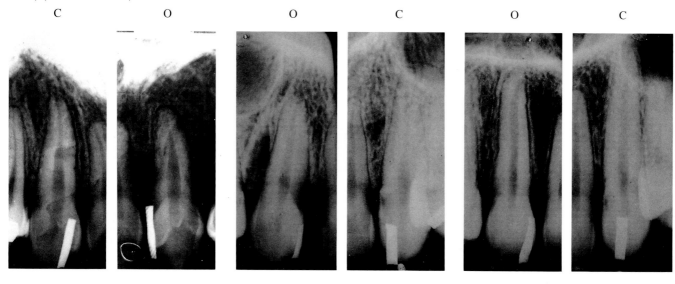

Autotransplantation of canines

Maxillary canine impaction is usually not detected before root development is complete. As shown in the statistics in Chapter 6, the long-term survival of autotransplantation of canines with mature root formation is not especially good. However, if transplantation is carried out early, preferably before completion of root development, the prognosis is favorable (see Chapter 6, p. 202). Before transplantation is decided upon, it is essential that a detailed analysis of the space conditions of the graft and the recipient site be made (see Chapter 6, p. 180).

The cases where autotransplantation could be considered include the following:

Ectopic placement where the canine's path of eruption has resulted in marked resorption of the lateral and/or central incisor root(s) (Fig. 10.12).

Ectopic placement of the canine, where surgical exposure and subsequent orthodontic realignment are difficult, impossible, or can seriously damage the supporting structures of adjacent teeth (Fig. 10.13).

Ectopic placement where surgical exposure and orthodontic repositioning have failed or were refused.

Canine transplantation should be planned as early as possible and preferably at 11 or 12 years of age, when root development is not yet complete. At that time, most ectopic canines can be diagnosed and still be transplanted with a very good chance of pulpal and periodontal healing[55,56]. It is, therefore, recommended that children whose canines have not erupted by 11-12 years of age should be examined radiographically in order to diagnose the presence and location of the unerupted teeth and to plan subsequent treatment[57-63].

Autotransplantation of premolars to the canine region

In cases of traumatic loss of a canine, autotransplantation of a premolar is possible. Mandibular premolars are particularly suitable because of the similarity of the root anatomy to that of the lost tooth.

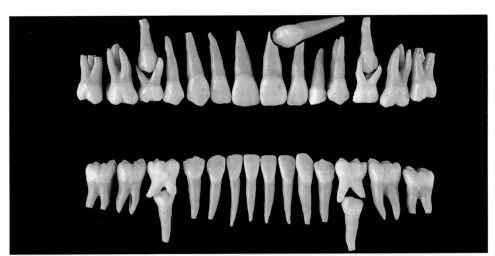

Fig. 10.12. Transplantation of an ectopically positioned canine which has caused root resorption of the lateral and central incisor.

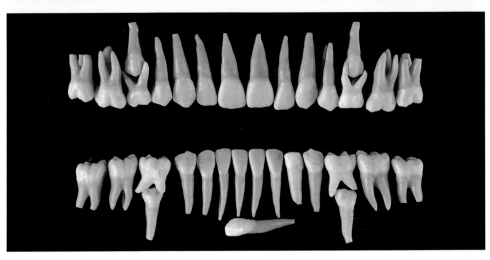

Fig. 10.13. Transplantation of an ectopically positioned mandibular canine

The incisor region

Absence of incisors in young persons frequently creates difficult treatment problems.[15,16] Aplasia of maxillary lateral incisors is relatively frequent, whereas other incisors are rarely congenitally absent. Among other causes of loss or extraction of incisors are traumatic injuries, malformation, advanced root resorption, and untreatable endodontic complications. The treatment possibilities usually available for dealing with these conditions include orthodontic space closure, prosthetic replacement, and autotransplantation.

In the following, each treatment procedure will be evaluated.

Orthodontic space closure

Suitable cases for orthodontic space closure include class I crowding and some cases of class II malocclusion. Such a solution could be considered when the lateral incisor is similar in crown dimension and morphology to a central incisor, when it is above average in root length, and when the crown of the adjacent canine lends itself to recontouring to the shape of a lateral incisor. On the other hand, anterior tooth loss in a class III malocclusion or a class I malocclusion with no space deficiency or even a surplus of space, with diminutive lateral incisors, and with pointed or yellowish canines, is best treated by autotransplantation or prosthetic replacement.

In the orthodontic replacement of anterior teeth, attention must be paid throughout treatment to the position of the midline, the axial inclination of the adjacent teeth, and the anchorage available.[99,101] Further clinical considerations in cases with maxillary incisors missing are discussed elsewhere.[99,101]

Prosthetic replacement

Because of the young age at which the need for prosthetic replacement usually arises, a temporary prosthetic appliance is often necessary prior to definitive restoration. There are several requirements to be met by this appliance. It should be an effective space maintainer and satisfactory from esthetic and hygienic points of view. It should not interfere with normal occlusal development or overload the permanent teeth; and it should not require any preparation of the permanent teeth.

Various removable and fixed prosthetic devices to which artificial teeth are added may be used as temporary replacements. The acid-etch technique also provides new possibilities. In some cases, the crown of the patient´s own tooth can be bonded to the adjacent teeth as an esthetic space maintainer. Experimentation with various forms of lingually bonded frameworks to which an artificial tooth is added is promising. Such devices include the Rochette and Maryland resin-retained bridges[64-68] and bonded spiral wire-supported acrylic teeth.[100]

Concerning the long-term prognosis of fixed prosthetics, several clinical studies have shown that gingival inflammatory changes adjacent to cast restorations are correlated to the location of crown margins (whether placed subgingivally, at the level of the gingiva or supragingivally[36,71,83-98]), to crown and bridge construction,[69-82,85-86,97] and to oral hygiene.[71,83,87-91,97]

The long-term prognosis with respect to restoration longevity has only been sparsely documented.[72-82] In a study of 1046 bridges, an average yearly failure rate of 4% was found. The risk of failure was particularly pronounced in the younger age groups (i.e., below 21 years of age).[73,74] Similar risks have been found with full crown restorations.[77,98] It should be added that in other long-term studies covering up to 10 years, a lower failure rate was found.[80,82,91] Pulp necrosis with subsequent periapical complication of the abutment teeth should also be mentioned. Thus, one study demonstrated a 4% frequency of pulp necrosis in a group of fully crowned teeth 10 years after restoration.[77]

Autotransplantation

Transplantation of teeth to the anterior region is a new treatment alternative (Figs. 10.14 and 10.15).[1,3,8,9] Although published materials are small, they indicate a favorable long-term prognosis when premolars are autotransplanted to the incisor region in young individuals.[1,3,102-104] The applicability of this method is dependent upon the availability of donor teeth and knowledge of growth and development of the jaws. In rare cases, supernumerary teeth can be used.[3] Premolars can be extracted in the same or opposite dental arch and be transplanted to the incisor region (Figs. 10.14 to 10.16). In some cases of multiple tooth loss a combination of orthodontic space closure and autotransplantation can be useful (Figs. 10.17 and 10.18). In this regard, the type of incisor to be replaced should be considered. A slender maxillary central incisor can thus be replaced by all premolars (except the maxillary first premolar, due to its root anatomy). In the case of broad maxillary incisors, the selected premolar (preferably the second maxillary premolar) can be rotated 90^0 in order to create a sufficient cervical dimension mesiodistally. When several clinical procedures are combined, such as rotation of the graft, selective grinding, and recontouring with composite resin, they can provide a more satisfactory solution than most other treatment alternatives (Fig. 10.17). The use of porcelain laminate veneer restorations can also provide esthetically acceptable results in these cases. As the development of most premolars is complete by 12 years of age, the indication for transplantation to the anterior region must be evaluated and determined at an early age.

Orthodontic movement of transplanted teeth

If orthodontic movement of the graft is necessary, this can be done about 3 months after transplantation, when there is complete and maximal revascularization of the graft (see Chapter 1, p. 36). Orthodontic movement should, if possible, and depending upon the stage of root development, be completed by 6-9 months after transplantation, before the onset of extensive pulp canal obliteration. Orthodontic movement of transplanted teeth does not appear to lead to excessive root resorption.[8,9,105] To close the extraction site, fixed appliance therapy can be instituted immediately after extraction of the maxillary or mandibular premolars. If there are large maxillary sinus recesses, or one or both jaws are retrognathic, it may be an advantage to use a reverse headgear to supplement the intraorally fixed appliance.

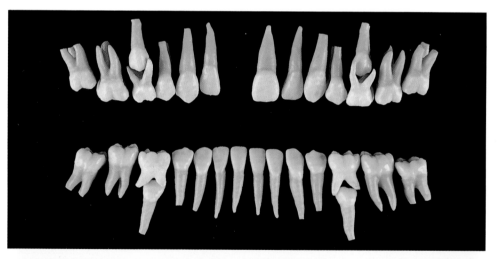

Fig. 10.14. Transplantation of a premolar as a replacement for a central maxillary incisor.

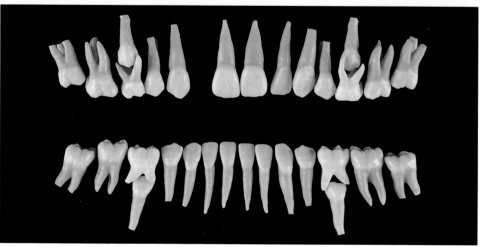

Fig. 10.15. Transplantation of a premolar as a replacement for a lateral maxillary incisor.

Fig. 10.16. Autotransplantation of a second maxillary premolar as a replacement for a lost central incisor

The patient is a 13-year-old boy who lost his right central incisor due to trauma at the age of 9. Note the atrophy of the alveolar process. The donor tooth is erupted but has a wide open apex.

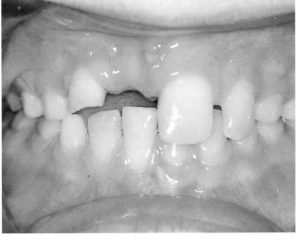 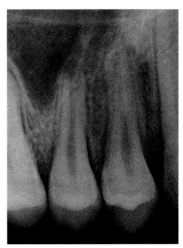

Condition after transplantation
The graft was rotated 45⁰ in order to accommodate the narrow alveolar process.

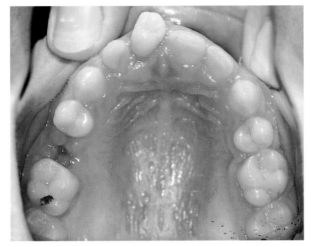 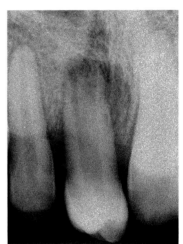

Orthodontic rotation of graft
Three months after transplantation space was created and rotation of the graft was initiated. The mesial rotation resulted in proximal contact of the graft´s labial and palatal surface. The treatment time for the orthodontic therapy was 1 year.

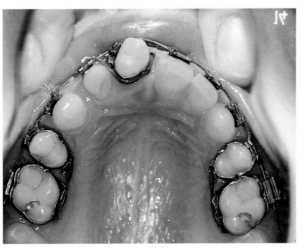 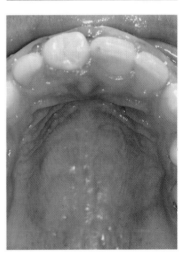

Restoring the graft
After a slight grinding of the "labial" and "palatal" surface of the graft the tooth was restored with composite one year after the transplantation.

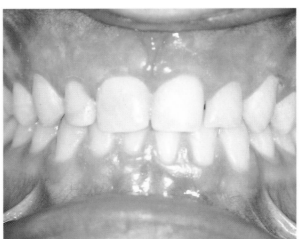 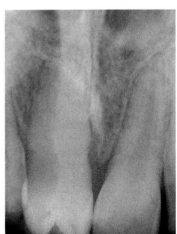

269

Fig. 10.17. Combined orthodontic treatment and transplantation in a case with anterior tooth loss

Two incisors have been avulsed in a 9-year-old girl.

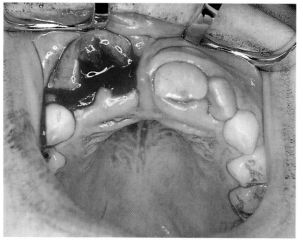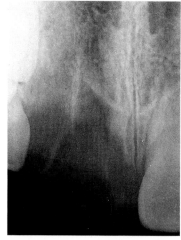

Treatment plan

The treatment plan is to move orthodontically the canine into the lateral incisor region and the first premolar into the canine region, and finally to transplant the mandibular second premolar into the central incisor region.

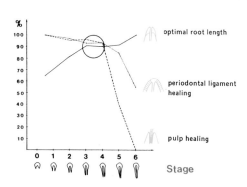

CHANCE OF SUCCESFUL HEALING RELATED TO STAGE OF ROOT DEVELOPMENT OF AUTOTRANSPLANTED PREMOLARS

optimal root length

periodontal ligament healing

pulp healing

Stage

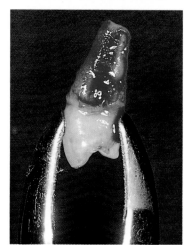

Transplantation and orthodontic treatment

The canine has been moved into the lateral incisor region.

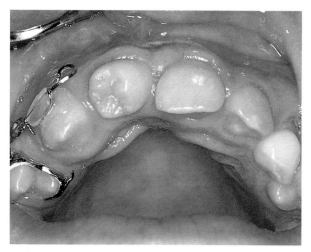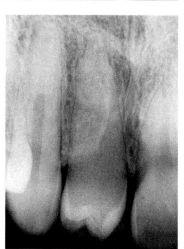

Restoration of the anterior segment

The premolar has been moved into the canine region and 45° rotated and the palatal cusp reduced. The canine has been moved into the lateral incisor region and its cusp and the proximal surfaces have been reduced. The transplanted premolar has been restored with composite. From Andreasen & al., 1989.[102]

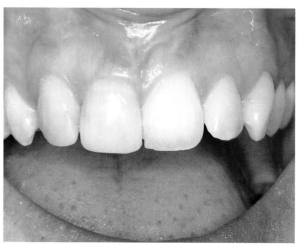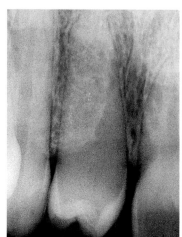

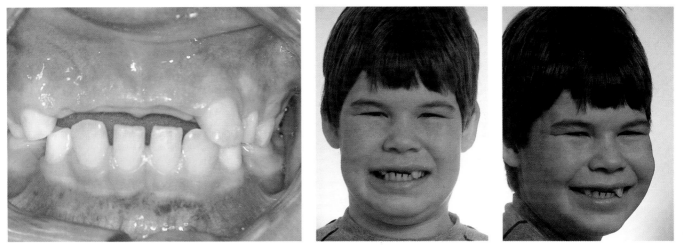

Fig. 10.18. Autotransplantation of two first mandibular premolars as replacements for three lost maxillary incisors

This 10-year-old boy has lost three incisors in an accident. The treatment plan is to treat the tooth loss with a combination of autotransplantation of premolars in the central incisor region and orthodontic closure in the right lateral maxillary region.

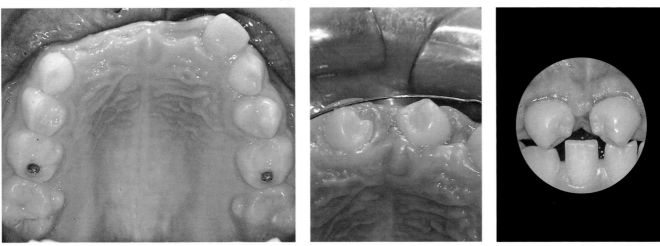

Autotransplantation to the central incisor region
Two first mandibular premolars were grafted to the central incisor region. Both teeth were rotated 90⁰ to give the graft more cervical width.

Orthodontic space closure and composite restoration of grafts
Orthodontic space closure was performed in both arches. The right canine was moved mesially to replace the lateral incisor. The two transplanted premolars were restored with composite after grinding. The treatment time for orthodontic therapy was 2 years and 8 months.

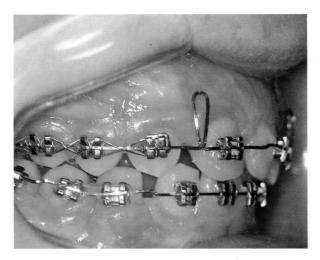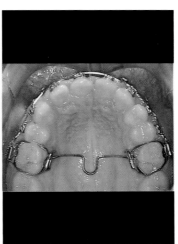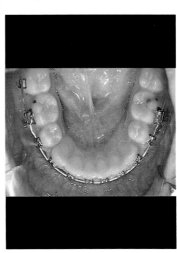

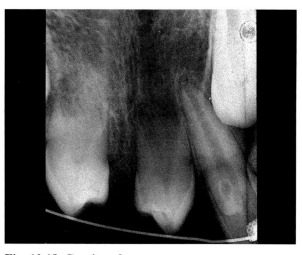 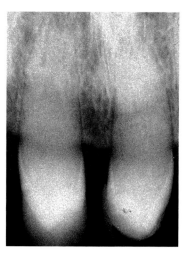

Fig. 10.18. Continued

Radiographic appearance of graft region

Radiographs show the condition at the time of transplantation at the age of 10 and follow-ups at the age of 12 and 14 years. Two roots have developed in both grafts.

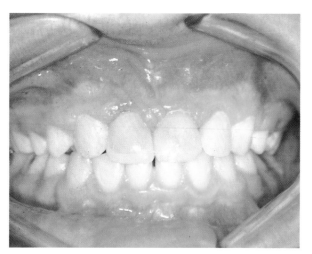 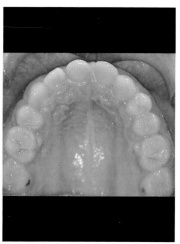 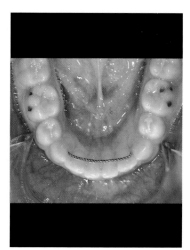

The clinical condition is shown at the age of 16. A banded retainer has been applied in the mandible.

Clinical appearance after treatment

The final treatment result appears from intra- and extraoral photographs. Note the reconstruction of both dental and alveolar bone anatomy.

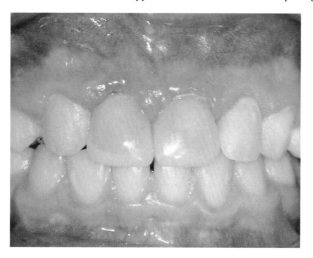 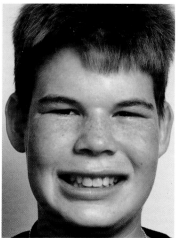 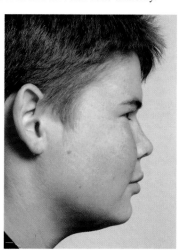

Essentials

Premolar region
Indications
Concomitant premolar impaction in one jaw segment and premolar aplasia in another (Fig. 10.3)
Uni- or bilateral absence of mandibular second premolars, when orthodontic space closure is not accepted or difficult , e.g., (1) profile is weak, (2) crowding is mild, and (3) bite is deep (Fig. 10.4)
Unevenly distributed multiple aplasias (Figs. 10.5 and 10.8)

Graft selection
Usually premolars

Stage of graft development
2/3-4/4 root formation with open apex

Molar region
Indication
Primarily to replace first molars (Figs. 10.9-10.10)

Graft selection
Usually third molars

Stage of graft development
3/4-4/4 root formation with open apex

Canine region
Indication
Ectopic position of the canine, where conventional surgical exposure and orthodontic repositioning is not feasible (Figs. 10.12 and 10.13)
Graft selection
Canines; sometimes premolars

Stage of graft development
3/4-4/4 root formation with open apex

Incisor region
Indication
Loss of one or more permanent incisor(s) (Figs. 10.14 and 10.18)

Graft selection
Premolars

Stage of graft development
3/4-4/4 root formation with open apex

Orthodontic movement of transplanted teeth
3-9 months after transplantation

References

1. Slagsvold O, Bjercke B. Autotransplantation of premolars in cases of missing anterior teeth. Trans Eur Orthod Soc 1970; 66: 473-85.

2. Slagsvold O, Bjercke B. Autotransplantation of premolars with partly formed roots. A radiographic study of root growth. Am J Orthod 1974; 66: 355-66.

3. Slagsvold O, Bjercke B. Applicability of autotransplantation in cases of missing upper anterior teeth. Am J Orthod 1978; 74: 410-21.

4. Slagsvold O, Bjercke B. Indications for autotransplantations in cases of missing premolars. Am J Orthod 1978; 74: 241-57.

5. Kristerson L. Autotransplantation of human premolars. A clinical and radiographic study of 100 teeth. Int J Oral Surg 1985; 14: 200-13.

6. Schwartz O, Bergmann P, Klausen B. Autotransplantation of human teeth. A life table analysis of prognostic factors. Int J Oral Surg 1985; 14: 245-58.

7. Schwartz O, Bergmann P, Klausen B. Resorption of autotransplanted human teeth: a retrospective study of 291 transplantations over a period of 25 years. Int Endod J 1985; 18: 119-31.

8. Paulsen HU, Andreasen JO. Autotransplantation in orthodontic treatment. Nederlandse Vereniging Woor Orthodontische Studie. Studieweek: 248-64, 1985.

9. Paulsen HU. L'autotransplantation de prémolaires lors des traitments orthodontiques. Une nouvelle possibilite therapeuque. Rev Orthop Dento Faciale 1989; 23: 209-23.

10. Zachrisson BU. In search of excellence in orthodontics. Course synopsis, 1984.

11. Andreasen JO, Paulsen HU, Yu Z, Ahlquist R, Bayer T, Schwartz O. A long term study of 370 autotransplanted premolars. Part I. Surgical procedure and standardized techniques for monitoring healing. Eur J Orthod 1990; 12: 3-13

12. Andreasen JO, Paulsen HU, Yu Z, Bayer T, Schwartz O. A long term study of 370 autotransplanted premolars. Part II. Tooth survival and pulp healing subsequent to transplantation. Eur J Orthod 1990; 12: 14-24

13. Andreasen JO, Paulsen HU, Yu Z, Schwartz O. A long term study of 370 autotransplanted premolars. Part III. Periodontal healing subsequent to transplantation. Eur J Orthod 1990; 12: 25-37.

14. Andreasen JO, Paulsen HU, Yu Z, Bayer T. A long term study of 370 autotransplanted premolars. Part IV. Root development subsequent to transplantation. Eur J Orthod 1990; 12: 38-50.

15. Ravn JJ, Almer Nielsen, L. Overtal og aplasier hos 1530 Københavnske skolebørn. Tandlægebladet 1973; 77: 12-22.

16. Rølling S. Hypodontia of permanent teeth in Danish schoolchildren. Scand J Dent Res 1980; 88: 365-69.

17. Hidasi G. Der Verhalten der persistierender Milchmolaren. Zahn Mund Kieferheilkd 1976; 64: 28-31.

18. Rune B, Sarnäs KV. Rootresorption and submergence in retained deciduous second molars. A mixed-longitudinal study of 77 children with developmental absence of second premolars. Eur J Orthod 1984; 6: 123-31.

19. Kurol J, Thilander B. Infraocclusion of primary molars with aplasia of the permanent successor. A longitudinal study. Angle Orthod 1984; 54: 283-94.

20. Björk A, Skieller V. Facial development and tooth eruption. An implant study at the age of puberty. Am J Orthod 1972; 62: 339-83.

21. Rönnermann A. Early loss of primary molars. Thesis. Department of Orthodontics, Faculty of Odontology, University of Göteborg, Sweden 1977.

22. Havikko K. The formation and the alveolar and clinical eruption of the permanent teeth. Thesis. Department of Pedodontics and Orthodontics of the Institute of Dentistry, University of Helsinki, Finland 1971.

23. Daugaard-Jensen I. Extraction of first molars in discrepancy cases. Am J Orthod 1973; 64: 115-36.

24. Rantanen AV. The age of eruption of the third molar teeth. A clinical study based on Finnish university students. Thesis. Department of Operative Dentistry, Institute of Dentistry, University of Helsinki, Finland 1967.

25. Helmore FE. Surgical aid to eruption for orthodontic treatment. Aust Dent J 1967; 12: 372-78.

26. Hagerström L, Björlin G. Kirurgisk-ortodontisk behandling av retinerade hörntänder i överkäken. Swed J 1967; 60: 129-33.

27. Prescot M, Goldberg M. Controlled eruption on impacted teeth with treaded pins. J Oral Surg 1969; 27: 615-18.

28. Andreasen GF. A review of the approaches to treatment of impacted maxillary cuspids. Oral Surg Oral Med Oral Pathol 1987; 31: 479-84.

29. Thilander H, Thilander B, Persson G. Treatment of impacted teeth by surgical exposure. A survey study. Swed Dent J 1973; 66: 519-25.

30. von der Heydt K. The surgical uncovering and orthodontic positioning of unerupted maxillary canines. Am J Orthod 1975; 68: 256-76.

31. Alling CC. Impacted canine teeth. Dent Clin North Am 1979; 23: 439-42.

32. Eskici A. Präorthodontisch-chirurgische Behandlung retinierter bzw. verlagerter Zähne bei jugendlichen Gebissen. Dtsch Zahnärztl Z 1979; 34: 133-35.

33. Levine B, Skope L. Direct bonding of unerupted teeth for orthodontic movement. J Am Dent Assoc 1979; 98: 55-57.

34. Hunter SB. Treatment of the unerupted maxillary canine. Part 1. Preliminary considerations and surgical methods. Br Dent J 1983; 154: 294-96.

35. Hunter SB. Treatment of the unerupted maxillary canine. Part 2. Orthodontic methods. Br Dent J 1983; 154: 324-26.

36. Valderhaug J, Birkeland JM. Periodontal conditions in patients 5 years following insertion of fixed protheses. Pocket depth and loss of attachment. J Oral Rehabil 1976; 3: 237-43.

37. Vanarsdall RL, Corn H. Soft tissue management of labially positioned unerupted teeth. Am J Orthod 1977; 72: 53-64.

38. Gaulis RP. Parodonte marginal de canines superieures incluses. Evaluation suite a différentes méthodes d'accés chirurgical et de systeme orthodontique. Thesis. Geneve: Zurich Imprimerie Berichthaus 1978.

39. Gaulis RP, Joho JP. Parodonte marginal de canines superieures incluses. Evaluation suite a differentes methodes d'acces chirurgical et de systéme orthodontique. Rev Mens Suisse Odontostomatol 1978; 88: 1249-319.

40. Heaney TG, Atherton JD. Periodontal problems associated with the surgical exposure of unerupted teeth. Br J Orthod 1985; 3: 79-85.

41. Shiloah J, Kopczyk RA. Mucogingival considerations in surgical exposure of maxillary impacted canines. J Dent Child. 1978; 45: 79-81.

42. Azaz B, Steiman Z, Koyoumdijisky-Kaye E, Lewin-Epstein J. The sequelae of surgical exposure of unerupted teeth. J Oral Surg 1980; 38: 121-27.

43. Modéer T, Odenrick L. Post-treatment periodontal status of labially erupted maxillary canines. Acta Odontol Scand 1980; 38: 253-56.

44. Smith RG. A longitudinal study into the depth of the clinical gingival sulcus of human canine teeth during and after eruption. J Periodont Res 1982; 17: 427-33.

45. Becker A, Kohavi D, Zilberman Y. Periodontal status following the alignment of palatally impacted canine teeth. Am J Orthod 1983; 84: 332-36.

46. Kohavi D, Zilberman Y, Becker A. Periodontal status following the alignment of buccally ectopic maxillary canine teeth. Am J Orthod 1984; 85: 78-82.

47. Kohavi D, Becker A, Zilberman Y. Surgical exposure, orthodontic movement, and final tooth position as factors in periodontal breakdown of treated palatally impacted canines. Am J Orthod 1984; 85: 72-77.

48. Ericsson I, Linde J. Recession in sites with inadequate width of the keratinized gingiva. An experimental study in the dog. J Clin Periodontol 1984; 11: 95-103.

49. Hagerström L, Björlin G. Kirurgisk-ortodontisk behandling av retinerade hörntänder i överkäken. Sven Tandläk Tidskr 1967; 60: 129-33.

50. Buchhorn I. Følger efter behandling af palatinalt retinerede hjørnetænder. Thesis, Copenhagen 1985.

51. Howard RD. The displaced maxillary canine: Positional variations associated with incisor resorption. Dental Pract Dent Rec 1972; 22: 279-81.

52. Chevallier E. Réflexions sur la résorption coronaire des canines incluses. Rev Stomatol 1974; 75: 320-21.

53. Kisling E, Ravn E. To tilfælde med anormal trykresorption på overkæbeincisiver. Tandlægebladet 1977; 81: 153-55.

54. Sasakura H, Yoshida T, Murayama K, Hanada K, Nakajima T. Root resorption of upper permanent incisor caused by impacted canine. Int J Oral Surg 1984; 13: 299-306.

55. Rud J. Transplantation of canines. Tandlægebladet 1985; 89: 399-413.

56. Andreasen JO. Ectopic eruption of permanent canines electing resorption of incisors: Treatment by autotransplantation of the canine. Tandlægebladet 1987; 91: 487-92.

57. Ericson S, Kurol J. Radiographic assessment of maxillary canine eruption in children with clinical signs of eruption disturbance. Eur J Orthod 1986; 8: 133-40.

58. Ericson S, Kurol J. Longitudinal study and analysis of clinical supervision of maxillary canine eruption. Community Dent Oral Epidemiol 1986; 14: 172-76.

59. Ericson S, Kurol J. Radiographic examination of ectopically erupting maxillary canines. Am J Orthod Dentofacial Orthop 1987; 91: 483-92.

60. Ericson S, Kurol J. Incisor resorption caused by maxillary cuspids. A radiographic study. Angle Orthodont 1987; 57: 332-46.

61. Ericson S, Kurol J. Resorption of maxillary lateral incisors due to ectopic eruption of the canines. A clinical and radiographic analysis of predisposing factors. Am J Orthod Dentofacial Orthop 1988; 94: 503-13.

62. Ericson S, Kurol J. Early treatment of palatally erupting maxillary canines by extraction of the primary canines. Eur J Orthod 1988; 10: 283-95.

63. Williams BH. Diagnosis and prevention of maxillary cuspid impaction. Angle Orthod 1981; 51: 30-40.

64. Livaditis GJ, Thompson VP. Etched castings: An improved retentive mechanism for resin-bonded retainers. J Prosthet Dent 1982; 47: 52-54.

65. Holm B. Marylandbro - et alternativ til den konventionelle broprotetik. Tandlægebladet 1986; 90: 669-77.

66. Ekstrand K. Erfarenheter av 120 kompositretinerede påläggsbroar. Swed Dent J 1984; 18: 987-93.

67. Bergendal B, Hallonsten A-L, Koch G, Ludvigsson N, Olgart K. Composite retained onlay bridges. A follow-up study in adolescents. Swed Dent J 1983; 7: 217-25.

68. Villiams VD, Denehy GE, Thayer KE, Boyer DB. Acid-etch retained cast metal prostheses: a seven-year retrospective study. J Am Dent Assoc 1984; 108: 629-31.

69. Randow K. On the functional deformation of extensive fixed partial dentures. An experimental clinical and epidemiological study. Thesis. Swed Dent J suppl.34, 1986.

70. Bäcklund N, Åkesson N-Å. Efterundersökning av kron- och broarbeten. Odontol Rev 1957; 8: 121-33.

71. Ericsson SG, Marken K-E. Effect of fixed partial dentures on surrounding tissues. J Prosthet Dent 1968; 20: 517-25.

72. Kantorowich GF. Bridges. An analysis of failures. Dent Pract Dent Rec 1968; 18: 176-78.

73. Robert DH. The failure of retainers in bridge prostheses. An analysis of 2000 retainers. Br Dent J 1970; 128: 117-24.

74. Roberts DH. Relationship between age and the failure rate of bridge prostheses. Br Dent J 1970; 128: 175-81.

75. Schwartz NL, Whitsett LD, Berry TG, Stewart JL. Unserviceable crowns and fixed partial dentures: Lifespan and causes for loss of serviceability. J Am Dent Assoc 1970; 81: 1395-1401.

76. Fuhr K, Kares K, Siebert G. Nachuntersuchungen festsitzende Ersatzes. Dtsch Zahnärztl Z 1971; 26: 716-24.

77. Kerschbaum T, Voss R. Zum Risiko durch Überkronung. Dtsch Zahnärztl Z 1979; 34: 740-43.

78. Kerschbaum T, Voss R. Die praktische Bewahrung von Krone und Inlay. Dtsch Zahnärztl Z 1981; 36: 243-49.

79. Glantz P-O, Ryge G, Jendresen MD, Nilner K. Quality of extensive fixed prosthodontics after five years. J Prosthet Dent 1984; 52: 475-79.

80. Reuter J E, Brose MO. Failures in full crown retained dental bridges. Br Dent J 1984; 157: 61-66.

81. Karlsson S, Hedegård B. Efterundersökning av patienter med större brokonstruktioner. Swed Dent J 1984; 24: 1425-30.

82. Maryniuk GA. In search of treatment longevity. - A 30 year perspective. J Am Dent Assoc 1984; 109: 739-44.

83. Leempoel PJB, Eschen S, De Haan AFJ, Van't Hof MA. An evaluation of crowns and bridges in a general dental practice. J Oral Rehabil 1985; 12: 515-28.

84. Silness J. Periodontal conditions in patients treated with dental bridges. J Periodont Res 1970; 5: 60-68.

85. Hüttner G. Nachuntersuchungen von Kronen und Brücken-zahnersatz in bezug auf den Kronenrand und das marginale Paro-dontium. Dtsch Zahnärztl Z 1971; 26: 724-29.

86. Groop HP, Schwindling R. Statistische Feststellungen über feh-lerhafte Kronengestaltung mit Folgen auf Zahn, Parodont und Gingiva. Dtsch Zahnärztl Z 1971; 26: 734-42.

87. Bergman B, Hugoson A, Olsson C-O. Periodontal and prosthetic conditions in patients treated with removable partial dentures and artificial crowns. A longitudinal two-year study. Acta Odontol Scand 1971; 29: 621-38.

88. Silness J, Hunsbeth J, Figenschou B. Effects of tooth loss on the periodontal condition of neighbouring teeth. J Periodont Res 1973; 8: 237-42.

89. Silness J, Ohm E. Periodontal conditions in patients treated with dental bridges. V. Effect of splinting adjacent abutment teeth. J Peridont Res 1974; 9: 121-26.

90. Silness J, Gustavsen F, Mangersnes K. The relationship between pontic hygiene and mucosal inflammation in fixed bridge recipients. J Periodont Res 1982; 17: 434-39.

91. Valderhaug J, Heløe LA. Oral hygiene in a group of supervised patients with fixed prostheses. J Periodontol 1977; 48: 221-24.

92. Valderhaug J. Periodontal conditions and carious lesions fol-lowing the insertion of fixed prostheses: a 10 year follow-up study. Int Dent J 1980; 30: 296-304.

93. Janenko C, Smales RJ. Anterior crowns and gingival health. Aust Dent J 1979; 24: 225-31.

94. Ariely E. Vergleichende Untersuchungen der Beziehung zwi-schen Kronenrand und freier Gingiva. Dtsch Zahnärztl Z 1979; 34: 206-11.

95. Meyer E, Eichner K. Klinische Untersuchungsergebnisse zu verblendeten Kronen und Brücken. (Vergleich Kunststoff/ Keramik). Dtsch Zahnärztl Z 1980; 35: 864-69.

96. Nyman S, Ericsson I. The capacity of reduced periodontal tis-sues to support fixed bridgework. J Clin Periodontol 1982; 9: 409-14.

97. Ullman S, Arnold M. Periodontalreaktionen an überkronten Zähnen im Vergleich zu korrespondierenden Zæhnen. Stomatol DDR 1982; 32: 421-6.

98. Karlsson S, Hedegård B. Efterundersökning av patienter med större brokonstruk-tioner. Del II: Klinisk undersökning på patienter behandlade under 1974-1975 av privattändläkare. Swed Dent J 1984; 76: 1425-34.

99. Zachrisson BU. Improving orthodontic results in cases with maxillary incisors missing. Am J Orthodont 1978; 73: 274-289.

100. Årtum J, Zachrisson BU. New technique for semipermanent replacement of missing incisors. Am J Orthodont 1984; 85: 367-375.

101. Zachrisson BU, Thilander B. Treatment of dento-alveolar ano-malies. In: Thilander B, Rönning O (eds). Introduction to Ortho-dontics. Tandläkarförlaget, Stockholm 1985: 135-184.

102. Andreasen JO, Paulsen HU, Fjellvang H, Barfod K. Autotrans-plantation af præmolarer til behandling af tandtab i overkæbefronten. Tandlægebladet 1989; 93: 435-40.

103. Paulsen HU, Andreasen JO, Schwartz O. Behandling af tab i fronten med autotransplantation af præmolarer. Tandlægernes nye Tidskrift 1990; 5: 70-75.

104. Joho JP, Schatz JP. Autotransplantation et planification ortho-dontique. Rev Mens Suisse Odontostomatol 1990; 100: 174-87.

105. Deplagne H. Autotransplantation de germes de prémolaires. Résultats. Rev Orthop Dento Faciale 1984; 18: 495-506.

106. Lagerström L, Kristerson L. Influence of orthodontic treatment on root development of autotransplantated premolars. Am J Orthodont 1986; 89: 146-49.

Chapter 11
Restoration of transplanted teeth

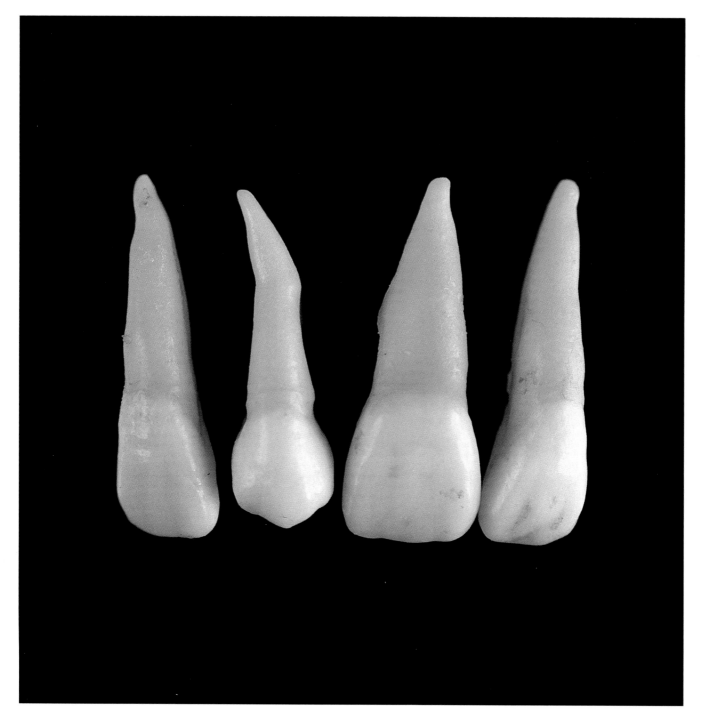

Transplantation of teeth to other sites may entail restoration in order to achieve an esthetically acceptable result. The need for restoration primarily involves teeth transplanted to the maxillary incisor and canine region (Fig. 11.1). However, before the different restorative principles are described, it might be worthwhile to consider how transplanted teeth can differ from other teeth in their response to restorative procedures.

Fig. 11.1. A central incisor which has been avulsed is replaced with a second maxillary premolar. The transplanted premolar has been restored with a composite restoration.

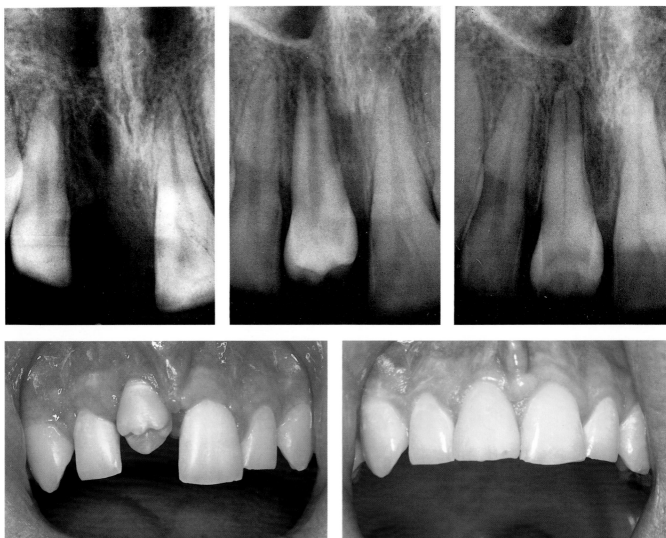

Treatment planning

In a tooth transplanted with an incompletely formed root, revascularization of the pulp normally occurs, but usually with pulp canal obliteration to follow. Pulp canal obliteration usually can be diagnosed 3 to 6 months after transplantation. This newly formed dentin differs from normal dentin by virtue of its cellular content and many vascular inclusions (Fig. 11.2). A preparation which exposes dentin may thus lead to bacterial invasion into the vascular canals with subsequent development of pulp necrosis (Fig. 11.3).[1] However, use of the new dentin bonding agents may help to eliminate this problem.

Safe restoration of transplanted teeth therefore requires the following considerations: (1) The pulp status should be known before restoration, i.e., a positive sensibility response should be elicited. (2) The restoration should be made so that no or only a minimum of dentin is exposed. At least no post-transplantation dentin must be exposed. (3) The restorative procedure used should prevent or limit microleakage, which leads to bacterial invasion. (4) Finally, the restoration should stay clear of the gingival margin in order to maintain optimal gingival health.

If the tooth has been endodontically treated, the first two considerations can be ignored.

In the following, various restorative principles will be described for different regions, according to the type of transplant used.

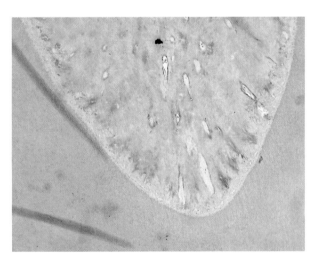
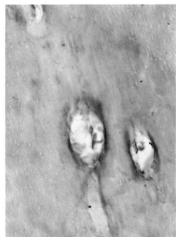

Fig. 11.2. Transplanted maxillary incisor with vascular inclusions in dentin formed after transplantation. Note that the vascular inclusions extend deep into dentin.

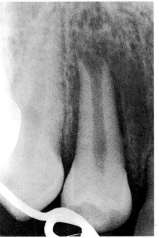
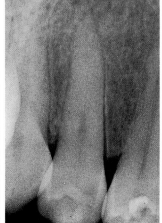
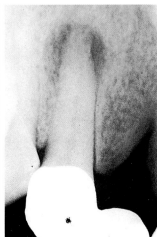

Fig. 11.3. Pulpal complications developed subsequent to crown preparation. One year after crown preparation, a periapical radiolucency is seen. From Kristerson, 1985.[1]

Maxillary central incisor region

In this region, a wide range of transplant possibilities exist. Thus, premolars, cuspids, and even third molars can be used. In the following, typical restorative procedures will be described for each of these types of transplant.

Mandibular premolars

Second premolars are preferred over first premolars because of their slightly larger coronal dimensions. Depending on esthetic requirements, these teeth are placed either in normal orientation or rotated 90° mesially, if larger cervical dimensions are required mesiodistally (Fig. 11.4).

For mandibular premolars placed in *normal graft position*, the following changes in crown anatomy will be required (Fig. 11.4): a slight reduction in the curvature of the labial surface and reduction of the lingual cusp. These reductions should be made without exposing posttransplantation dentin. In some cases, accidental bulges have to be accepted in order not to expose posttransplantation dentin. However, harmony of the incisal edges will often compensate for this defect and still yield an acceptable esthetic result. Furthermore, the fissure system of the occlusal surface should be opened to ensure that no caries is left under the composite restoration. After these changes, the tooth is restored using an acid-etch/composite resin technique (Fig. 11.5).

In the case of 90° *mesial rotation* the "labial" and "lingual" surfaces must be reduced and a gingivectomy performed before restoration according to the guidelines already described on p. 279.

Maxillary premolars

These transplants are placed either in normal position or rotated 45° or 90°, depending on space conditions in that region or broad or narrow cervical dimensions. In the case of *normal graft position* restoration begins with an analysis of necessary changes in crown anatomy which will transform the graft to a central incisor (Fig. 11.6). For this purpose, the graft should be viewed horizontally and axially. The following changes are usually necessary: (a) the labial surface should be slightly flattened and (b) the lingual cusp should be reduced. When these changes have been made, the tooth is then restored with an acid-etch/composite resin technique (Fig. 11.5).

In the case of 90° *mesial rotation* of a premolar transplant, the following changes in crown anatomy will be necessary (Fig. 11.7) (a) slight reduction of the incisal part of the "facial" surface of the tooth, (b) similar reduction of the palatal surface, and (c) gingivectomy labially to create symmetry.

A gingivectomy should be performed prior to restorative procedures. In this regard, it should be kept in mind that creeping reattachment will usually occur after such a procedure, implying that tissue should be removed at a level 1 mm higher than what is anticipated to be the future gingival level.[2]

When the above-mentioned changes in crown anatomy have been made the crown is restored using the techniques described above.

Fig. 11.4. Second mandibular premolar transplanted to the central incisor region on a model. The double exposure illustrates where reduction of the transplant is necessary.

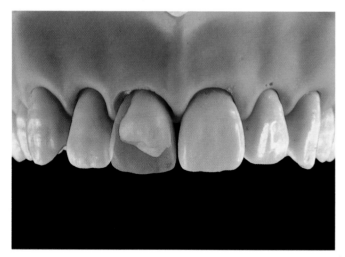
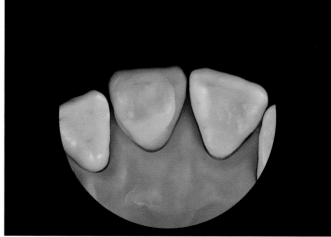

Fig. 11.5. Composite restoration of a transplanted second mandibular premolar

A frontal and axial inspection is performed in order to determine the necessary areas of crown reduction.

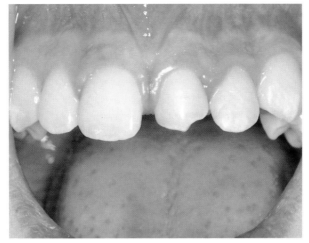 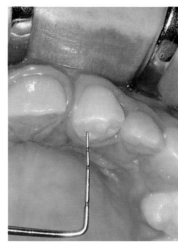

Reduction of the crown

The labial surface is reduced slightly. Thereafter the lingual cusp is partly removed and the fissure system is expanded. Preferably dentin is not exposed.

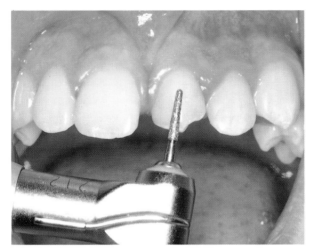 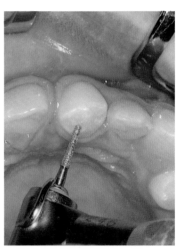

Choosing a crown form

A crown form is selected which matches the homologous incisor (e.g., Odus Pella, Dentairs SA, 18 Rue de Bosquets, CH 1800 Vevey, Switzerland). Thereafter the enamel is etched, rinsed in water, and dried.

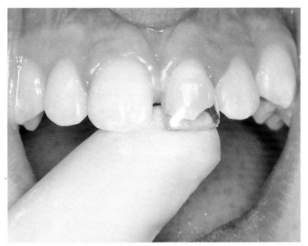 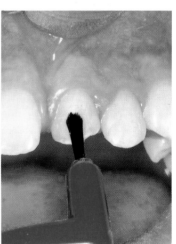

Seating the crown

After selection of a shade which matches the middle and cervical part of the tooth, the crown form is seated with composite on the prepared transplant.

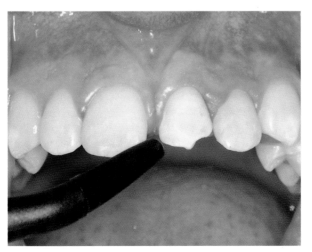 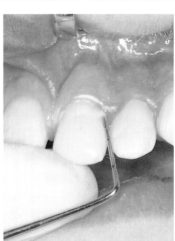

Fig. 11.5. Continued

Creating the labial surface
After polymerization of the composite the surface layer of the labial surface is removed with a bur.

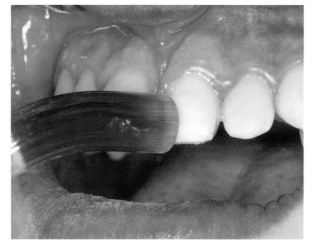

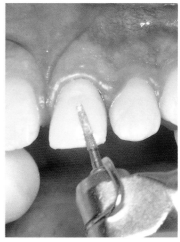

Contouring the labial surface
The labial surface is restored with translucent composite which matches the different sites on the crown. At this time small irregularities in color can be painted on using tinting material. The rough contouring of the crown is performed with a tapered diamond bur. Polishing is carried out with abrasive disks.

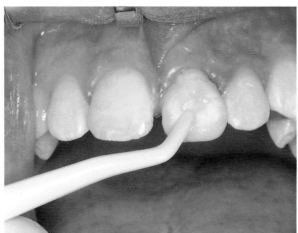

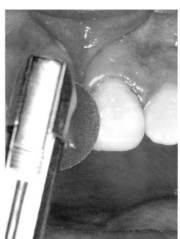

Contouring the palatal surface
The concave contour of the lingual surface is performed with a wheel-shaped diamond. The proximal and palatal margins are polished with small abrasive disks.

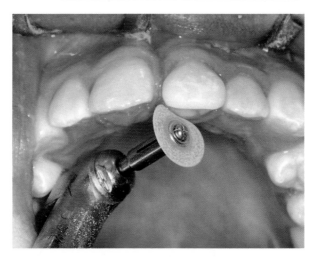

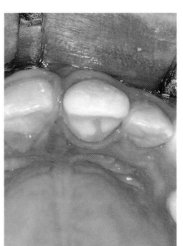

Final restoration
Clinical and radiographic appearance after restoration.

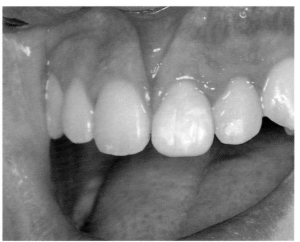

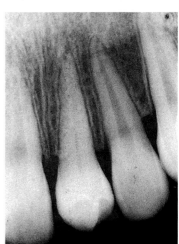

Maxillary third molars

In rare cases, maxillary third molars are so diminutive that they can be used as a replacement for lost central incisors. In these cases, the crown has to be reduced considerably on the labial and lingual aspects, whereafter it can be restored using the acid-etch/composite restoration technique (Fig. 11.8).

Fig. 11.6. Maxillary second premolar transplanted to the central incisor region on a model. The double exposure shows the necessary anatomic alterations.

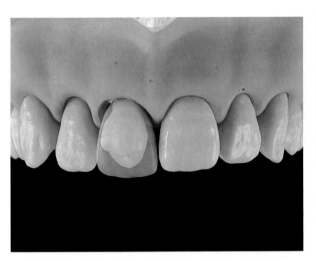

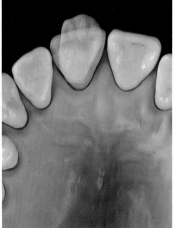

Fig. 11.7. Maxillary second premolar transplantation to the central incisor region and rotated 90° on a model. The double exposure shows the necessary crown reduction.

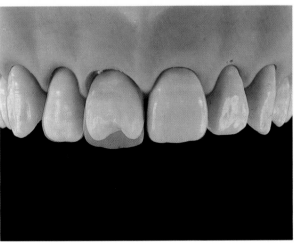

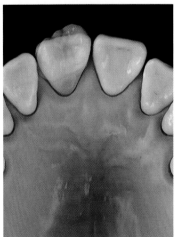

Fig. 11.8. Maxillary third molar transplant to the central incisor region

This 23-year-old man had lost his central incisor due to trauma at the age of 20. Note the marked atrophy of the alveolar process.

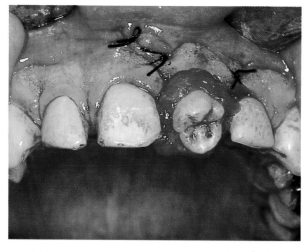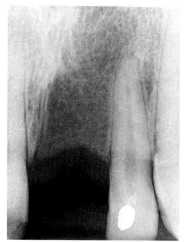

Radiographic examination

A panoramic exposure shows that a nonerupted maxillary third molar was available as a possible graft.

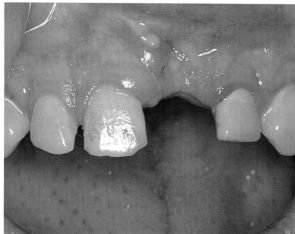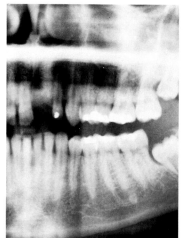

Transplanting the third molar

Due to atrophy of the alveolar process it was necessary to remove and replant the labial bone plate in order to make room for the graft.

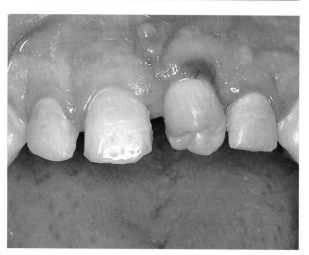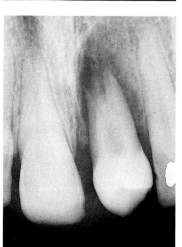

Restoring the transplant

The labial and palatal surfaces have been reduced prior to restoration with composite.

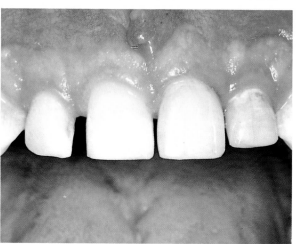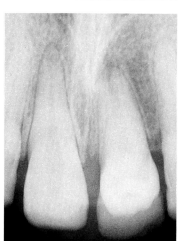

Maxillary lateral incisor region

In this region, the optimal replacement tooth is the mandibular first premolar from the opposite side of the arch. In these cases, the only restorative procedure necessary is slight reduction of the labial and lingual cusps (Fig. 11.9).

Maxillary cuspid region

In order to replace a missing maxillary canine, mandibular first or second premolars can be used (Fig. 11.10). The restorative procedures in these cases are minimal, consisting only of reduction of the lingual cusp. In order to create symmetry, it is sometimes necessary to augment the labial cusp with composite resin (Fig. 11.11).

Fig. 11.9. Mandibular first premolar transplanted to the lateral incisor region on a model. The double exposure illustrates where reduction of the transplant is necessary.

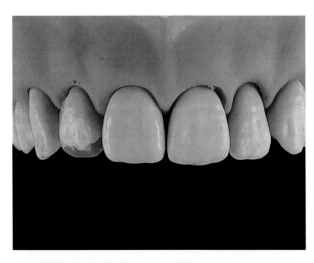
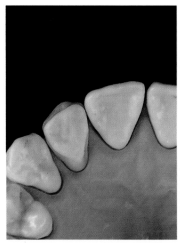

Fig. 11.10. Transplantation of a mandibular premolar as a replacement for a lost canine.

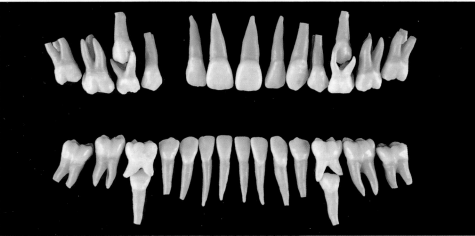

Fig. 11.11. Mandibular second premolar transplanted to the canine region. The cusp has been augmented with composite resin.

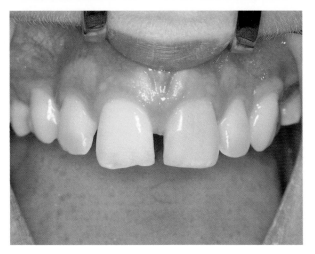
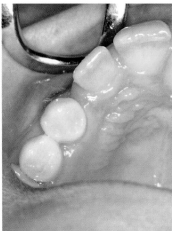

Maxillary premolar region

In cases of multiple aplasia of premolars, transplantation of maxillary third molars may be indicated. In these cases, the augmentation of the mesiobuccal cusp may give the appearance of a premolar, especially when the maxillary arch is viewed frontally (Fig. 11.12).

Fig. 11.12. Maxillary third molar transplanted to the premolar region. The transplant has been augmented with composite in order to simulate a labial premolar cusp.

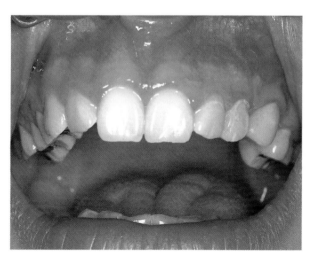
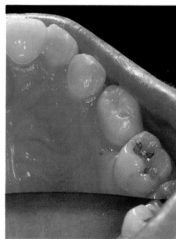

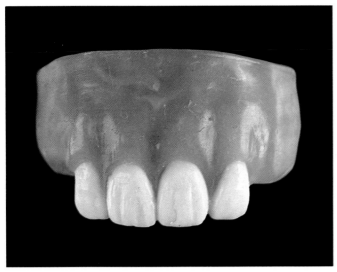
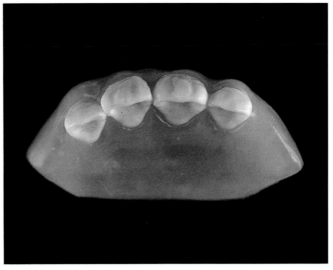

Fig. 11.13. Restorative procedures used to "broaden" a transplant to the anterior region. In this simulation, there is a 2-mm difference in crown diameter between the two central incisors. The labial surface is kept flat with maximum separation between mamelons and with acute proximal angles. The incisal edges should end with square mesial and distal corners.

Special cases
Asymmetric space conditions in the anterior region

In cases where adjacent teeth have drifted into the extraction site and for various reasons orthodontic realignment is not possible, the problem arises as to how to restore a transplanted premolar whose mesiodistal dimension is less than the contralateral (Fig. 11.13).[3] In these cases, slight grinding of the proximal surface of the adjacent central incisor may compensate for some of the space loss. The length of the restored tranplanted tooth should be maximal to enhance the illusion of symmetry. The labial surface should be flattened, with maximum separation between mamelons, and acute proximal angles to suggest a broader tooth. Finally, the incisal edge should end with square mesial and distal corners.

Another situation can arise where a maxillary premolar has been transplanted and rotated 90⁰. In these cases, the mesiodistal dimension of the transplant is usually slightly greater than the contralateral central incisor (Fig. 11.14). In this situation, the opposite optical effect can be used to minimize asymmetry.[3] First, the contralateral central incisor can be slightly enlarged mesially. Secondly, the crown length of the transplant restoration should be as large as possible. To reduce the impression of the larger mesiodistal dimension, it can also be useful to round the labial surface and narrow the separation between mamelons. This tends to deflect light, giving the illusion of smaller dimensions. Finally, the mesial and distal corners of the incisal edge should be rounded. All these optical illusions will help reduce the mesiodistal width and suggest symmetry.

Fig. 11.14. Restorative procedures used to "narrow" a transplant to the anterior region. There is a 2-mm difference between the two central incisors. The labial surface is kept rounded with minimal separation between mamelons and with rounded proximal angles. The incisal edges end with rounded mesial and distal corners.

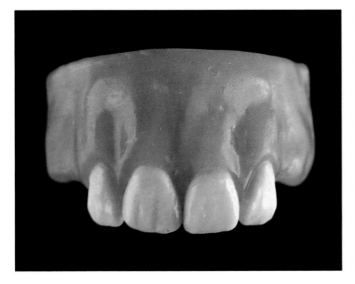
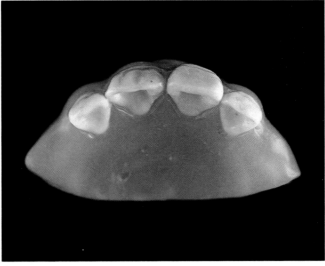

Essentials

Prerequisites before restoration

Pulp status should be known.
The labial gingival level should be in harmony with the contralateral homologue; if it is not, a gingivectomy should be performed.

When to restore

3 to 6 months after transplantation

Principles of restoration

Reduction of the crown to accommodate the new crown anatomy.
No or minimal dentin exposure.
Microleakage should be prevented.
The restoration should preferably stay clear of the gingiva

References

1. Kristerson L. Autotransplantation of human premolars. A clinical and radiographic study of 100 teeth. Int J Oral Surg 1985; 14: 200-213.

2. Monefeldt I, Zachrisson BU. Adjustment of clinical crown height by gingivectomy following orthodontic space closure. Angle Orthod 1977; 47: 256-64.

3. Goldstein RE. Esthetics in dentistry. Philadelphia: JB Lippincott Company, 1976: 425-40.

Appendix 1
Follow-up schedule for replanted teeth

Post-replantation interval

1 week	Pulp extirpation and calcium hydroxide dressing in cases with completed root formation. Removal of splint in uncomplicated cases (complete and incomplete root development).
2-3 weeks	Radiographic and clinical control at 2 weeks in replanted teeth with incomplete root formation and 3 weeks in cases with complete root formation.
4 weeks	Optional: for high-risk cases for root resorption. Removal of splints in cases with extensive bone damage. Revision of calcium hydroxide root canal dressing.
6 weeks	Radiographic and clinical control including sensibility testing in teeth with incomplete root formation.
6 months	Radiographic and clinical control including sensibility testing. Revision of calcium hydroxide dressing or gutta-percha root filling.
1 year	Radiographic and clinical control including sensibility testing. Revision of calcium hydroxide dressing or gutta percha root filling.

Appendix 2
Follow-up schedule for autotransplanted teeth

Posttransplantation interval

1 week   Removal of sutures.

3 weeks   Radiographic and clinical control. Removal of splint. Pulp extirpation and calcium hydroxide dressing in teeth with completed root formation.

4 weeks   Optional: for high risk cases of root resorption.

8 weeks   Radiographic and clinical control including sensibility testing.

6 months   Radiographic and clinical control including sensibility testing. Revision of calcium hydroxide dressing or gutta-percha root filling.

1 year   Radiographic and clinical control including sensibility testing. Revision of calcium hydroxide dressing or gutta-percha root filling.

Appendix 3
Follow-up schedule for allotransplanted teeth

Posttransplantation interval

1 week   Removal of sutures.

3-4 weeks   Optional: pulp extirpation and calcium hydroxide dressing if the tooth has not been root filled extra-orally and has complete root formation.

6 weeks   Radiographic and clinical control. Removal of splint.

6 months   Revision of calcium hydroxide dressing or gutta-percha root filling. Radiographic and clinical control.

1 year   Radiographic and clinical control.

Appendix 4
Dimensions of maxillary and mandibular permanent teeth

After Björndal & al., 1974*.

Tooth		Overall length	Crown height	Root length	Mesio-distal crown diameter	Labio-lingual crown diameter
Maxillary	Mean	23.7	11.2	12.5	9.0	7.4
central	SD	1.5	0.9	1.5	0.6	0.4
incisor	Max	27.3	12.7	15.2	10.3	8.3
	Min	21.5	9.3	9.1	8.0	6.7
Maxillary	Mean	23.1	9.9	13.0	6.9	6.6
central	SD	1.7	0.8	1.6	0.9	0.4
incisor	Max	26.0	11.7	15.8	8.2	7.5
	Min	19.2	8.1	9.8	5.0	5.5
Maxillary	Mean	27.3	11.0	16.3	7.7	8.4
canine	SD	2.6	1.0	2.0	0.4	0.6
	Max	33.3	13.8	20.9	8.3	9.6
	Min	23.3	8.7	12.2	6.8	6.9
Maxillary	Mean	23.3	9.1	13.7	7.0	9.5
first	SD	1.7	0.8	1.5	0.2	0.5
premolar	Max	25.8	11.5	17.2	7.6	10.5
	Min	18.8	7.8	10.7	6.8	8.5
Maxillary	Mean	22.3	8.5	14.4	7.2	9.4
second	SD	2.1	0.8	1.9	0.6	0.6
premolar	Max	26.4	10.1	18.9	8.5	10.7
	Min	16.7	7.0	9.7	6.3	8.5
Maxillary	Mean	22.3	8.4	14.2	10.9	11.8
first	SD	2.1	0.8	1.3	0.7	0.4
molar	Max	25.0	9.6	17.1	11.9	12.5
	Min	19.6	7.3	11.9	9.9	10.7
Maxillary	Mean-	22.2	8.4	13.8	10.2	11.8
second	SD	1.2	0.6	1.1	0.7	0.7
molar	Max	25.2	9.6	15.8	11.1	13.2
	Min	20.1	7.3	10.9	8.9	10.5

Tooth		Overall length	Crown height	Root length	Mesio-distal crown diameter	Labio-lingual crown diameter
Mandibular central incisor	Mean	21.8	9.7	12.8	5.7	5.9
	SD	1.7	1.0	1.0	0.3	0.2
	Max	25.1	11.5	15.0	6.2	6.3
	Min	19.4	7.6	10.7	5.4	5.5
Mandibular lateral incisor	Mean	23.3	10.4	13.5	6.0	6.2
	SD	1.2	0.5	1.2	0.4	0.3
	Max	25.0	11.3	16.0	6.6	6.8
	Min	21.0	9.2	10.3	5.5	5.5
Mandibular canine	Mean	26.0	11.6	15.7	6.7	7.8
	SD	1.4	0.8	1.4	0.5	1.0
	Max	27.4	12.2	18.0	7.1	8.7
	Min	24.6	10.1	13.6	5.9	6.0
Mandibular first premolar	Mean	22.9	8.9	15.0	7.2	7.9
	SD	0.9	0.6	1.1	0.2	0.3
	Max	24.2	9.6	16.7	7.6	8.5
	Min	21.2	7.7	12.9	6.9	7.4
Mandibular second premolar	Mean	22.3	8.6	14.4	7.4	8.6
	SD	2.1	0.5	1.8	0.4	0.5
	Max	25.0	9.7	17.0	8.0	9.5
	Min	19.3	8.0	11.0	6.9	7.7
Mandibular first molar	Mean	22.0	8.3	15.1	11.8	10.8
	SD	1.4	0.7	1.2	0.5	0.7
	Max	25.0	10..2	17.3	12.8	12.4
	Min	19.3	6.4	11.9	11.1	9.4
Mandibular second molar	Mean	21.7	8.7	13.8	11.4	10.3
	SD	1.5	0.9	1.3	0.7	0.4
	Max	25.8	13.1	17.6	13.2	11.5
	Min	19.0	6.8	10.3	10.0	9.5

* Björndal AM, Henderson WG, Skidmore AE, Kellner FH. Anatomic measurements of human teeth extracted from males between the ages of 17 and 21 years. Oral Surg Oral Med Oral Pathol 1974; 38: 791-803.

Appendix 5
Relationship between radiographic and actual tooth dimensions in the mandible according to film-focus distance

Measurement on radiograph in mm	Film-focus distance in cm					
	15	20	25	30	35	40
	Actual tooth dimensions in mm					
5.0	4.5	4.6	4.7	4.8	4.8	4.8
6.0	5.4	5.5	5.6	5.7	5.8	5.8
7.0	6.3	6.4	6.5	6.7	6.7	6.7
8.0	7.2	7.4	7.5	7.6	7.7	7.7
9.0	8.1	8.3	8.4	8.6	8.6	8.7
10.0	9.0	9.2	9.4	9.5	9.6	9.6
11.0	9.9	10.1	10.3	10.5	10.6	10.6
12.0	10.8	11.1	11.2	11.4	11.5	11.6
13.0	11.7	12.0	12.2	12.4	12.5	12.5
14.0	12.6	12.9	13.1	13.3	13.4	13.5
15.0	13.5	13.8	14.0	14.3	14.4	14.5
16.0	14.4	14.8	15.0	15.2	15.4	15.4
17.0	15.3	15.7	15.9	16.2	16.3	16.4
18.0	16.2	16.6	16.8	17.2	17.3	17.4
19.0	17.1	17.5	17.8	18.1	18.2	18.3
20.0	18.0	18.4	18.7	19.1	19.2	19.3
21.0	18.9	19.4	19.7	20.0	20.2	20.2
22.0	19.8	20.3	20.6	21.0	21.1	21.2
23.0	20.7	21.2	21.5	21.9	22.1	22.2
24.0	21.6	22.1	22.5	22.9	23.0	23.1
25.0	22.5	23.0	23.4	23.8	24.0	24.1

Measurements based on a film-tooth distance of 1.5 cm and a right angle technique.

Appendix 6

Relationship between radiographic and actual tooth dimensions in the maxilla according to film-focus distance

Measurement on radiograph in mm	Film-focus distance in cm					
	15	20	25	30	35	40
	Actual tooth dimensions in mm					
5.0	4.2	4.4	4.5	4.6	4.7	4.7
6.0	5.0	5.2	5.4	5.5	5.6	5.7
7.0	5.9	6.1	6.3	6.5	6.5	6.6
8.0	6.7	7.0	7.2	7.4	7.5	7.5
9.0	7.5	7.9	8.0	8.3	8.4	8.5
10.0	8.3	8.7	8.9	9.2	9.4	9.4
11.0	9.1	9.6	9.8	10.2	10.3	10.4
12.0	10.0	10.5	10.7	11.1	11.2	11.3
13.0	10.8	11.3	11.6	12.0	12.1	12.2
14.0	11.7	12.2	12.5	12.9	13.1	13.2
15.0	12.5	13.1	13.4	13.8	14.0	14.1
16.0	13.3	14.0	14.8	14.8	14.9	15.1
17.0	14.2	14.8	15.3	15.7	15.9	16.0
18.0	15.0	15.7	16.1	16.6	16.8	16.9
19.0	15.8	16.5	17.0	17.5	17.7	17.9
20.0	16.7	17.4	17.9	18.5	18.7	18.8
21.0	17.5	18.3	18.8	19.4	19.6	19.8
22.0	18.7	19.2	19.6	20.3	20.5	20.7
23.0	19.2	20.0	20.5	21.2	21.5	21.6
24.0	20.0	20.9	21.4	22.2	22.4	22.6
25.0	20.9	21.8	22.3	23.1	23.3	23.5

Measurements based on a film-tooth distance of 1.5 cm and a right angle technique.

Appendix 7
Surgical instruments for tooth transplantation

1. Contra-angle handpiece with internal cooling (model Intra 3552) for socket preparation in premolar and molar regions. **KaVo**, D-7950 Biberach/Riss 1, Germany.

2. Handpiece with internal cooling (model Intra 6) for socket preparation in canine and incisor regions. **KaVo**, D-7950 Biberach/Riss 1, Germany.

3. Surgical bur with internal cooling (model Kirschner 167 IK) for *general* bone removal during socket preparation. **KOMET**, Gebr. Brasseler, Postfach 160, D-4920 Lemgo, Germany.

4. Surgical bur with internal cooling (model Kirschner 81 IK, 4 mm) for *localized* bone removal during socket preparation. **KOMET**, Gebr. Brasseler, Postfach 169, D-4920 Lemgo, Germany.

5. Surgical blade (no. 15) used generally for incisions. **Swann-Morton & Co. Ltd**, Sheffield 6, England.

6. Surgical blade (no. 12) used for incisions in the removal of maxillary third molars. **Swann-Morton & Co. Ltd**, Sheffield 6, England.

7. Surgical blade (no. 11) used for periosteal flap extension. **Swann-Morton & Co. Ltd**, Sheffield 6, England.

8. Surgical blade (no. 11) specially ground to the shape of a stylet, which permits high apical incision of the periodontal ligament or follicle during graft removal. **Swann-Morton & Co. Ltd**, Sheffield 6, England.

9. Punch biopsy instrument (6 mm) for access incision on edentulous alveolar ridge. **Simonsen & Weel**, Roskildevej 14, DK- 2620 Copenhagen, Denmark.

10. Sliding caliper (model Züricher, no. 042-752) for pre- and peroperative measurements. **Dentaurum**, D-7530 Pforzheim, Germany.

11. Periosteal elevator (model Obwegeser, 6 mm, no. 68.02.01) for general use and for loosening of the graft. **MEDICON**, D-7200 Tuttlingen, Germany.

12. Narrow double-ended rougine (model Nordberg) for shielding the graft during surgical bone removal as well as separation of the follicle from the bony crypt. **LØCO**, B-W Dental Aps, Finsensvej 39 A, DK-2000 Copenhagen F., Denmark.

13. Tissue retractor (model Sörensen Hein, no. 68.18.60) for use in the removal of palatally and lingually impacted premolars. **MEDICON**, D-7200 Tuttlingen, Germany.

14. Amalgam carver (model Nyström) for separating the graft from the bony crypt. **LØCO**, B-W Dental Aps, Finsensvej 39 A, DK-2000 Copenhagen F., Denmark.

15. Narrow unibeveled chisel (model Stille 23, 3 mm, no. 260.03) for *localized* bone removal. **Simonsen & Weel**, Roskildevej 14, DK-2620 Copenhagen, Denmark.

16. Broad unibeveled chisel (model Stille 23, 6 mm, no. 260.06) for *general* bone removal. **Simonsen & Weel**, Roskildevej 14, DK-2620 Copenhagen, Denmark.

17. Osteotome (model Stille 23, 6 mm, no. 270.06) for removal of proximal bone (septum) and the labial bone plate. **Simonsen & Weel**, Roskildevej 14, DK-2620 Copenhagen, Denmark.

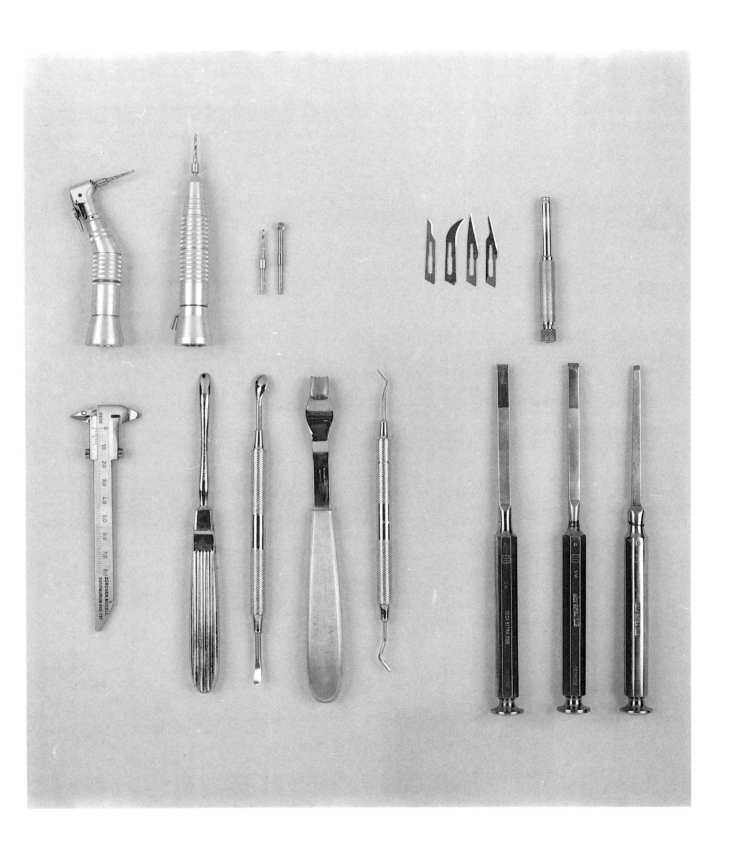

Index

Surgical procedure
- allotransplantation 230
- autotransplantation
- - canines 183
- - incisors 208
- - molars 115
- - premolars 144
- replantation
- - intentional 101
- - of avulsed teeth 61
- repositioning 122
- tilting of molars 122
Suture splint 160

T

Tap water storage of avulsed teeth 59, 81
Tetanus prophylaxis 61
Thawing 247
- curve 252
Tissue typing 228
T killer cells 225

U

Undifferentiated mesenchymal pulp cells, role of 35

V

Vitality testing (see sensibility testing)

W

Wire splint 160
Wound healing 16